T0401889

# Femoroacetabular Impingement

Óliver Marín-Peña

Editor

# Femoroacetabular Impingement

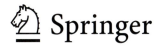

*Editor*
Óliver Marín-Peña
Department of Orthopedic and Traumatology
Hospital Infanta Leonor
Madrid, Spain

Originally published: Choque Femoroacetabular
© Oliver Marín-Peña et al.. Instituto de Cirugía de Cadera, 2010

Ediciones Díaz de Santos
www.diazdesantos.es/ediciones
ediciones@diazdesantos.es

ISBN 978-3-642-22768-4        e-ISBN 978-3-642-22769-1
DOI 10.1007/978-3-642-22769-1
Springer Heidelberg Dordrecht London New York

Library of Congress Control Number: 2011940838

© Springer-Verlag Berlin Heidelberg 2012

Printed on acid-free paper

Springer is part of Springer Science+Business Media (www.springer.com)

# Foreword

Femoroacetabular impingement is one of the areas of greatest interest to specialists in the hip joint. This pathology first attracted attention at the beginning of the twenty-first century, after passing unnoticed for a considerable time. Building on the experiences of the Berne school, recent publications have contributed to our understanding of the physiopathology and diagnosis of this condition, of related biomechanical disorders and their development, as well as the need and indications for early non-aggressive treatment.

In Spain, a group of young orthopedic surgeons took an interest in this pathology and acquired considerable clinical experience comparable to that of the best centers worldwide. For this reason, and particularly given the fact that this is a new area, even though it is undoubtedly essential to make the results of such work known through the most influential journals of our specialty, it is also important to gather together these experiences and the principles that underlie our work in a volume like the present one.

I have been involved in the preparation of this book from the outset, since Dr. Oliver Marín first started to plan its publication; the challenge, as always, was to avoid last-minute haste. The result has well repaid us for all our time and effort. This book deals with all the most pressing issues in hip surgery, laying the foundations for future developments. The field outlined and the techniques discussed here must then be left to pass the test of time.

Be this as it may, the first stone has been laid, and it remains for us to congratulate the authors, Springer editorial and Spanish orthopedic surgery as a whole and to thank them for all their work. We hope it will be useful for hip surgeons and enable them to offer better treatment to their patients.

Francisco Forriol

# Preface

*Femoroacetabular Impingement* (FAI) is a compilation of the work of many hip surgeons interested in this pathology. The ultimate goal of this work is to provide an updated knowledge of diagnostic and treatment aspects of this disease, collecting different points of view from experts around the world.

The classical publication of Smith Petersen in 1936, inadvertently favored the birth of a disease. Professor Reinhold Ganz in Berne became the father of FAI, clearly describing the mechanisms of injury and treatment. Since the first articles of Bern group, hundreds of publications have deepened in diagnostic and therapeutic aspects and have contributed to a rapid advance in knowledge of FAI. This book involves many of these FAI experts, who described different approaches to the injured hip joint. I greatly appreciate all their generous collaboration and patience with the difficulties in publishing the work. This book would not have been published without the invaluable support of MAPFRE Foundation. It would be a great satisfaction if the effort made by all authors, finally serves to facilitate understanding of femoroacetabular impingement.

Madrid, Spain                                                                                                    Óliver Marín-Peña

# Acknowledgements

I would like to thank Fernando Corella for his collaboration in the illustrations of the book and Alejandro Caffarini for the excellent translation. Also thanks to the Spanish Society of Hip Surgery (SECCA) and the Spanish Society of Orthopedic Surgery and Traumatology (SECOT), especially to Professor Francisco Forriol, for their support. Finally, I would like to thank my wife Marta and my son Pablo for their infinite comprehension.

Madrid, Spain                                                                      Óliver Marín-Peña

# Contents

# Part I

# Concept and Physical Exam in FAI

# Historical Evolution of the Concept of Femoroacetabular Impingement as a Cause of Hip Osteoarthritis

Martin Lavigne, Laffosse Jean-Michel,
and Vendittoli Pascal-André

Nowadays, discoveries of the pathomechanisms responsible for disease development are made mostly at the molecular level. The potential biomechanisms evoking primary degenerative hip joint changes are still being investigated intensively. With improved imaging techniques and novel treatment modalities, accumulating evidence supports the hypothesis that a simple mechanical conflict is the primary instigator in a large proportion of cases labeled as primary hip joint osteoarthritis (OA), without primary dysfunction at the molecular level. This chapter examines the series of events that have resulted in femoroacetabular impingement (FAI), being nowadays considered a cause of secondary hip joint OA.

There is still much debate about the etiology of hip OA [1]. The term secondary OA applies to degenerative hip joint disease attributable to a known cause, such as trauma, septic arthritis, and acetabular dysplasia, among others. Although the relationship of hip OA with a specific etiological factor can sometimes be established, the reverse is even more frequent, and most patients suffering from hip joint OA are left with no precise cause. In this situation, hip OA is categorized as primary or idiopathic. In the absence of a precise identifiable cause, the osteoarthritic process is felt to result from primary dysfunction at the subchondral bone and/or cartilage levels, although it may involve several other factors, some related to the patient (e.g., age, gender, hormone levels, genetics, and nutrition), the joint (subtle anatomical variants, muscle weakness, misalignment, and joint laxity), or lifestyle (repetitive physical activities and obesity).

As early as 1933, Elmslie [2] observed that although several causes of hip joint OA were well established in certain patients, in many of them, the disease was not accompanied by any identifiable factors. He postulated that people who developed hip OA by the age of 40–50 may have had undiscovered preexisting hip joint deformity. In particular, he drew attention to femoral head changes resembling *coxa plana* in early adult life that may produce degenerative alterations due to a mechanical misfit in the joint and felt that the best way of avoiding these was to keep the mechanics as normal as possible. Elmslie's findings seemed to pave the way for a quest to better understand the pathomechanisms, or abnormal mechanics, involved in the development of hip OA. It is somewhat surprising to realize that despite Elmslie's hypothesis dating back more than seven decades, the etiology of so-called primary or idiopathic hip OA is still not fully grasped.

In accordance with Elmslie's findings, four studies published between 1947 and 1961 were not able to identify the cause of radiographic hip OA in 24.3–65% of cases [3–7]. However, several subsequent studies shed more light on the potential etiology of some hip OA cases labeled as "idiopathic." In 1965, Murray [6] revisited the concept of primary hip joint OA, postulating that most primary hip OA cases were, in fact, secondary to minimal anatomical variations "so slight that their radiological appearance was regarded as being

M. Lavigne (✉) • V. Pascal-André
Service de Chirurgie Orthopédique,
Hôpital Maisonneuve – Rosemont, Montréal, QC, Canada
e-mail: lavigma2@hotmail.com

L. Jean-Michel
Service de Chirurgie Orthopédique,
Hôpital Maisonneuve – Rosemont, Montréal, QC, Canada

Service de Chirurgie Orthopédique, Institut Locomoteur,
Centre Hospitalier Toulouse – Rangueil, Toulouse, France

Ó. Marín-Peña (ed.), *Femoroacetabular Impingement*,
DOI 10.1007/978-3-642-22769-1_1, © Springer-Verlag Berlin Heidelberg 2012

within normal limits." He described what he called "tilt deformity" of the femoral head as its abnormal relationship to the femoral neck, characterized by a residual varus tilt of the femoral head vis-à-vis the femoral neck, shortening of the femoral neck, and remodeling of the lateral part of the femoral head. After reviewing 200 anteroposterior radiographs of patients with primary OA, he concluded that 65% of cases were, in fact, secondary to preexisting, asymptomatic anatomical abnormalities: acetabular dysplasia identified in 25.5% and tilt deformity in 39.5%. He postulated that tilt deformity could be the result of premature femoral head epiphyseal plate fusion, mild trauma, transient synovitis, or minor epiphysiolysis. Murray considered that tilt deformity rendered patients prone to hip OA development because of joint incongruity and concluded that early intervention could be a valuable treatment strategy to arrest joint deterioration.

These hallmark findings by Murray were supported in the mid-1970s by three other studies. In 1974, Stulberg and Harris [8] reported subtle forms of acetabular dysplasia in more than 40% of patients with so-called idiopathic arthritis. In 1975, Stulberg et al. [9] described the "pistol-grip deformity" of the proximal femur, similar to the tilt deformity of Murray, characterized by flattening of the lateral neck surface, hooking at the inferomedial femoral head–neck junction, and loss of height with widening of the femoral head. After reviewing 75 radiographs of primary hip OA, Murray found 39% of cases with subtle acetabular dysplasia and 40% of cases with pistol-grip deformity. Finally, in 1976, Solomon [10] hypothesized that hip joint OA was always secondary to some underlying abnormality of the hip joint, after finding a predisposing factor in all but 27 of 327 cases of hip OA. Besides known secondary causes of OA, he also found evidence of subtle acetabular dysplasia, tilt deformity, and postinflammatory OA in most cases of idiopathic or primary hip joint OA. He stated that "OA occurs in joints to which other things happen first." He concluded that studies on the natural history of these predisposing joint abnormalities and the precise manner in which they sensitize to cartilage degeneration were important to define in which patients surgical correction of the deformity would be justified to prevent OA from developing.

Decades before subtle femoral and acetabular changes were considered potential etiologies of primary idiopathic hip OA, painful conditions were described in

relation to gross hip joint deformity with restriction of motion. Smith-Petersen observed that the pathological anatomy of the acetabulum and/or the proximal femur may produce pain with hip joint motion [11]. He proposed a plastic procedure for the relief of hip joint conditions resulting from interference with normal hip joint mechanics. Such conditions were described as *malum coxae senilis*, intrapelvic protrusion of the acetabulum, old slipped upper femoral epiphysis, femoral neck fractures with malunion, Legg–Calvé–Perthes disease, and acetabular fractures [11]. Smith-Petersen postulated that the source of pain was "impingement of the femoral neck on the anterior acetabular margin." Such impingement would result in "traumatic arthritis with characteristic alterations of the joint surfaces as well as of the synovia."

Therefore, by the mid-1970s, many authors adopted the concept that mechanical conflict (due to subtle femoral or acetabular deformity) was the pathomechanism responsible for many cases of pain in the hip joint with or without OA rather than a primary dysfunction at the molecular level. However, the relationship between the subtle acetabular and femoral deformities described by Stulberg and Harris [8], Solomon [10], and Murray [6] and the development of hip joint OA was still not clearly established. The drawback of Stulberg's, Solomon's, and Murray's studies was their retrospective review of radiographs, which showed already damaged hip joints. This led Resnick [12] to propose in 1976 that the tilt deformity described by Murray could simply be the consequence of the osteoarthritic process rather than its cause.

Primary OA usually occurs later in life, and a defect in cartilage structure or function might play a role. However, if primary hip joint OA resulted from a defect in cartilage structure and/or function, it would be intuitive to assume an association between hip joint OA and OA at other locations. The fact that joints such as the ankle and elbow rarely develop OA unless they are traumatized tends to go against this assumption. To confirm that subtle joint deformities do contribute to the development of hip OA, more clinical evidence was clearly needed.

In the 1980s and 1990s, acetabular labral tears were frequently described in the orthopedics literature. The role of the acetabular labrum in normal and abnormal hip joint mechanics was not yet fully understood. Most labral tears were related to traumatic events [13], but tears occurring without a history of injury were also encountered and felt to predispose to coxarthrosis [14–16]. With the further development of hip arthroscopy, the diagnosis of labral tears became easier [17], and its association with hip joint articular damage was reported. Up to 95% of labral tears were identified by Santori and Villar [18] and Farjo et al. [19] along with substantial damage to acetabular cartilage. Labral pathology was addressed at the time of hip arthroscopy without clearly understanding the pathogenesis of joint damage. Based on their experience with hip arthroscopy and cadaver dissections, McCarthy et al. [20] proposed that labral tears alter the biomechanical environment of the hip, leading to articular cartilage degeneration and eventually to OA. Thus, until a decade ago, the pathomechanism by which labral tears and cartilage damage occurred was still not elucidated.

In the last 10 years, clinical tests and imaging techniques have been refined to facilitate the detection of morphologies at risk of FAI. In particular, magnetic resonance imaging (MRI) has become the preferred modality for investigating labrum, cartilage, and joint space pathology by multiplanar image acquisition, such as radial imaging. Magnetic resonance arthrography permits the identification of the associated femoral head–neck junction abnormalities frequently seen in FAI [21]. However, the pathomechanism involved in FAI could not be recognized until after the technique of surgical hip dislocation could be executed without morbidity. With the development of safe access to the hip joint, avoiding avascular necrosis of the femoral head and allowing a full view of the hip joint, Ganz et al. [22] were able to better define the pathogenic mechanism involved in FAI.

A series of observations by Ganz further supported the concept that mild deformation of the proximal femur or acetabulum could be responsible for a clinical syndrome characterized by pain, reduced range of motion, and damage to the acetabular labrum and articular cartilage. The term pincer FAI was first described in 1999 [23] as a complication observed in some patients after periacetabular osteotomy (PAO) performed for acetabular dysplasia. Groin pain and limited range of motion were noted in five patients following pelvic osteotomy. MRI in some patients revealed labral tears and cartilage damage not present before PAO. These patients were reoperated to improve reduced head–neck offset with clinical amelioration. In 2000, Leunig [24] noted the presence of early OA changes related to varying degrees of slipped capital femoral epiphysis (SCFE) in 13 patients treated by open hip

joint dislocation. All patients demonstrated evidence of acetabular labrum and acetabular cartilage damage on direct inspection of the joint. The deformed anterior femoral head and neck junction was seen entering the hip joint and pressing against the labrum and articular cartilage. These were the first two studies that intuitively led Ganz and collaborators to postulate that FAI played a role in the development of hip joint OA [25]. In a cadaveric investigation, Goodman et al. [26] observed that mild slipped-like deformity of the femoral head was associated with arthritic hip joint changes. With computer modeling, Rab [27] further illustrated the concept of FAI secondary to SCFE which predicted hip joint damage. Finally, in 2003, Ganz et al. proposed that many cases of idiopathic hip joint OA may be explained by the FAI concept [25]. Based on dynamic evaluation and direct observation of more than 600 cases undergoing surgical hip joint dislocation, they postulated that the pathomechanics of FAI lead to OA. Since then, there has been an exponential increase in the number of studies published on FAI.

Several studies have reported detailed direct or arthroscopic visualization of joint damage in FAI patients [28–34]. In a series of 30 cases of FAI operated with surgical dislocation, Peters and Erickson [34] found damage to the acetabular labrum or the underlying articular cartilage in 26 cases located in the anterior-superior quadrant of the acetabulum. Tannast et al. [35] demonstrated that the labral and cartilage lesions observed intraoperatively in a group of patients correlated with the damage predicted by computer simulation. Joint damage was greatest in the anterosuperior area of the labrum–cartilage complex. In his computer model, Rab [27] showed that abutment of the deformed metaphysis typical of SCFE against the acetabular rim was responsible for increased intra-articular pressure, which, in turn, ultimately led to irreversible joint damage. This has come to be called cam impingement, which is characterized by deep chondral injuries and secondary damage to the labrum. The other FAI form, pincer impingement, first attacks the labrum, with subsequent lesions occurring in articular cartilage.

The concept of hyaline cartilage damage as a consequence of mechanical conflict is not unique to the hip joint, and pathological mechanical conflicts during motion of other joints have prompted the description of well-accepted clinical syndromes. For example, in 1957, O'Donoghue [36] reported a condition called impingement exostosis of the talus and tibia. In a normal ankle joint, the concavity of the neck of the talus provides impingement-free dorsiflexion until the anterior tibial articular surface comes in contact with the neck of the talus. This is much like what is found in extreme hip joint motion, when the femoral neck comes into contact with the acetabular rim. O'Donoghue observed patients who developed reactive bone on the anterior surface of the tibia and talar neck secondary to mild chronic trauma caused by forceful dorsiflexion. With continuing trauma, more osteophytes were produced, which further increased pain and limited motion. A surgical procedure was described to remove osteophytes to restore impingement-free range of motion. In all but 1 case, the articular surface showed degenerative changes.

With accumulating knowledge on the pathomechanisms involved in FAI, various treatment methods have become available, and the positive clinical outcome of patients who have undergone surgery to restore normal joint mechanics has further supported the relationship between hip OA and FAI. Prospective longitudinal studies of normal subjects and patients suffering from FAI would confirm that FAI leads to hip joint OA. These investigations may also help to define the origin of the abnormal anatomies involved in FAI, such as suboptimal femoral head-to-neck offset and anterior acetabular overcoverage. Prospective studies of patients treated for FAI should demonstrate if the disease can be arrested by restoring normal hip joint mechanics. Animal experiments may help determine if FAI and its consequences can be reproduced. Based on accumulating clinical evidence, it seems reasonable to affirm that FAI is among the most frequent causes of degenerative hip joint disease.

# References

1. Mankin H, Brandt K, Shulman L (1986) Workshop on etiopathogenesis of osteoarthritis. Proceedings and recommendations. J Rheumatol 13(6):1130–1160
2. Elmslie R (1933) Aetiological factors in osteoarthritis of hip joint. Br Med J 1(1):1–4
3. Gade E (1947) A contribution to the surgical treatment of osteoarthritis of the hip joint. Acta Chir Scand 95(suppl 120):1
4. Lloyd-Roberts G (1955) Osteoarthritis of the hip: a study of the clinical pathology. J Bone Joint Surg Br 37(1):4–47
5. Adam A, Spence A (1958) Intertrochanteric osteotomy for osteoarthritis of the hip: a review of fifty-eight operations. J Bone Joint Surg Br 40(2):219–226
6. Murray R (1965) The aetiology of primary osteoarthritis of the hip. Br J Radiol 38(455):810–824
7. Nicoll EA, Holden NT (1961) Displacement osteotomy in the treatment of osteoarthritis of the hip. J Bone Joint Surg Br 43(1):50–60
8. Stulberg S, Harris W (1974) Acetabular dysplasia and development of osteoarthritis of the hip. In: The hip: Proceedings of the Second Open Scientific Meeting of the Hip Society. C.V. Mosby, St. Louis, pp 82–93
9. Stulberg S, Cordell L, Harris W et al (1975) Unrecognized childhood hip disease: a major cause of idiopathic osteoarthritis of the hip. In: The hip: Proceedings of the Third Meeting of the Hip Society. C.V. Mosby, St. Louis, pp 212–228
10. Solomon L (1976) Patterns of osteoarthritis of the hip. J Bone Joint Surg Br 58(2):176–183
11. Smith-Petersen M (2009) The classic: treatment of malum coxae senilis, old slipped upper femoral epiphysis, intrapelvic protrusion of the acetabulum, and coxa plana by means of acetabuloplasty. Clin Orthop Relat Res 467(7):608–615
12. Resnick D (1976) The "tilt deformity" of the femoral head in osteoarthritis of the hip: a poor indicator of previous epiphysiolysis. Clin Radiol 27(3):355–363
13. Fitzgerald RJ (1995) Acetabular labrum tears. Diagnosis and treatment. Clin Orthop Relat Res 311:60–68
14. Altenberg A (1977) Acetabular labrum tears: a cause of hip pain and degenerative arthritis. South Med J 70(2):174–175
15. Ueo T, Hamabuchi M (1984) Hip pain caused by cystic deformation of the labrum acetabulare. Arthritis Rheum 27(8):947–950
16. Currier BL, Fitzgerald RJ (1988) Acetabular labrum tears of the hip. Transaction of the AAOS 55th Annual Meeting, Atlanta
17. Ikeda T, Awaya G, Suzuki S et al (1988) Torn acetabular labrum in young patients. Arthroscopic diagnosis and management. J Bone Joint Surg Br 70(1):13–16
18. Santori N, Villar R (2000) Acetabular labral tears: result of arthroscopic partial limbectomy. Arthroscopy 16(1):11–15
19. Farjo L, Glick J, Sampson T (1999) Hip arthroscopy for acetabular labral tears. Arthroscopy 15(2):132–137
20. McCarthy J, Noble P, Schuck M et al (2001) The watershed labral lesion: its relationship to early arthritis of the hip. J Arthroplasty 16(8 Suppl 1):81–87
21. Leunig M, Werlen S, Ungersböck A et al (1997) Evaluation of the acetabular labrum by MR arthrography. J Bone Joint Surg Br 79(2):230–234
22. Ganz R, Gill T, Gautier E et al (2001) Surgical dislocation of the adult hip: a technique with full access to the femoral head and acetabulum without the risk of avascular necrosis. J Bone Joint Surg Br 83(8):1119–1124
23. Myers SR, Eijer H, Ganz R (1999) Anterior femoroacetabular impingement after periacetabular osteotomy. Clin Orthop Relat Res 363:93–99
24. Leunig M, Casillas MM, Hamlet M et al (2000) Slipped capital femoral epiphysis: early mechanical damage to the acetabular cartilage by a prominent femoral metaphysis. Acta Orthop Scand 71(4):370–375
25. Ganz R, Parvizi J, Beck M et al (2003) Femoroacetabular impingement: a cause for osteoarthritis of the hip. Clin Orthop Relat Res 417:112–120
26. Goodman D, Feighan J, Smith A et al (1997) Subclinical slipped capital femoral epiphysis. Relationship to osteoarthrosis of the hip. J Bone Joint Surg Am 79(10):1489–1497

27. Rab GT (1999) The geometry of slipped capital femoral epiphysis: implications for movement, impingement, and corrective osteotomy. J Pediatr Orthop 19(4):419–424

28. Beck M, Kalhor M, Leunig M et al (2005) Hip morphology influences the pattern of damage to the acetabular cartilage: femoroacetabular impingement as a cause of early osteoarthritis of the hip. J Bone Joint Surg Br 87(7):1012–1018

29. Guanche CA, Bare AA (2006) Arthroscopic treatment of femoroacetabular impingement. Arthroscopy 22(1):95–106

30. Philippon MJ, Schenker ML (2006) Arthroscopy for the treatment of femoroacetabular impingement in the athlete. Clin Sports Med 25(2):299–308, ix

31. Wettstein M, Dienst M (2006) Hip arthroscopy for femoroacetabular impingement. Orthopade 35(1):85–93

32. Espinosa N, Rothenfluh DA, Beck M et al (2006) Treatment of femoro-acetabular impingement: preliminary results of labral refixation. J Bone Joint Surg Am 88(5):925–935

33. Beck M, Leunig M, Parvizi J et al (2004) Anterior femoro-acetabular impingement: part II. Midterm results of surgical treatment. Clin Orthop Relat Res 418:67–73

34. Peters CL, Erickson JA (2006) Treatment of femoro-acetabular impingement with surgical dislocation and debridement in young adults. J Bone Joint Surg Am 88(8):1735–1741

35. Tannast M, Goricki D, Beck M et al (2008) Hip damage occurs at the zone of femoroacetabular impingement. Clin Orthop Relat Res 466(2):273–280

36. O'Donoghue D (1957) Impingement exostoses of the talus and tibia. J Bone Joint Surg Am 39(4):835–920

# Mechanism of Femoroacetabular Impingement

Martin Beck, Slaman Chegini, Stephen Ferguson, and Harish S. Hosalkar

## Historical Background

In 1965, Murray [1] suggested for the first time the relation of the so-called tilt deformity, a rather subtle deformity of the proximal femur, to the subsequent development of osteoarthritis of the hip. Sometime later, Solomon and his team from South Africa [2, 3] as well as Harris and his coworkers [4, 5] from the United States performed some additional work on the theory that subtle deformities of the proximal femur are responsible for later degeneration of the hip joint. However, the causative factor that eventually leads to joint degeneration remained unrecognized until the work of Ganz and coworkers [6–8]. The development of the technique of surgical dislocation of the hip [6], based on recent anatomical data on the blood supply to the femoral head [9], made it possible to examine hip joint degeneration at early stages of the disease. All of these observations eventually led to a new hypothesis on the etiology of hip osteoarthritis (OA), one proposing that these previously unrecognized or ignored developmental deformities or abnormalities

in morphology lead to arthritis through the mechanism of femoroacetabular impingement (FAI) [7].

Femoroacetabular impingement is currently recognized as a precursor to osteoarthritis of the hip. It is characterized by an abnormal morphology of the hip leading to abutment of the proximal femur against the acetabulum during joint motion (flexion and internal rotation in particular). This repeated pathologic contact eventually leads to the development of symptomatic FAI, a precursor to osteoarthritis [7].

## Evidence in Support of the Theory

Two key facts that support the theory are (1) the recognition of the mechanism leading to hip OA and (2) the possibility that correction of that mechanism could delay the development of the OA [7].

First pioneered and stimulated by Ganz and coworkers and subsequently confirmed by a variety of observations from several centers across the world, a mechanism as to how these often subtle developmental abnormalities adversely affect the joint and lead to OA in many cases has been described [7]. The principal mechanism is a femoroacetabular impingement induced by motion of the well-constrained hip.

The recognition of this pathomechanism could not be proven until after the technique of surgical dislocation of the hip had been developed to the extent that it could be executed without risk of avascular necrosis or other morbidities [6, 9]. Surgical dislocation of the hip subsequently allowed for in situ observation of the FAI process and also for the attribution of the various damage patterns within the joint to different FAI morphologies [10]. Although FAI can take place anywhere

M. Beck (✉)
Department of Orthopedic Surgery,
Kantonspital, Luzern, Switzerland
e-mail: martin.beck@ksl.ch

S. Chegini • S. Ferguson
ARTORG Center for Biomedical Engineering Research,
Institute for Surgical Technology and
Biomechanics, University of Bern,
Bern, Switzerland

H.S. Hosalkar
Department of Orthopaedic Surgery,
School of Medicine, University of Pennsylvania,
Philadelphia, PA, USA

around the femoroacetabular joint, the most common site is anterolateral and is produced by flexion and variable degrees of internal rotation of the hip.

## Types of FAI

Two distinct types of FAI have been identified [8]. The first type occurs with the jamming of a nonspherical protrusion of the femoral head into the acetabular cavity; it is therefore named cam FAI. The second type is characterized by the linear impact of the acetabular rim against the head–neck junction in a local (e.g., acetabular retroversion) or global (e.g., coxa profunda or protrusio) overcoverage of the acetabulum; it is therefore named pincer FAI.

## Clinical Examination and Findings

Patients with femoroacetabular impingement are young, usually in their 20s–40s. The estimated prevalence is 10–15% [11]. Patients present with groin pain during or after sports activities that can irradiate distally and medially toward the knee. Groin pain can occur after prolonged sitting with the flexed hip. Occasionally, the impingement is accompanied by locking or catching with a sharp pain that starts in the groin. Some patients describe trochanteric pain irradiating from the lateral thigh. Typically, they are aware of their limited hip mobility long before symptoms appear. On clinical examination, patients with femoroacetabular impingement demonstrate a restricted range of motion, particularly internal rotation in flexion [8, 12]. Occasionally, unavoidable passive external rotation of the hip while performing a hip flexion is present. This has been described previously and is termed a positive "Drehmann's" sign [13] The impingement test is almost always positive [8]. This test is done with the patient supine; the hip is rotated internally as it is flexed passively to approximately 90° and adducted. Flexion and adduction leads to the approximation of the femoral neck to the acetabular rim. Additional internal rotation induces shearing forces at the labrum, creating pain when there is a labral lesion. Occasionally, posterior impingement can also occur. In this situation, the pain can be produced by external rotation of the flexed hip if the impinging area is posterosuperior. Another provocative test to elicit posterior impingement

is done by having the patient lie supine on the edge of the bed with the legs hanging free from the end of the bed to create extension. External rotation in extension giving rise to posterior pain, often perceived in the buttock, is indicative of posteroinferior impingement [6, 8]. A positive impingement test has been correlated closely to acetabular rim lesions as seen on specific modern MRI arthrograms of the hip [14].

## Cam Impingement

Cam impingement is more common in young men, occurring commonly in the third decade of life (average age of 32 years). Cam impingement is the femoral cause of FAI and is caused by an aspherical femoral head where the aspherical portion gets jammed into the acetabulum (Fig. 2.1).

The asphericity, which can manifest itself as flattening of the anterior contour of the femoral head–neck junction or even an osseous bump, creates a decreased femoral head–neck offset, which is defined by the distance between the widest diameter of the femoral head and the most prominent part of the femoral neck [15]. The recurrent irritation during flexion and internal rotation leads to abrasion of the acetabular cartilage or its avulsion from the subchondral bone (Fig. 2.2) [16]. Cam impingement can be caused by an asphericity of the femoral head–neck junction or by a retroverted femoral neck or head. Osseous bumps are typically located either in the lateral femoral head–neck junction (so-called pistol grip, seen on an anteroposterior pelvic radiograph) or in the anterosuperior (seen on an axial cross-table view) location of proximal femoral head–neck junction. A pistol-grip deformity is characterized on radiographs by flattening of the usually concave surface of the lateral aspect of the femoral head due to an abnormal extension of the more horizontally oriented femoral epiphysis [4, 17–19].

Cam impingement is usually caused by a primary osseous variant of the head–neck junction that is considered to be caused by a growth abnormality of the capital femoral epiphysis, but it can also be the result of several known causes, such as a subclinical slipped capital femoral epiphysis or Legg–Calvé–Perthes disease, or it can occur after femoral neck fractures; it may also be idiopathic [20–22].

Quantification of the amount of asphericity can be accomplished by the angle α, the femoral offset, or the

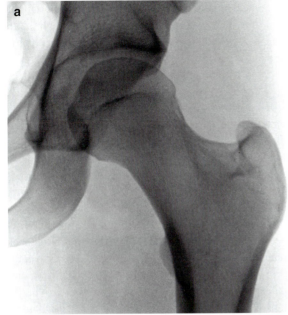

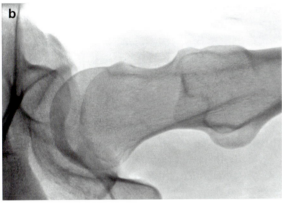

**Fig. 2.1** Radiographs of a hip with cam impingement presenting as a pistol-grip deformity. (**a**) The anteroposterior view showing asphericity of the femoral head as the area which extrudes from the circle laterally. (**b**) The lateral cross-table view showing asphericity of the femoral head extending from the circle

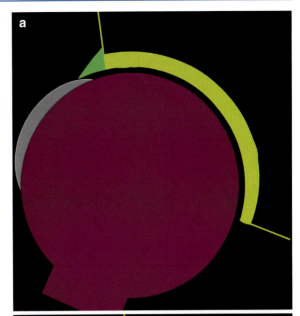

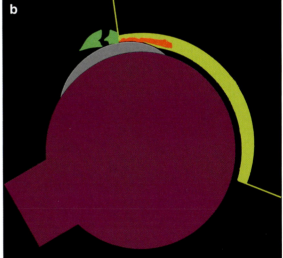

**Fig. 2.2** Diagram of the mechanism of damage in cam impingement on a lateral view of the hip. (**a**) During flexion, the aspherical part of the femoral head is jammed into the acetabulum, (**b**) compressing the cartilage and pushing it centrally at the same time until the cartilage is sheared off the subchondral bone

offset ratio. Angle $\alpha$ is the angle between the femoral neck axis and a line connecting the head center with the point of beginning asphericity of the head–neck contour [23] (Fig. 2.3a). It can be measured on radiographs. There is some debate about the normal upper value of the normal angle $\alpha$. Several studies state that the normal angle $\alpha$ value is of 42–43° [23–25]. Unfortunately, the lower limit of the pathological range is often considered a normal angle $\alpha$ (Fig. 2.3b). Another parameter for quantification of cam impingement is anterior offset, which is defined as the difference

in radius between the anterior femoral head and the anterior femoral neck on a cross-table axial view of the proximal femur [15]. In asymptomatic hips, anterior offset is $11.6 \pm 0.7$ mm; hips with cam impingement have a decreased anterior offset of $7.2 \pm 0.7$ mm. As a general rule for clinical practice, an anterior offset less than 10 mm is a strong indicator for cam impingement. In addition, the so-called offset ratio can be calculated, which is defined as the ratio between the anterior offset

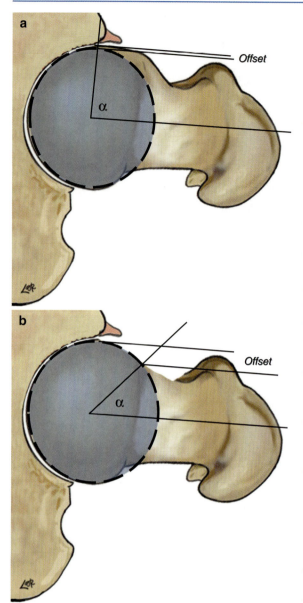

**Fig. 2.3** Cam impingement. (**a**) Axial view of normal hip with normal offset and normal alpha angle (normal angle $\alpha = 43°$). (**b**) Decreased femoral head–neck offset with consecutive increased alpha angle ($\alpha'$)

calculated reliably only on CT scans involving the proximal and distal parts of the femur [28]. In addition, a coxa vara (defined by a centrum collum diaphyseal angle [CCD] of less than 125°) has been recognized as a cause of cam impingement [29].

## Pincer Impingement

Pincer impingement is more common in middle-aged women, occurring around age 40. It can occur with various disorders. Pincer impingement is the result of overcoverage of the hip and can lead to osteoarthritis [30]. Pincer impingement is also the result of a linear contact between the acetabular rim and the femoral head–neck junction due to general or focal acetabular overcoverage (Fig. 2.4). In contrast to cam impingement, cartilage damage of the acetabular cartilage is restricted in pincer hips to a small thin strip near the labrum that is more circumferentially located (Fig. 2.5) [10].

## Causes of Pincer FAI

(a) *Deep socket*
   i. Coxa profunda
   ii. Protrusio
(b) *Maloriented socket*
   i. Retroversion (idiopathic, DDH, Perthes, overcorrection, post-traumatic dysplasia, bladder extrophy, PFFD)

## General Acetabular Overcoverage

Normally, general or comprehensive acetabular overcoverage is correlated with the radiologic depth of the acetabular fossa. In a normal hip joint with an appropriately seated acetabulum, the acetabular fossa line lies lateral to the ilioischial line on an anteroposterior pelvic radiograph. When the floor of the fossa acetabuli touches or overlaps the ilioischial line medially, the condition is defined as "coxa profunda." Protrusio acetabuli is present when the femoral head overlaps the ilioischial line medially [31]. Both of these abnormal morphological variants relate to an increased acetabular depth. However, there is currently no evidence that protrusion is a natural progression of coxa profunda.

and the diameter of the head. The offset ratio is $0.21 \pm 0.03$ in asymptomatic patients and $0.13 \pm 0.05$ in hips with cam impingement [26].

Another notable cause for cam impingement is femoral retrotorsion, which can occur as a primary entity or post-traumatically following femoral neck fracture healing [22, 27]. Femoral retrotorsion can be

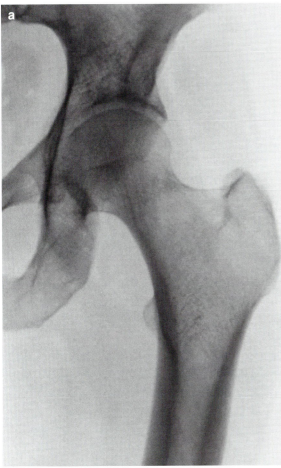

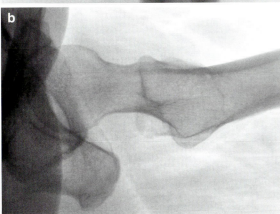

**Fig. 2.4** Radiographs of a hip with pincer impingement showing coxa profunda with ossification of the acetabular labrum (**a**) anteroposterior and (**b**) lateral views. The head is spherical in both planes

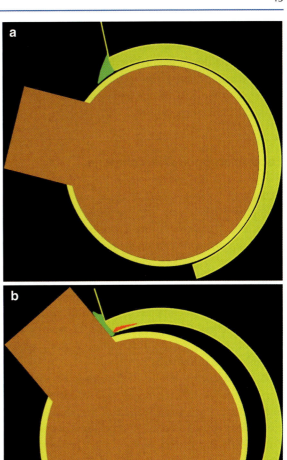

**Fig. 2.5** Diagram of the mechanism of damage in pincer impingement on a lateral view of the hip. (**a**) During flexion, the labrum acts as a buffer between the femoral neck and the acetabulum. Only a small area of acetabular cartilage is subject to compression along the rim. (**b**) Posteriorly, the femoral head is levered out, creating a contrecoup lesion

Generally, a deep acetabulum is associated with excessive acetabular coverage that can be quantified with the lateral center edge angle or the acetabular index [32]. The lateral center edge angle is the angle formed by a vertical line and a line connecting the femoral head center with the lateral edge of the acetabulum. The acetabular index is the angle formed by a horizontal line and a line connecting the medial point of the sclerotic zone with the lateral center of the acetabulum. In hips with coxa profunda or protrusio acetabuli, the acetabular index (also called "acetabular roof angle") is typically 0° or even negative. Another parameter for quantification of femoral coverage is the femoral head extrusion index, which defines the percentage of femoral head that is uncovered when a horizontal line is drawn parallel to the inter-teardrop line [33]. A normal extrusion index is less than 25%; although to the best of our knowledge no study has defined a minimum extrusion.

## Focal Acetabular Overcoverage

Acetabular version is best assessed on an AP pelvic radiograph, taken with the standards defined previously [34]. Focal overcoverage can occur in the anterior or the posterior part of the acetabulum. Anterior overcoverage is called "cranial acetabular retroversion" or "anterior focal acetabular retroversion" and causes anterior femoroacetabular impingement that can be reproduced clinically with painful flexion and internal rotation. By carefully tracing the anterior and posterior acetabular rims, different acetabular configurations can be identified.

A normal acetabulum is anteverted and has the anterior rim line projected medially to the posterior wall line [34, 35]. Focal overcoverage of the anterosuperior acetabulum causes a cranially retroverted acetabulum. This is defined with the anterior rim line being lateral to the posterior rim in the cranial part of the acetabulum and crossing the latter in the distal part of the acetabulum. This figure-of-8 configuration is called the "crossover" sign (Fig. 2.6).

To distinguish between a too-prominent anterior wall and a deficient posterior wall, the posterior wall must be depicted in greater detail. Therefore, the "posterior wall" sign was introduced as an indicator for a prominent posterior wall. This can cause posterior impingement with reproducible pain in hip extension and external rotation. In a normal hip, the visible outline of the posterior rim descends approximately through the center point of the femoral head. If the posterior line lies laterally to the femoral center, a more prominent posterior wall is present. In contrast, a deficient posterior wall has the posterior rim medial to the femoral head center. A deficient posterior wall is often correlated with acetabular retroversion or dysplasia [36]; an excessive posterior wall can often be seen in hips with coxa profunda or protrusio acetabuli but can also occur as an isolated entity. Acetabular retroversion can also be caused by acetabular reorientation procedures if the configuration of the acetabular rims is not taken into consideration [37, 38].

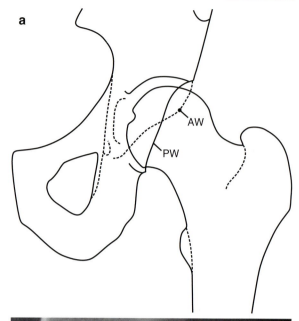

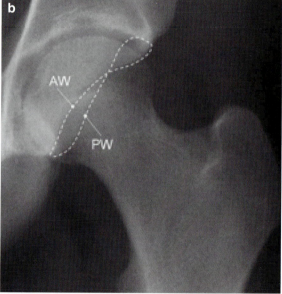

**Fig. 2.6** Diagrammatic illustration (*left*) and radiographic (*right*) presentations of focal anterior overcoverage of hip. Acetabular retroversion is defined as anterior wall (AW) being more lateral than posterior wall (PW), whereas in normal hip, anterior wall lies more medially. This cranial acetabular retroversion can also be described by "figure-of-8" configuration

This persistent abutment in the anterior part of the joint can lead to a slight subluxation posteroinferiorly. The increased pressure between the posteroinferior acetabulum and the posteromedial aspect of the femoral head can cause chondral damage to the posteroinferior part of the acetabulum as a contrecoup lesion, which occurs in approximately one-third of pincer cases [8, 10]. The resulting loss of joint space can be visualized on a faux profile and is a bad prognostic sign.

In certain hips, distinguishing between the two lines of the acetabular rim is difficult. As a helpful guideline, the posterior rim line can always be readily identified when starting from the inferior edge of the acetabulum. An anteroposterior radiograph centered over the hip is not usable for reliable diagnosis of acetabular retroversion. This projection will imply a discrepancy in the appearance of the acetabular rim compared with a standard pelvic radiograph on which the anterior rim will be displayed more prominently because it lies closer to the X-ray beam source [39]. Therefore, acetabular version is generally overestimated when interpreting an anteroposterior radiograph centered over the hip. In addition, a cross-over sign can even be missed if only an anteroposterior radiograph of the hip is available.

The appearance of acetabular morphology depends on the individual pelvic orientation, which can vary considerably in terms of tilt and rotation. Increased pelvic tilt or a rotation to the ipsilateral hip leads to a more pronounced retroversion sign and vice versa [34, 39]. A neutral pelvic rotation is defined as the tip of the coccyx pointing toward the midpoint of the superior aspect of the symphysis pubis. As a general rule, a neutral pelvic tilt is defined as the distance of 3.2 cm between the upper border of the symphysis and the midportion of the sacrococcygeal joint for men and 4.7 cm for women [23]. With the help of one additional lateral radiograph, the radiographs of extensively rotated or tilted pelves can be calculated back with recently developed software Hip2Norm to ensure a tilt and rotation independent of anatomically based interpretation of the acetabular morphologic configuration [39, 40]. If obtained, the lateral pelvic view must be taken after the anteroposterior projection without motion of the patient and with the central beam directed to the upper tip of the greater trochanter. In addition to acetabular pathomorphologies, pincer impingement can also be caused by excessive hip motion in patients in whom no obvious acetabular disorder is present. It occurs typically in hypermobile young women (e.g., ballet dancers).

## Typical Articular Damage Pattern in Different Types of FAI

Pattern of damage to the acetabular cartilage and the labrum does depend upon the shape and morphology of the hip. We have previously reported on details of damage patterns in acetabular cartilage in different types of FAI [10].

In all hips with a cam impingement, the acetabular cartilage was noted to be damaged in the anterosuperior area of the acetabulum, and all these cases also involved separation of the acetabular cartilage from the labrum. The labrum usually had a stable attachment to the bone, but the acetabular cartilage was torn off the labrum which, in some cases, showed additional degenerative changes (Fig. 2.7a). In a normal hip, the

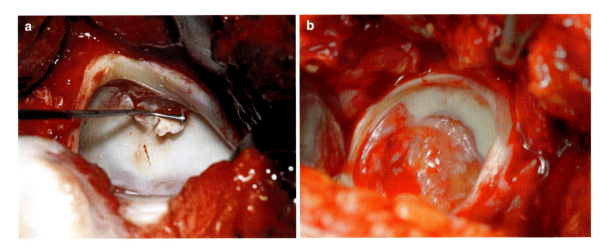

**Fig. 2.7** (**a**) Characteristic damage pattern in a cam type lesion. (**b**) Characteristic damage pattern in a pincer type lesion

acetabular labrum merges with the acetabular cartilage through a transition zone without any gap [41].

In hips with a pincer impingement, the damage was located more circumferentially, usually including only a narrow strip of the acetabular cartilage (Fig. 2.7b). The changes in the labrum were colocated with the damage to the cartilage, often presenting as ossification of the labrum.

The patterns of damage in the cam and pincer impingements differ considerably and require a different pathomechanical explanation. The principal problem in the hip with a cam impingement is absent anterior-to-anterolateral waisting of the junction of the femoral neck and head. This is equivalent to a cam, which is an eccentric part added to a rotating device. During flexion, the eccentric part slides into the anterosuperior acetabulum and induces compression and shear stresses at the junction between the labrum and the cartilage and at the subchondral tidemark. The labrum is stretched and pushed outward, and the cartilage is compressed and pushed centrally (Fig. 2.2), causing a separation between the labrum and cartilage. Therefore, for so-called undersurface tears of the labrum, the correct terminology would be "separation of the acetabular cartilage from the labrum." This theory is supported by the observation that in all hips with a cam impingement, the labrum had a stable fixation to the acetabular rim, but in half of the hips, the cartilage was separated from it or was missing. If the labrum was torn off the acetabular rim, the acetabular cartilage could be expected to be intact.

The "pincer" does not cause an impingement because of asphericity of the femoral head. The dominant feature is that of a deep socket in which the range of movement of the hip is limited by the overcovering acetabular rim. At the limit of movement, the femoral neck abuts against the labrum, which acts like a bumper. The labrum is compressed between the femoral neck and the underlying bone, and the force is further transmitted to the acetabular cartilage. The transmission of force to the cartilage is restricted to a narrow band along the acetabular rim (Fig. 2.5). Repeated microtrauma induces bone growth at the base of the labrum, which subsequently ossifies. In cam impingement, the damage to the acetabular joint is located anterosuperiorly.

In coxa profunda, the prototype for pincer impingement, the deep socket limits movement in all directions and leads to a more circumferential pattern of damage. Since the principal direction of movement is flexion, most of the lesions are located at the anterosuperior acetabular rim. When impingement occurs at the anterosuperior rim and further flexion is enforced, the femoral head begins to sublux posteriorly and, because of the constrained nature of the hip, increased pressure between the posteromedial aspect of the femoral head and the posteroinferior acetabulum occurs. This contrecoup lesion was observed in the femoral head in 62% and in the posteroinferior acetabulum in 31% of our previously reported series.

Protrusio, acetabular retroversion, ossification of the labrum, and a negative acetabular index angle also lead to a pincer impingement. Cam and pincer impingement are two basic mechanisms and rarely occur in isolation; in our study, only 26 of 149 hips presented with an isolated aspherical head and 16 with an isolated coxa profunda. Most have a combination of these two basic mechanisms and are classified as mixed cam–pincer impingement. The damage to the cartilage in these cases is usually a combination of the two patterns of damage.

## Biomechanical Studies Analyzing FAI

### Effect of Impingement on Stress Distributions in the Hip Joint

Hip joint function is closely related to its anatomical form. The healthy joint provides three rotational degrees of freedom (flexion–extension, adduction–abduction, and internal–external rotation), allowing extensive and painless mobility. The morphology of the hip joint varies for different individuals depending on age, gender, race, and developmental changes [42].

Abnormal morphology of the joint, either on the femoral head or acetabulum, is often observed in patients with symptomatic FAI. Besides the morphology of the joint, the load and motion patterns that induce impingement are critical points to be investigated. FAI is believed to occur due to motion, rather than through axial overloading of the hip. Furthermore, impingement is a problem of morphological variations of the hip joint and is not observed within the range of "normal" acetabular and femoral geometry. This hypothesis is well supported by clinical observations and by recently published biomechanical data [43]. Biomechanical investigations of the impingement phenomenon have the potential to provide quantitative information on the mechanical response of the joint, which may facilitate diagnosis and improved treatment.

## Computational Simulation of Impingement

### Hip Joint Morphological Variation

The anatomical parameters of the human hip that affect the extent of impingement can be described by selected parameters on the femoral head and the acetabulum. The key parameter on the acetabulum is the measure of acetabular coverage, defined by the center-edge (CE) angle. The CE angle, also called angle of Wiberg [44], is defined as the angle formed by the line passing from the center of the femoral head to the lateral edge of the acetabulum and a vertical line drawn through the center of the femoral head (Fig. 2.8).

A relevant anatomical parameter on the femoral head for impinging joints has been defined recently by Nötzli et al. [23] as the angle α, which describes the relationship between femoral head and neck geometry (Fig. 2.3a, b). By altering these two parameters, it is possible to create computational models representing a normal joint (CE=20°, α=50°), dysplastic joint (CE=0°, α=50°), cam type joint (CE=20°, α=80°), pincer type joint (CE=40°, α=50°), or combination of both cam and pincer (CE=40°, α=80°).

Since the morphological parameters of a patient may fall within these extreme cases, it is important to create joint models that cover the full range between these extremes. Computer-aided design software provides a versatile tool for the creation of joint models with a broad range of morphological parameters: anterior CE angles of 0°, 10°, 20°, 30°, and 40° and femoral alpha angles of 40°, 50°, 60°, 70°, and 80°, creating a matrix of 25 different idealized joints. Examples of a normal joint and a typical cam type joint are shown in Fig. 2.9.

### Material Properties

The internal stresses developed during locomotion and impingement depend heavily on the properties of the articulating surfaces. Representative cartilage material properties have been selected as linear elastic, with an elastic modulus and Poisson ratio of E=12 MPa and ν=0.45, respectively [45]. Appropriate material properties of labrum tissue have been determined in our own previous work as E=20 MPa and ν=0.4 [46]. The

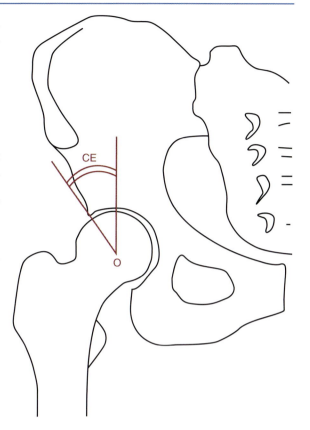

**Fig. 2.8** Definition of the CE angle as an indication of femoral head coverage

compliance of the underlying bony structures of the hip joint is often neglected, as its influence on the calculated contact pressures and stresses is negligible, and therefore, these may be considered rigid bodies. It has been experimentally verified that the contact between cartilage layers has a very low friction coefficient, providing an almost frictionless articulation of the joint; hence, the contact between the femoral and acetabular cartilage is defined as surface-based, finite sliding, and frictionless contact.

### Loads and Activities

The forces and motions occurring during different daily activities induce internal deformations and stresses in the soft tissues of the hip joint, for both the normal and pathological hip. Some activities like walking apply high axial forces on the hip joint over a rather limited range of motion, while other activities, like the transition from standing to sitting, are associated with a higher motion range but a lower peak force. The frequency of the activity that a joint experiences through

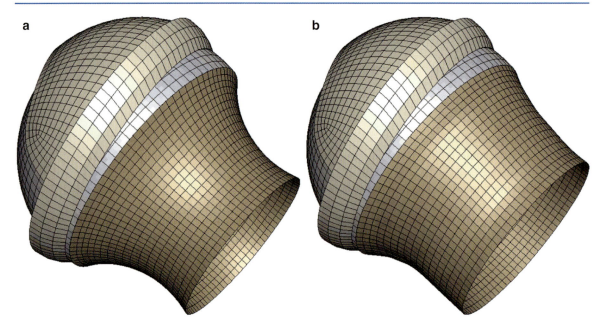

**Fig. 2.9** (**a**) A typical normal hip joint and (**b**) a cam type impinging joint

daily life should also be considered as an important factor. Standing-to-sitting and walking have been chosen as frequently occurring repetitive activities of a routine daily life, with a substantial influence on overall joint loading.

For the determination of appropriate kinetic and kinematic boundary conditions for such simulations, the in vivo studies conducted by Bergmann et al. [47] can be considered a gold standard, as they provide direct in situ dynamic force and motion measurements from a relatively large selection of patient volunteers during a variety of activities. For these novel measurements, an instrumented joint endoprosthesis and a telemetry system have been developed. The force and motion data for standing to sitting and normal walking was applied to the matrix of 25 different joints, and the response of the joints was calculated using a three-dimensional finite element analysis. In these simulations, time-synchronized force and motion was applied to the center of femoral head, which was free to translate and relocate itself within the hip joint. An average body weight was assumed as 836 N, taken as a composite of the patient volunteers.

### Internal Joint Mechanics

Biomechanical simulation allows the calculation of the local contact pressure between the soft tissues of the hip joint, as well as internal von Mises stresses, a measure of internal distortion energy and tissue deformation. These values were calculated during the whole cycle of walking and standing-to-sitting for all 25 joints. A typical von Mises stress distribution in a cam type joint is shown in Fig. 2.10.

To evaluate the influence of joint morphology on the internal mechanical environment within the joint, it is illustrative to calculate the peak von Mises stresses for each joint conformation from the cycle of both walking and standing-to-sitting, then to plot the maximum value for each representative joint geometry (Fig. 2.11). Elevated stresses for low CE angles generally correspond to rim overloading during walking for the dysplastic hip, whereas hip joints with acetabular overcoverage or femoral head–neck deformity ("pincer" and "cam" joints) demonstrate a substantial increase in stresses during activities with large motions. Of particular importance, the blue zone of Fig. 2.11 shows a range of CE and alpha angle values for which the stresses are minimized for both types of activity ($20° \leq CE \leq 30°$ and $\alpha \leq 50°$).

### Discussion

Nowadays, FAI is an established mechanism leading to osteoarthritis of the hip in young adult patients without dysplasia. This concept is based on extensive

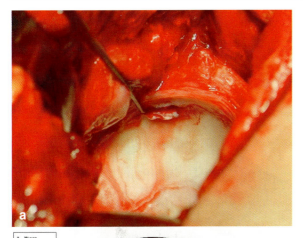

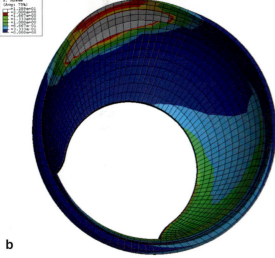

**Fig. 2.10** (**a**) A clinical case with cam type impingement. (**b**) Results of the finite element simulation for the case of standing-to-sitting

these often subtle deformities resulted in OA of the hip. Of notice is also that the secondary deformities of the femoral neck have been described [50, 51]. It was only the ability to dislocate the hip safely that enabled us to examine the joint dynamically and to match damage patterns with deformities and thus establish the concept of FAI [6–8].

At the acetabular rim, there is almost always a colocation of labral and acetabular cartilage pathology [8, 10]. To the observer unfamiliar with the pathomechanism of FAI, it would seem unclear whether the cartilage damage is secondary to labral pathology, vice versa, or if both are part of the impingement process. As shown previously, the damage pattern in cam and pincer FAI is different [10]. In pincer FAI, the labrum is squeezed between the acetabular rim and the femoral neck and acts more as a bumper. In the initial stages of the disease, macroscopically no damage is observed, and it is only in the later stages that fibrillations and fissuring become visible. The pathological changes occur in the substance of the labrum and have been previously described as cleavage planes within the substance of the labrum [41]. The ongoing microtrauma finally induces bone formation at the base of the labrum until the entire labrum becomes ossified [8]. The acetabular cartilage damage is restricted to only a narrow band and is observed at late stages of the disease. In cam FAI, the problem is different. Here, the labrum dodges the asphericity because of its elasticity. The acetabular cartilage, however, is comparably stiff and pushed away toward the depth of the acetabulum. Eventually, the transition zone between the hyaline acetabular cartilage and the fibrocartilage of the labrum fails. On superficial observation, this may appear as an undersurface tear of the labrum; in fact, it is the hyaline cartilage that is ripped off and displaced. The labrum in its substance remains unchanged, certainly in the early stages of the process. This concept is supported by the intraoperative observation and also by the histological study of Seldes et al. [41] who described this as one of the two possible cartilage damage patterns. Therefore, it can be summarized that pincer FAI first affects the labrum, whereas cam FAI first affects the acetabular cartilage. Solitary labral tears arising from an acute traumatic event are rare and are more common in societies with violent sport activities like football or rugby. Labral tears seen during arthroscopic examination of the hip [52], particularly in the anterosuperior region of the acetabulum, most

clinical observations made by Ganz et al. [8] who have performed surgical dislocations of the hip on more than a 1,000 patients suspected of having FAI. More recently, the concept has also been supported by biomechanical studies [40, 48] and by the sophisticated FE analysis of Chegini et al. [43].

Even before the development of the concept of FAI, several studies suggested that milder deformities of the proximal femur in patients without a history of developmental disease were a cause of osteoarthritis [1, 19, 49]. It was shown that a so-called "pistol-grip deformity" is present in 40% of patients who develop osteoarthritis of the hip [19]. Except for Goodmann et al. [49], who mentioned motion as a possible initiator of joint damage, no indication was given of how

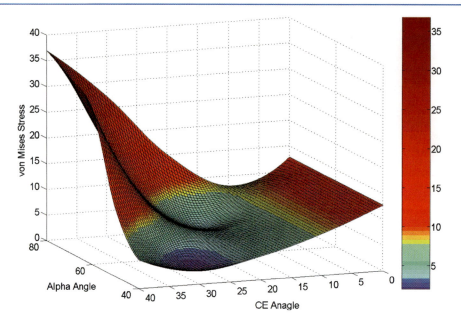

**Fig. 2.11** Maximum of peak von Mises stress from walking and standing-to-sitting

likely represent FAI. This premise is supported by the observation that most labral tears seen during hip arthroscopy also are associated with chondral injury [52]. McCarthy et al. reporting on more than 400 hip arthroscopies, noted a highly significant association between the presence of labral lesions and degeneration of the articular surface. Approximately two-thirds of their patients with fraying or a tear of the labrum had evidence of chondral damage.

Although detailed analysis of the outcome of surgical intervention is still ongoing, the preliminary results indicate that surgical dislocation of the hip and improvement of the head and neck offset are successful in addressing the symptoms arising from the underlying impingement. Surgical intervention is more successful in patients with early FAI [14, 16]. In patients with moderate to severe loss of joint space, the outcome is likely to be less than optimal. Therefore, early diagnosis and timely delivery of care are likely to retard the degenerative process and delay the need for hip arthroplasty. Although long-term results are awaited, surgical treatment of patients with FAI has been encouraging to date. As hypothesized, pathological morphology of the hip joint leads to high contact pressures and internal cartilage stresses that may be contributing factors for degeneration, delamination, or hypertrophy of the soft tissues within the hip joint.

The results of biomechanical studies with hip simulation (described above) suggest that the optimum morphological parameters for low-stress function of the hip joint are a CE angle between 20° and 30° and an angle α of less than 50°. The location of high-stress zones in the impinging joint corresponds well with clinically observed damage zones, yet the limitations of such simulations should also be considered. The in vivo load and motion data are derived from patients who have experienced major reconstructive surgery on their joints and therefore provided a lower bound for what may be considered physiological joint forces and motions. Idealized hip joint models provide a convenient and consistent simulation tool for completing a parametric study of morphological factors contributing to joint degeneration; however, these simulations could be further improved with the use of patient-specific finite element models. The high-stress zones predicted by the simulations are relevant to clinical practice; the range of the morphological parameters that minimize the stresses may be considered a guideline for joint preservation surgery and is within the range recommend by surgeons, based on their own clinical experience.

The current advancements in the ability of MRI to identify chondral pathology will likely help in our understanding of the natural history of FAI. Better understanding of the pathophysiology of impingement as a cause of arthritis of the hip will enable additional therapeutic interventions to be developed. Finally, further refinements of surgical procedures should not only enhance outcome but also allow surgeons to better determine the indications for these impingement procedures.

**Acknowledgment**   Nina Agrawal, BA, Clinical Research Coordinator, Children's Hospital of Philadelphia, PA.

# References

1. Murray RO (1965) The aetiology of primary osteoarthritis of the hip. Br J Radiol 38(455):810–824
2. Solomon L (1976) Patterns of osteoarthritis of the hip. J Bone Joint Surg Br 58(2):176–183
3. Solomon L, Beighton P, Lawrence JS (1976) Osteoarthrosis in a rural South African Negro population. Ann Rheum Dis 35(3):274–278
4. Harris WH (1986) Etiology of osteoarthritis of the hip. Clin Orthop Relat Res 213:20–33
5. Harris WH, Bourne RB, Oh I (1979) Intra-articular acetabular labrum: a possible etiological factor in certain cases of osteoarthritis of the hip. J Bone Joint Surg Am 61(4):510–514
6. Ganz R, Gill TJ, Gautier E, Ganz K, Krugel N, Berlemann U (2001) Surgical dislocation of the adult hip a technique with full access to the femoral head and acetabulum without the risk of avascular necrosis. J Bone Joint Surg Br 83(8):1119–1124
7. Ganz R, Leunig M, Leunig-Ganz K, Harris WH (2008) The etiology of osteoarthritis of the hip: an integrated mechanical concept. Clin Orthop Relat Res 466(2):264–272
8. Ganz R, Parvizi J, Beck M, Leunig M, Notzli H, Siebenrock KA (2003) Femoroacetabular impingement: a cause for osteoarthritis of the hip. Clin Orthop Relat Res 417:112–120
9. Gautier E, Ganz K, Krugel N, Gill T, Ganz R (2000) Anatomy of the medial femoral circumflex artery and its surgical implications. J Bone Joint Surg Br 82(5):679–683
10. Beck M, Kalhor M, Leunig M, Ganz R (2005) Hip morphology influences the pattern of damage to the acetabular cartilage: femoroacetabular impingement as a cause of early osteoarthritis of the hip. J Bone Joint Surg Br 87(7):1012–1018
11. Leunig M, Ganz R (2005) Femoroacetabular impingement. A common cause of hip complaints leading to arthrosis. Unfallchirurg 108(1):9–10, 12–17
12. Ito K, Leunig M, Ganz R (2004) Histopathologic features of the acetabular labrum in femoroacetabular impingement. Clin Orthop Relat Res 429:262–271
13. Drehmann F (1979) Drehmann's sign. A clinical examination method in epiphysiolysis (slipping of the upper femoral epiphysis). Description of signs, aetiopathogenetic considerations, clinical experience (author's transl). Z Orthop Ihre Grenzgeb 117(3):333–344
14. Parvizi J, Leunig M, Ganz R (2007) Femoroacetabular impingement. J Am Acad Orthop Surg 15(9):561–570
15. Eijer H, Leunig M, Mahomed M, Ganz R (2001) Cross-table lateral radiograph for screening of anterior femoral head-neck offset in patients with femoroacetabular impingement. Hip Int 11:37–41
16. Beck M, Leunig M, Parvizi J, Boutier V, Wyss D, Ganz R (2004) Anterior femoroacetabular impingement: part II. Midterm results of surgical treatment. Clin Orthop Relat Res 418:67–73
17. Resnick D (1976) The 'tilt deformity' of the femoral head in osteoarthritis of the hip: a poor indicator of previous epiphysiolysis. Clin Radiol 27(3):355–363
18. Siebenrock KA, Wahab KH, Werlen S, Kalhor M, Leunig M, Ganz R (2004) Abnormal extension of the femoral head epiphysis as a cause of cam impingement. Clin Orthop Relat Res 418:54–60
19. Stulberg S, Cordell L, Harris W, Ramsey P, MacEwen G (1975) Unrecognized childhood hip disease: a major cause of idiopathic osteoarthritis of the hip. Paper presented at: The hip: Proceedings of the Third Open Scientific Meeting of the Hip Society, St. Louis, MO
20. Leunig M, Casillas MM, Hamlet M et al (2000) Slipped capital femoral epiphysis: early mechanical damage to the acetabular cartilage by a prominent femoral metaphysis. Acta Orthop Scand 71(4):370–375
21. Snow SW, Keret D, Scarangella S, Bowen JR (1993) Anterior impingement of the femoral head: a late phenomenon of Legg-Calve-Perthes' disease. J Pediatr Orthop 13(3):286–289
22. Strehl A, Ganz R (2005) Anterior femoroacetabular impingement after healed femoral neck fractures. Unfallchirurg 108(4):263–273
23. Notzli HP, Wyss TF, Stoecklin CH, Schmid MR, Treiber K, Hodler J (2002) The contour of the femoral head-neck junction as a predictor for the risk of anterior impingement. J Bone Joint Surg Br 84(4):556–560
24. Beaule PE, Zaragoza E, Motamedi K, Copelan N, Dorey FJ (2005) Three-dimensional computed tomography of the hip in the assessment of femoroacetabular impingement. J Orthop Res 23(6):1286–1292
25. Neumann M, Cui Q, Siebenrock KA, Beck M (2009) Impingement-free hip motion: the 'normal' angle alpha after osteochondroplasty. Clin Orthop Relat Res 467:699–703, Epub Nov 19, 2008
26. Tannast M, Siebenrock KA, Anderson SE (2007) Femoroacetabular impingement: radiographic diagnosis – what the radiologist should know. AJR Am J Roentgenol 188(6):1540–1552
27. Tschauner C, Fock CM, Hofmann S, Raith J (2002) Rotational abnormalities of the hip joint. Radiologe 42(6):457–466
28. Murphy SB, Simon SR, Kijewski PK, Wilkinson RH, Griscom NT (1987) Femoral anteversion. J Bone Joint Surg Am 69(8):1169–1176
29. Millis M, Kim Y, Kocher M (2004) Hip joint-preserving surgery for the mature hip: the Children's Hospital experience. Orthop J HMS 6:84–87
30. Giori NJ, Trousdale RT (2003) Acetabular retroversion is associated with osteoarthritis of the hip. Clin Orthop Relat Res 417:263–269
31. Ruelle M, Dubois JL (1962) The protrusive malformation and its arthrosic complication. I. Radiological and clinical symptoms. Etiopathogenesis. Rev Rhum Mal Osteoartic 29:476–489
32. Murphy SB, Kijewski PK, Millis MB, Harless A (1990) Acetabular dysplasia in the adolescent and young adult. Clin Orthop Relat Res 261:214–223

33. Heyman CH, Herndon CH (1950) Legg-Perthes disease; a method for the measurement of the roentgenographic result. J Bone Joint Surg Am 32(A:4):767–778

34. Siebenrock KA, Kalbermatten DF, Ganz R (2003) Effect of pelvic tilt on acetabular retroversion: a study of pelves from cadavers. Clin Orthop Relat Res 407:241–248

35. Mast JW, Brunner RL, Zebrack J (2004) Recognizing acetabular version in the radiographic presentation of hip dysplasia. Clin Orthop Relat Res 418:48–53

36. Reynolds D, Lucas J, Klaue K (1999) Retroversion of the acetabulum. A cause of hip pain. J Bone Joint Surg Br 81(2): 281–288

37. Dora C, Mascard E, Mladenov K, Seringe R (2002) Retroversion of the acetabular dome after Salter and triple pelvic osteotomy for congenital dislocation of the hip. J Pediatr Orthop B 11(1):34–40

38. Myers SR, Eijer H, Ganz R (1999) Anterior femoroacetabular impingement after periacetabular osteotomy. Clin Orthop Relat Res 363:93–99

39. Tannast M, Zheng G, Anderegg C et al (2005) Tilt and rotation correction of acetabular version on pelvic radiographs. Clin Orthop Relat Res 438:182–190

40. Tannast M, Goricki D, Beck M, Murphy SB, Siebenrock KA (2008) Hip damage occurs at the zone of femoroacetabular impingement. Clin Orthop Relat Res 466(2):273–280

41. Seldes RM, Tan V, Hunt J, Katz M, Winiarsky R, Fitzgerald RH Jr (2001) Anatomy, histologic features, and vascularity of the adult acetabular labrum. Clin Orthop Relat Res 382:232–240

42. Than P, Sillinger T, Kranicz J, Bellyei A (2004) Radiographic parameters of the hip joint from birth to adolescence. Pediatr Radiol 34(3):237–244

43. Chegini S, Beck M, Ferguson SJ (2009) The effects of impingement and dysplasia on stress distributions in the hip joint during sitting and walking: a finite element analysis. J Orthop Res 27(2):195–201

44. Wiberg G (1939) Studies on dysplastic acetabular and congenital subluxation of the hip joint. With special reference to the complication of osteo-arthritis. Acta Chir Scand 83 (Suppl 58):5–135

45. Moglo KE, Shirazi-Adl A (2003) On the coupling between anterior and posterior cruciate ligaments, and knee joint response under anterior femoral drawer in flexion: a finite element study. Clin Biomech (Bristol, Avon) 18(8): 751–759

46. Ferguson SJ, Bryant JT, Ito K (2001) The material properties of the bovine acetabular labrum. J Orthop Res 19(5):887–896

47. Bergmann G, Deuretzbacher G, Heller M et al (2001) Hip contact forces and gait patterns from routine activities. J Biomech 34(7):859–871

48. Kubiak-Langer M, Tannast M, Murphy SB, Siebenrock KA, Langlotz F (2007) Range of motion in anterior femoroacetabular impingement. Clin Orthop Relat Res 458:117–124

49. Goodman DA, Feighan JE, Smith AD, Latimer B, Buly RL, Cooperman DR (1997) Subclinical slipped capital femoral epiphysis. Relationship to osteoarthrosis of the hip. J Bone Joint Surg Am 79(10):1489–1497

50. Angel JL (1964) The reaction area of the femoral neck. Clin Orthop Relat Res 32:130–142

51. Odgers PN (1931) Two details about the neck of the femur. (1) The Eminentia. (2) The Empreinte. J Anat 65(Pt 3): 352–362.3

52. McCarthy JC, Noble PC, Schuck MR, Wright J, Lee J (2001) The Otto E. Aufranc Award: the role of labral lesions to development of early degenerative hip disease. Clin Orthop Relat Res 393:25–37

# Physical Exam in FAI

Óliver Marín-Peña

The patient with FAI is typically a 20–50-year-old male with insidious hip pain but with no traumatic injury [1, 2]. In the first appointment, the focus must be placed on the etiology of the symptoms. These symptoms could be divided into pain that is referred to the hip (lumbar pain, pelvic pain), extra-articular pain (piriformis syndrome, trochanteric bursitis, psoas bursitis), intra-articular pain without bone deformity (labral lesion, chondral defects, loose bodies, synovitis), intra-articular pain with bone deformity (dysplasia, femoro-acetabular impingement, Perthes-type deformity, avascular necrosis), and advanced joint degeneration.

Onset of symptoms in male FAI patients usually occurs at ages 25–38, whereas in females, presentation tends to be bimodal (first at puberty and subsequently toward the end of the third decade) [1, 2].

If hip pain is observed in a teenager, Perthes' disease or SCFE must be ruled out. Although FAI is the most frequent cause of hip pain in athletes involved in sports requiring extreme ranges of motion [3], non-athlete patients also suffer hip pain during occupational activities or weekend sport practice, albeit later in life.

Patients should be asked about any previous surgeries and other hip pathologies as well as about their current occupation and daily sport activities [1, 2]. Information about the characteristics of the pain and its provoking and alleviating factors can also be useful. Duration of pain is usually over 6 months, and persistence of symptoms is generally directly proportional to the extent of chondrolabral damage [2]. Most patients complain about groin pain that migrates to the greater trochanter, buttocks, and even radiates to the knee secondary to abnormal gait biomechanics [4]. Patients may indicate the location of pain by gripping their lateral hip, just above the greater trochanter, between the thumb and index finger. This is known as the C-sign. Initially, the pain is intermittent and increases with activities such as long walks and hyperflexion (sitting down and leg-crossing, hitting a ball, jumping fences, doing martial arts, and driving). Catching or locking is usually related to an intra-articular lesion such as a labral tear or a chondral flap [5, 6]. Sometimes pain can present after prolonged sitting or minor trauma [7, 8]. Before an accurate diagnosis is finally made, it is not unusual for the patient's symptoms to have been evaluated by multiple clinicians and mistakenly associated with adductor lesions, inguinal hernias, or pubic osteopathy. Some authors have described cases of patients undergoing abdominal surgery, lumbar decompression surgery, or knee arthroscopies when their symptoms had in fact been caused by FAI [9]. Burnett et al. [10] presented a series of 66 patients with labral lesions, some of whom had undergone different kinds of surgery (1 inguinal herniorrhaphy, 1 psoas tenotomy, 2 diagnostic laparoscopies) before the condition was eventually identified.

A proper physical examination must evaluate for abductor weakness, coxa saltans, and bursitis. Full range of motion must be assessed, differentiating the true limits of hip motion from pelvic motion. In FAI patients, limitation of motion tends to affect mainly flexion, adduction, and internal rotation [11, 12], being more pronounced if the hip is flexed to 90° [6, 10, 13]. Philippon et al. [8] found significant differences in the

Ó. Marín-Peña
Department of Orthopedic and Traumatology,
University Hospital Infanta Leonor (Madrid-Spain),
e-mail: olivermarin@yahoo.es

Ó. Marín-Peña (ed.), *Femoroacetabular Impingement*,
DOI 10.1007/978-3-642-22769-1_3, © Springer-Verlag Berlin Heidelberg 2012

**Fig. 3.1** Impingement Test. (**a**) Maneuver is initiated at 90° of flexion, (**b**) which is continuous with a slight internal rotation

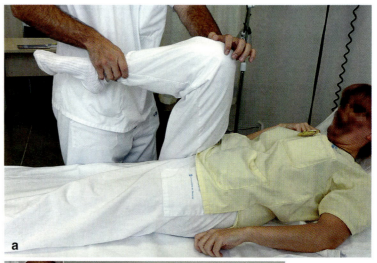

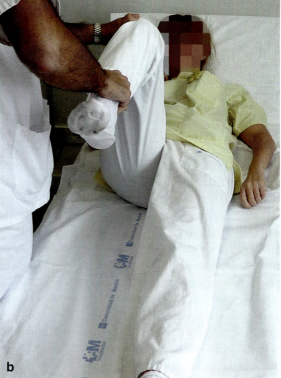

internal rotation and flexion of the symptomatic vis-à-vis the contralateral hip.

Physical evaluation for FAI should comprise the following specific tests:

- Impingement test. This test is performed with the patient supine and produces groin pain when the femur is internally rotated and adducted at 90° of hip flexion. In this position, the bone bump impinges on the acetabular rim leading to excessive shear stress [9, 14]. This maneuver is not specific to FAI but must be positive for an accurate diagnosis of FAI. When the impingement test is positive, the test must be repeated following an intra-articular injection of local anesthetic to prove the intra-articular origin of the pain (Figs. 3.1 and 3.2).

- Apprehension test. With the patient lying supine, the symptomatic leg is placed in extension. The test is positive when application of gentle external rotation elicits moderate pain. Although not specified, a positive apprehension test is related to an injury in

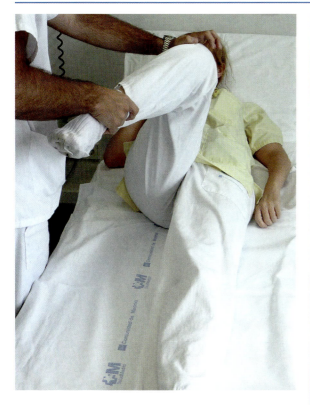

**Fig. 3.2** Final part of the maneuver with a mild hip adduction

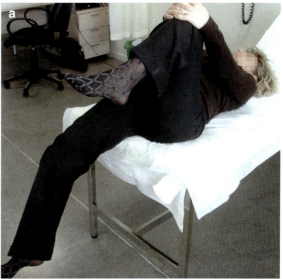

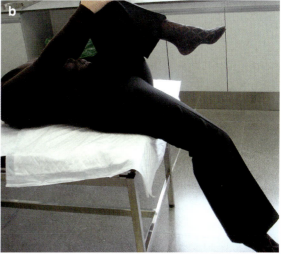

**Fig. 3.3** Apprehension Test in (**a**) extension and external rotation of the hip. (**b**) Patient should be placed at the edge of the table

the acetabular labrum in cases of mild acetabular dysplasia (Figs. 3.3 and 3.4).

- Flexion, Abduction, and External Rotation of the hip (FABER) test. With the patient in a figure-four position, the clinician applies slight pressure on the knee and measures the vertical distance from the knee to the edge of the examination table. The result is considered positive if the measured distance is longer in the affected than in the contralateral limb [8, 15–18] (Fig. 3.5).
- Dial test. The patient lies supine with the knee of the affected limb extended and relaxed. The clinician gently rotates the knee on the examination table from full external rotation to full internal rotation. The test is positive if groin pain appears during full internal rotation (Figs. 3.6 and 3.7).
- Leg roll test. The patient is placed supine, with the knee of the symptomatic limb extended and relaxed. The examiner stands in front of the patient, holds the patient's heels, and internally rotates his/her feet, holding this position for a few seconds. The feet are subsequently released, and both symmetry in external rotation and range of rotation on both sides are noted. The test is

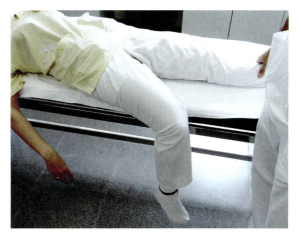

**Fig. 3.4** Apprehension Test with the patient at the lateral edge of the couch

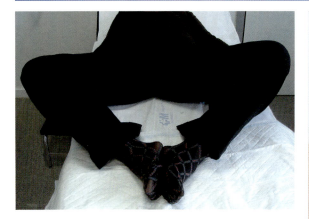

**Fig. 3.5** FABER test showing the symmetry of the lower limbs

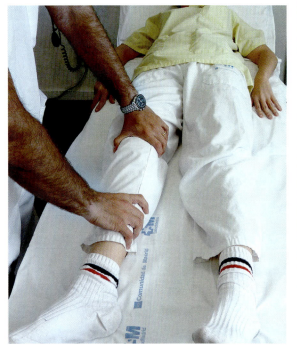

**Fig. 3.6** Maximum external rotation as the beginning of the dial test

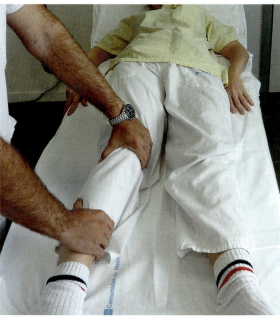

**Fig. 3.7** Final position at internal rotation in dial test

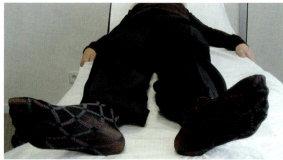

**Fig. 3.8** Final asymmetric position after rolling test, with greater external rotation on the healthy limb(right one) than on the pathologic limb (left one)

positive for FAI when a limitation to external rotation can be observed on the affected side, and it is positive for dysplasia or hyperlaxity when extended external rotation is observed (Fig. 3.8). In conclusion, overdiagnosis of FAI can be prevented through a thorough analysis of hip pain history and a meticulous physical exam. We should beware of the internet as the copiousness of information it provides could prove counterproductive and lead to an unsuccessful surgery if the origin of clinical findings is not taken into account.

## References

1. Clohisy JC, Knaus ER, Hunt DM, Lesher JM, Harris-Hayes M, Prather H (2009) Clinical presentation of patients with symptomatic anterior hip impingement. Clin Orthop Relat Res 467(3):638–644
2. Peters CL, Schabel K, Anderson L, Erickson J (2010) Open treatment of femoroacetabular impingement is associated with clinical improvement and low complication rate at short-term follow-up. Clin Orthop Relat Res 468(2): 504–510

3. Philippon MJ, Schenker ML (2006) Arthroscopy for the treatment of femoroacetabular impingement in the athlete. Clin Sports Med 25:299–308

4. Sierra RJ, Trousdale RT, Ganz R, Leunig M (2008) Hip disease in the young, active patient: evaluation and nonarthroplasty surgical options. J Am Acad Orthop Surg 1612: 689–703

5. Peelle MW, la Rocca GJ, Maloney WJ, Curry MC, Clohisy JC (2005) Acetabular and femoral radiographic abnormalities associated with labral tears. Clin Orthop Relat Res 441:327–333

6. Wenger DE, Kendell KR, Miner MR, Trousdale RT (2004) Acetabular labral tears rarely occur in the absence of bony abnormalities. Clin Orthop Relat Res 426:145–150

7. Parvizi J, Leunig M, Ganz R (2007) Femoroacetabular impingement. J Am Acad Orthop Surg 15(9):561–570

8. Philippon MJ, Maxwell RB, Johnston TL, Schenker M, Briggs KK (2007) Clinical presentation of femoroacetabular impingement. Knee Surg Sports Traumatol Arthrosc 15(8):1041–1047, 1021

9. Ganz R, Parvizi J, Beck M, Leunig M, Notzli H, Siebenrock KA (2003) Femoroacetabular impingement: a cause for osteoarthritis of the hip. Clin Orthop Relat Res 417:112–120

10. Burnett RS, Della Rocca GJ, Prather H, Curry M, Maloney WJ, Clohisy JC (2006) Clinical presentation of patients with tears of the acetabular labrum. J Bone Joint Surg Am 88:1448–1457

11. Klaue K, Durnin CW, Ganz R (1991) The acetabular rim syndrome. A clinical presentation of dysplasia of the hip. J Bone Joint Surg Br 733:423–429

12. Clohisy JC, Beaule PE, O'Malley A, Safran MR, Schoenecker P (2008) AOA symposium. Hip disease in the young adult: current concepts of etiology and surgical treatment. J Bone Joint Surg Am 9010:2267–2281

13. Jäger M, Wild A, Westhoff B, Krauspe R (2004) Femoroacetabular impingement caused by a femoral osseous head-neck bump deformity: clinical, radiological, and experimental results. J Orthop Sci 9:256–263

14. Klaue K, Durnin CW, Ganz R (1991) The acetabular rim syndrome. A clinical presentation of dysplasia of the hip. J Bone Joint Surg Br 73:423–429

15. Beall DP, Sweet CF, Martin HD (2005) Imaging findings of femoroacetabular impingement syndrome. Skeletal Radiol 34:691–701

16. Ribas-Fernández M, Marín-Peña O, Ledesma R, Vilarrubias JM (2007) Estudio de los primeros 100 casos mediante abordaje mini-anterior. Rev Ortop Traumatol 51(Suppl 2):57

17. Ribas M, Marín-Peña O, Regenbrecht B, De la Torre B, Vilarrubias JM (2007) Femoroacetabular osteochondroplasty by means of an anterior minimally invasive approach. Hip Int 2:91–98

18. Marin-Peña O, Gebhard C, Velev K, Ribas-Fernandez M, Plasencia-Arriba MA (2006) Femoroacetabular impingement: first step on the way to hip arthroplasty in young patients. J Bone Joint Surg Br 88:329

# Part II

# Imaging in FAI

# X-Ray Examination in FAI

## Klaus A. Siebenrock and Philipp Henle

The role of imaging in femoroacetabular impingement is to evaluate the hip for abnormalities associated with impingement and to exclude arthritis, avascular necrosis, or other joint problems on radiographs.

X-ray examination is in most circumstances the easiest available diagnostic technique to assess osseous pathologies of the hip joint. It allows identification of the pathomorphological characteristics of FAI as well as of other important causes of hip pain such as osteoarthritis, hip dysplasia, or avascular necrosis of the femoral head.

Standard conventional imaging comprises at least two radiographs:

- An anteroposterior pelvic view
- An axial cross-table view (or Dunn/Rippstein view at 45° of hip flexion)

In addition, a false profile view can be used to assess the posteroinferior part of the hip joint and anterior coverage.

## Imaging Technique

### Anteroposterior Pelvic View

The patient is placed in the supine position with 15° of internal rotation of both legs to compensate for femoral antetorsion and to provide better visualiza-

tion of the contour of the lateral femoral head–neck junction [1]. The central beam points to the midpoint between a line connecting both anterosuperior iliac spines and the superior border of the symphysis (Fig. 4.1).

### Axial Cross Table View

Accordingly, the cross-table view is taken with the affected leg internally rotated and the contralateral leg elevated. The central beam points to the inguinal fold (Fig. 4.1).

### False Profile

The false profile as described by Lequesne and de Sèze [2] constitutes a true lateral view of the hip. It is obtained with the patient standing and the pelvis rotated 65° relative to the film. The axis of the foot is parallel to the table. This view is technically appropriate when the distance between the two femoral heads is approximately the size of one femoral head.

## Radiographic Signs of FAI

Thorough analysis of radiographs is essential for a correct understanding of the pathomorphological characteristics of every patient, surgical decision-making and preoperative planning. There are several distinct morphological features in cam- and pincer-type FAI which can be identified on conventional radiographs.

K.A. Siebenrock (✉) • P. Henle
Department of Orthopaedic Surgery,
Inselspital, Bern University Hospital,
Bern, Switzerland
e-mail: monika.gempeler@insel.ch

Ó. Marín-Peña (ed.), *Femoroacetabular Impingement*,
DOI 10.1007/978-3-642-22769-1_4, © Springer-Verlag Berlin Heidelberg 2012

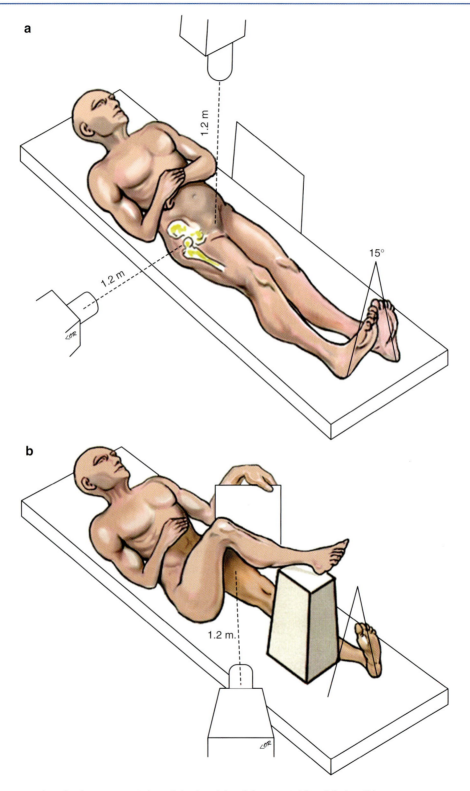

**Fig. 4.1** Correct settings for the anteroposterior pelvic view (**a**) and the cross table axial view (**b**)

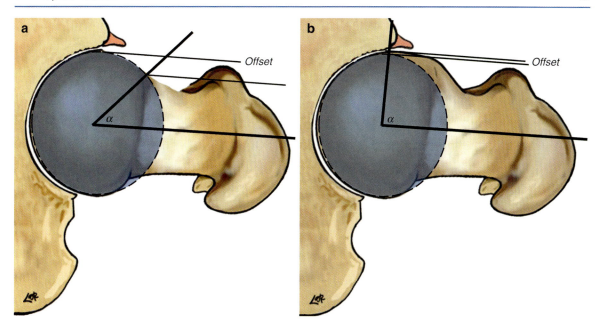

**Fig. 4.2** The α angle and anterior offset can be used for a quantitative description of the head–neck junction. (**a**) Normal hip. (**b**) Hip with cam impingement

## Cam Type FAI

### Pistol-Grip Deformity

A pistol-grip deformity is characterized on radiographs by a flattening of the usually concave surface of the lateral aspect of the femoral head due to an abnormal extension of the more horizontally oriented femoral epiphysis [3]. Several methods of quantifying this deformity exist:

### Alpha Angle

Quantification of the amount of asphericity can be accomplished by the angle α, the femoral offset, or the offset ratio [4]. The α angle is the angle between the femoral neck axis and a line connecting the head center with the point where the asphericity of the head–neck contour begins. It can be measured on axial (Fig. 4.2) and AP (Fig. 4.3) radiographs. On axial radiographs an α angle exceeding 50° is an indicator of an abnormally shaped femoral head–neck contour. The maximum normal α angle on the AP pelvic radiograph is 68° in men and 50° in women [5].

### Femoral Head–Neck Offset, Offset Ratio

Another parameter for quantification of cam impingement is anterior offset, which is defined as the difference in radius between the anterior femoral head and the anterior femoral neck on a cross-table axial view of the proximal femur (Fig. 4.2). In asymptomatic hips, the anterior offset is 11.6±0.7 mm; hips with cam impingement have a decreased anterior offset of 7.2±0.7 mm. As a general rule for clinical practice, an anterior offset less than 10 mm is a strong indicator for cam impingement.

In addition, the so-called offset ratio can be calculated, which is defined as the ratio between the anterior offset and the diameter of the head. The offset ratio is 0.21±0.03 in asymptomatic patients and 0.13±0.05 in hips with cam impingement [6].

### Triangular Index

The triangular index is constructed as follows: on the femoral neck axis, half of the radius ($r$) of the femoral head is measured. Then, a perpendicular line is drawn. The new radius ($R$) is defined as the distance between the femoral head center and the intersection point of the perpendicular line with the superior femoral head-neck contour (Fig. 4.3). The triangular index has better reproducibility than the α angle because it is constructed by clear geometric landmarks, whereas the α angle can sometimes be difficult to pinpoint. In addition, the triangular index is more independent from femoral rotation [5].

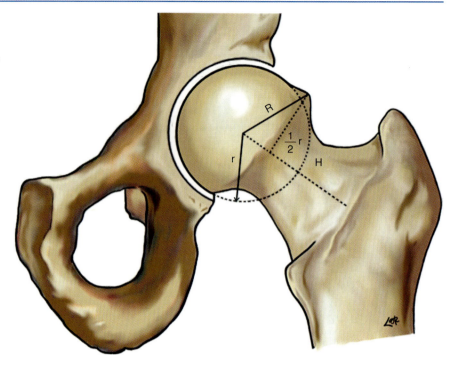

**Fig. 4.3** The triangular index is pathologic if the new radius $R$ is 2 mm or more longer than the radius $r$ of the spherical portion of the femoral head

## Femoral Retrotorsion and Coxa Vara

Another cause for cam impingement is femoral retrotorsion, which can occur as a primary entity [7] or posttraumatically after healed femoral neck fractures [8]. Femoral retrotorsion can be calculated reliably only on CT scans involving the proximal and distal parts of the femur [9]. In addition, a coxa vara (defined by a centrum collum diaphyseal angle [CCD] of less than 125°) has been recognized as a cause of cam impingement [10].

## Pincer-Type FAI

### Coxa Profunda, Protrusio Acetabuli

A normal hip appears on an anteroposterior pelvic radiograph with the acetabular fossa line lying laterally to the ilioischial line. A coxa profunda is defined when the floor of the acetabular fossa touches or overlaps the ilioischial line medially. Protrusio acetabuli is defined when even the femoral head overlaps the ilioischial line medially (Fig. 4.4).

### Lateral Center-Edge Angle, Acetabular Index

Generally, a deep acetabulum is associated with excessive acetabular coverage that can be quantified on an anteroposterior pelvic view with the lateral center edge angle or a particularly low or negative acetabular index.

The lateral center-edge angle is the angle formed by a vertical line and a line connecting the femoral head center with the lateral edge of the acetabulum. A "normal" lateral center edge angle has been described to range between 25° and 39° [11] (Fig. 4.5). The authors' feeling is that the LCE should ideally be between 25° and 30°.

The acetabular index (acetabular roof angle) is the angle formed by a horizontal line and a line connecting the medial point of the sclerotic zone with the lateral center of the acetabulum. In hips with coxa profunda or protrusio acetabuli, the acetabular index is typically 0° or even negative (Fig. 4.6).

### Extrusion Index

Another parameter for quantification of femoral coverage on an anteroposterior pelvic view is the femoral head extrusion index, which defines the percentage of femoral head that is uncovered when a horizontal line is drawn parallel to the inter-teardrop line. An extrusion index higher than 25% is associated with dysplasia [12] (Fig. 4.7).

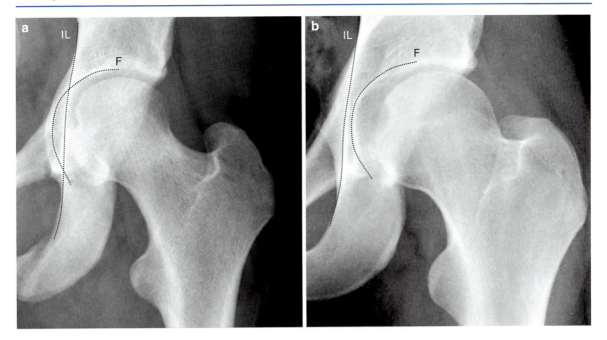

**Fig. 4.4** Ilioischial line (IL) and acetabular fossa (F) in a coxa profunda (**a**) and a normal hip (**b**)

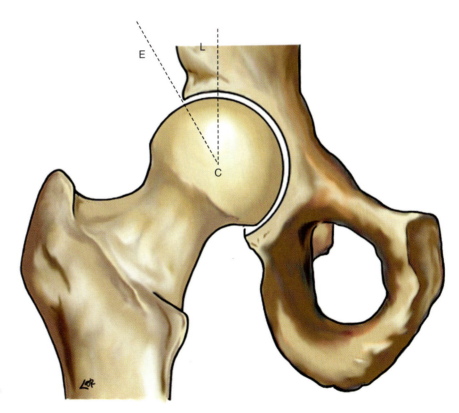

**Fig. 4.5** Lateral center edge (LCE) angle

**Fig. 4.6** The acetabular index (AI) varies between 0° and 10° in normal hips

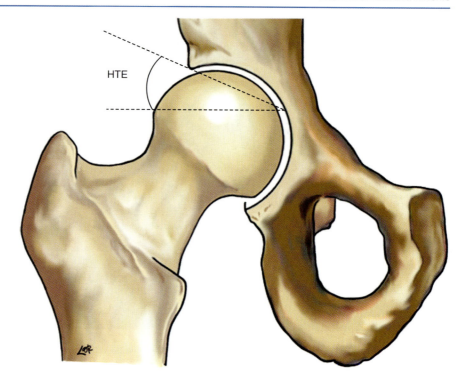

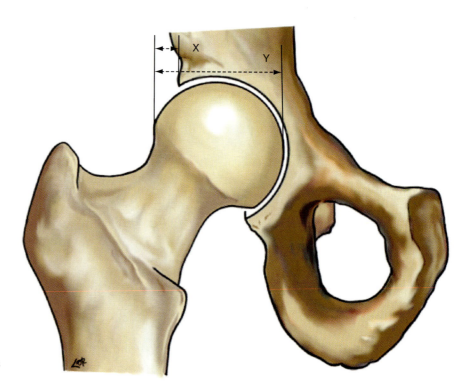

**Fig. 4.7** The femoral head extrusion index is defined as $X/Y \times 100\%$

## Linear Indentation Sign

On an axial cross table view, on the femoral side at the head–neck junction, a linear indentation may be observed in hips with pincer impingement and cortical thickening (Fig. 4.8).

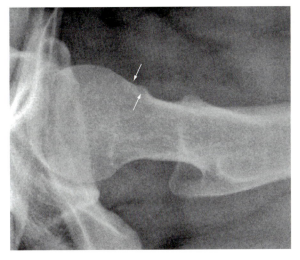

**Fig. 4.8** Cross table lateral view showing an indentation sign (*arrows*)

## Signs of Acetabular Retroversion

Retroversion of the acetabulum has been described as a posteriorly orientated acetabular opening with reference to the sagittal plane. Acetabular retroversion represents anterosuperior femoral head overcoverage that renders the hip prone to anterosuperior pincer-type impingement. It can be identified on technically correct anteroposterior pelvic views by three phenomena:

### Cross-Over Sign

A cross-over sign is caused by the anterior acetabular rim line being lateral to the posterior rim in the cranial part of the acetabulum and crossing the latter in its distal part (figure-of-8 configuration, Fig. 4.9).

### Posterior Wall Sign

The posterior wall sign is positive when the posterior wall descends medially to the center point of the femoral head indicating deficient posterior coverage. In normal hips, the posterior wall runs through the center of the femur (Fig. 4.10).

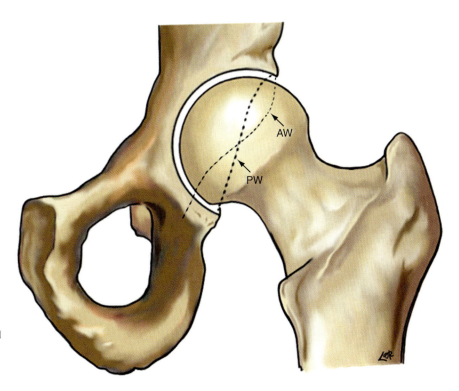

**Fig. 4.9** Cranial acetabular retroversion; the cross-over sign is positive when the projection of the anterior wall lies partly lateral to the posterior wall (*AW* anterior wall, *PW* posterior wall)

**Fig. 4.10** Acetabular retroversion; the posterior wall sign is positive when the center of the femoral head appears lateral to the posterior wall (*PW* posterior wall)

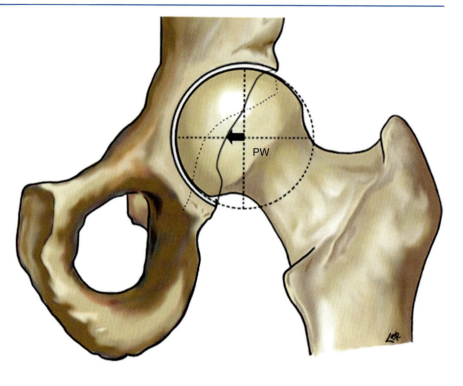

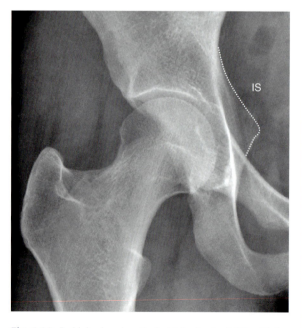

**Fig. 4.11** Ischial spine sign: the ischial spine is visible with the pelvic cavity

|  | Pincer | Cam |
|---|---|---|
| Radiographic signs on *anteroposterior* radiographs | Coxa profunda | Pistol – grip deformity |
|  | Protrusio acetabuli | α angle >50° (♀); >68° (♂) |
|  | Lateral center edge angle >39° | Triangular index ($R \geq r + 2$ mm) |
|  | Reduced extrusion index | CCD angle <125 |
|  | Acetabular index ≤0° |  |
|  | Posterior wall sign (acetabular retroversion) |  |
|  | Figure-of-8 configuration, cross-over sign (focal acetabular retroversion) |  |
|  | Ischial spine sign |  |
| Radiographic signs on cross-table radiographs | Linear indentation sign | α angle >50 |
|  |  | Femoral head–neck offset <8 mm |
|  |  | Offset ratio <0.18 |
|  |  | Femoral retrotorsion |

## Ischial Spine Sign

A retroverted acetabulum can also be suspected if the projection of the ischial spine is visible within the pelvic inlet. Kalberer et al. found this sign to have a positive predictive value of 98% for acetabular retroversion (Fig. 4.11) [13].

# References

1. Tannast M, Murphy SB, Langlotz F, Anderson SE, Siebenrock KA (2006) Estimation of pelvic tilt on antero-posterior X-rays: a comparison of six parameters. Skeletal Radiol 35:149–155
2. Lequesne M, de Séze S (1961) Le faux-profil du bassin. Rev Rhum 28:643–652
3. Siebenrock KA, Wahab KHA, Kalhor M, Leunig M, Ganz R (2004) Abnormal extension of the femoral head epiphysis as a cause of cam impingement. Clin Orthop Relat Res 418:54–60
4. Nötzli HP, Wyss TF, Stöcklin CH, Schmid MR, Treiber K, Hodler J (2002) The contour of the femoral head–neck junction as a predictor for the risk of anterior impingement. J Bone Joint Surg Br 84:556–560
5. Gosvig KK, Jacobsen S, Palm H, Sonne-Holm S, Magnusson E (2007) A new radiological index for assessing asphericity of the femoral head in cam impingement. J Bone Joint Surg Br 89(10):1309–1316
6. Eijer H, Leunig M, Mahomed MN, Ganz R (2001) Crosstable lateral radiograph for screening of anterior femoral head–neck offset in patients with femoro-acetabular impingement. Hip Int 11:37–41
7. Tschauner C, Fock CM, Hofmann S, Raith J (2002) Rotational abnormalities of the hip joint. Radiologe 42:457–466
8. Strehl A, Ganz R (2005) Anterior femoroacetabular impingement after healed femoral neck fractures. Unfallchirurg 108:263–273
9. Murphy SB, Simon SR, Kijewski PK, Wilkinson RH, Griscom T (1987) Femoral anteversion. J Bone Joint Surg Am 69:1169–1176
10. Millis MB, Kim YJ, Kocher MS (2004) Hip joint-preserving surgery for the mature hip: the Children's Hospital experience. Orthop J HMS 6:84–87
11. Murphy SB, Ganz R, Müller ME (1995) The prognosis in untreated dysplasia of the hip. J Bone Joint Surg Am 77:985–989
12. Li PLS, Ganz R (2003) Morphologic features of congenital acetabular dysplasia. Clin Orthop Relat Res 416:245–253
13. Kalberer F, Sierra RJ, Madan SS, Ganz R, Leunig M (2008) Ischial spine projection into the pelvis: a new sign for acetabular retroversion. Clin Orthop Relat Res 466(3):677–683

# MRI/CT in FAI

Kawan S. Rakhra

## Introduction

Femoroacetabular impingement (FAI) has become a well-recognized pathogenic factor in the evolution of hip osteoarthritis (OA). Impingement is secondary to anatomic abnormalities of the femoral head-neck junction and/or the acetabulum. These dysmorphisms lead to impaired, pathologic interaction of the femur with the acetabulum during motion of the hip joint, resulting in altered biomechanics, premature degeneration of hyaline cartilage, and eventually OA [1–5]. Given that impingement results from underlying structural aberrations, radiologic imaging is essential in the investigation of FAI. Imaging provides a visual presentation of the primary deformities of, as well as the secondary joint derangements that can result from, FAI, in both cam and pincer forms.

Radiography [1, 6, 7], computed tomography (CT) [5], and magnetic resonance imaging (MRI) [4, 8–11] are validated modalities for imaging the hip in the setting of FAI. Radiographs can demonstrate gross osseous alignment and morphology, although subtle osseous deformities may be underestimated. The shape, contour, and spatial relationship of the bones may not be demonstrated by radiography to the same degree as cross-sectional modalities such as CT and MRI [12–14]. Radiography is also limited by its poor demonstration of internal joint structures including the cartilage, labrum, capsule, and surrounding articular soft tissues [15–17].

K.S. Rakhra
Musculoskeletal Radiologist Department of Diagnostic Imaging, The Ottawa Hospital, University of Ottawa, 501 Smyth Road, Ottawa, Ontario, Canada
e-mail: krakhra@ottawahospital.on.ca

CT and MRI allow for the detection and quantification of primary anatomic abnormalities of the femur and acetabulum, with MRI also accurately depicting secondary changes to the cartilage, labrum, capsule, and joint space [5, 18–20].

## MRI and CT Investigation of FAI

### Overview

The MRI and CT modalities may contribute significantly to the investigation of FAI by:

1. Detection, characterization, and quantification of primary anatomic abnormalities of the femur and acetabulum
2. Detection and characterization of secondary derangements of the hip joint pertaining to the labrum, cartilage, subchondral bone, and joint space
3. Assistance in preoperative planning by providing an anatomic roadmap for primary

### Strengths and Weaknesses

Both MRI and CT can demonstrate a wide spectrum of findings of FAI, although MRI is the more robust and comprehensive modality. MRI offers exquisite contrast resolution allowing for distinction and characterization of the labrum, cartilage, joint space, capsule, compact and cancellous bone, and regional soft tissues [8, 14, 18]. Furthermore, unique to MRI is the multiplanar image acquisition capability. Images in the standard or oblique axial, sagittal, coronal, and radial planes can be directly acquired, or secondarily

Ó. Marín-Peña (ed.), *Femoroacetabular Impingement*,
DOI 10.1007/978-3-642-22769-1_5, © Springer-Verlag Berlin Heidelberg 2012

constructed, using post-processing reformation software. MRI does not involve ionizing radiation, which is important as many patients are diagnosed with FAI during their early, reproductive years of life. Drawbacks of MRI include relatively longer acquisition times, the susceptibility to motion artifacts, magnetic susceptibility artifacts due to regional metal prostheses and/or postsurgical artifacts, along with several other absolute and relative contraindications (claustrophobia, non-MR compatible prostheses, electronic implanted devices, cardiac pacer equipment, orbital metal bodies).

The combination of MRI with intra-articular injection of gadolinium-based contrast agents, direct magnetic resonance arthrography (MRA), is often used to facilitate evaluation of the small structures in the hip joint, including the labrum, hyaline cartilage, and loose bodies. The distension effect of the arthrogram may cause separation of the capsular, labral, and osteochondral structures resulting in increased spatial resolution. The injected contrast solution outlines both normal anatomic structures and abnormal pathologies, further improving contrast resolution and increasing the conspicuity of intra-articular pathology [9, 15, 21, 22].

Indirect MRA involves intravenous injection of gadolinium contrast, followed by a variable delay and/or physical activity regime. Gadolinium contrast will distribute within the joint space, diffusely enhancing the synovial fluid [22]. This will provide greater contrast resolution between the joint fluid and the labrum, cartilage, and capsule. The benefit of indirect MRA is that it is less invasive for the patient, and does not require fluoroscopically guided joint injection. However, the distension effect that direct MRA gives is not realized. There will also be enhancement of the background extra-articular soft tissues and vascular structures, both normal and pathologic. This may make articular pathology less conspicuous.

CT can be considered in patients for whom MRI is contraindicated. CT has very high spatial resolution providing detailed images of osseous morphology and alignment, although its relatively poor contrast resolution limits evaluation of the nonosseous articular structures and soft tissues. CT has been used to evaluate the osseous contour of the femur [5] and alignment of the acetabulum [23, 24]. CT may be combined with intra-articular injection of iodinated contrast agents to provide further assessment of labral and chondral integrity,

and to detect loose bodies [17, 25, 26]. CT acquires images in the axial plane, although images in the coronal, sagittal, oblique, or radial planes can be secondarily constructed by software reformations. Various post-processing algorithms and filters can be applied to optimize evaluation of the bones or soft tissues. The acquisition time is very short, and thus, motion artifacts are not significant. A major drawback of CT is the radiation dose which the patient receives, especially to the gonads. Thus, most centers will use MRI as the preferred cross-sectional modality of choice in the investigation of FAI.

## Imaging Protocols

Most clinical MRI scanners in practice are of 1.5 Tesla (T) field strength, although higher field strengths (3.0 T +) are now becoming increasingly used. Higher field strengths result in greater signal to noise and contrast to noise ratios [27] and allow for faster acquisitions and higher resolution.

MRI pulse-sequence selection depends on the technique used, with multiple, variable combinations of the sequence classes able to provide equally diagnostic studies. Spin echo, fast-spin echo, and gradient-recalled echo sequences can all be used in the MRI investigation of FAI. Three-dimensional (3D) volume, isotropic voxel acquisitions with multiplanar reformations have recently become feasible in terms of time and imaging quality, and can be applied to MRI and MRA of the hip [14]. Multiplanar imaging with at least one sequence or reformation in each plane should be standard.

For nonarthrographic MRI, the protocol should include T1 weighted imaging (WI) without fat suppression to demonstrate anatomy, joint alignment, marrow abnormality, or fractures. A fluid-sensitive sequence (T2 or proton density (PD), with fat suppression; short tau inversion recovery (STIR)) should always be part of any protocol to detect abnormal edema within marrow and soft tissues, and periarticular fluid collections or cysts [28]. In addition, fluid-sensitive sequences increase the contrast between joint fluid and adjacent labrum, cartilage, bone, and capsule. With nonarthrographic MRI studies, a higher resolution and increased number of sampling averages [8, 29] are used which may offset the lower contrast and spatial resolution of MRI compared to MRA.

With direct MRA, the most commonly used sequence is T1, with or without fat suppression, in addition to fluid sensitive sequences [22]. With indirect MRA the same sequence selection as for direct MRA is adequate, although with a few caveats. Fat suppression is strongly advised for maximal contrast resolution as the concentration of gadolinium within the joint may not be as high as with direct injection. As well, multiphasic imaging may be considered to understand the vascular physiology of the joint [22].

In both routine MRI and MRA, the hip in question is best imaged using a surface coil place around the joint. The patient is placed supine, and the feet may be fastened together to limit motion and to attempt to have a similar degree of rotation of the leg for all patients. A larger coil may also be simultaneously used in order to image a larger field of view including both hips. This can detect abnormalities in the contralateral hip which may also be symptomatic, or potentially have subclinical pathology. However, the hip is best evaluated when the field of view is smaller and targeted. For unilateral hip studies, there is a range of imaging parameters that are commonly used to adequately image the hip: field of view 14–18 cm, slice thickness 3–4 mm, matrix $512 \times 384$ to $256 \times 256$.

If using CT, the protocol should include thin, overlapping slices using a bone algorithm. The acquisition data should allow for high-resolution, multiplanar reformations. The CT parameters should be optimized to minimize radiation dose to the patient.

Regardless of the modality or technique being used, it is important to establish the acquisition/reformatting planes which allow for optimal visualization of the structures of interest. True axial, sagittal, and coronal planes allow for assessment of gross anatomy and joint alignment, although they are suboptimal for evaluation of smaller, variably located and oriented intra-articular structures due to variations in anatomy and positioning. Thus oblique plane imaging relative to specific landmarks is advised. The most commonly used approach is to obtain three oblique planes relative to the acetabulum, prescribing them from true axial plane images (Fig. 5.1). The oblique axial and coronal planes will be perpendicular to the anterior/posterior and superior/inferior margins of the acetabulum, respectively. The oblique axial plane is often prescribed, being parallel to the long axis of the femoral neck, which allows for more accurate assessment of the femoral head-neck junction. It is a very close,

sometimes exact, approximation, of the oblique axial acetabular plane (Fig. 5.2). Radial imaging has been recommended as a method for circumferentially evaluating the femoral head-neck junction over its full circumference [3–5, 11, 30, 31]. Radial images are based on a rotating plane using the center of the femoral neck as the axis of rotation, with images generated at defined intervals (Fig. 5.3). As such, each image is orthogonal to the femoral surface and visualizes the head-neck junction in profile [31].

## Primary Abnormalities of FAI (Anatomic)

There are known primary anatomic abnormalities of the femur and acetabulum which can predispose to femoroacetabular impingement.

### Femur

In the cam form of FAI, the main dysmorphism corresponds to the femoral head-neck junction. An excess of bone and/or cartilage bulk at the anterosuperior femoral head-neck junction, results in reduced offset of the femoral head over the neck and femoral head asphericity [1, 2, 4, 31, 32]. The abnormality can also been described as an osteochondral excrescence, a lack of head-neck concavity, or reduced waisting of the head-neck junction [3] (Fig. 5.4).

The oblique axial plane parallel to the long axis of the femoral neck is the most frequently used imaging plane to evaluate the femoral head-neck junction. This plane optimally images the anterior contour of the femoral head-neck junction. However, several recent studies have reported that, although present anteriorly, the diminished offset is most pronounced anterosuperiorly, and potentially at any location within the antero-superior quadrant [11, 30, 31]. Thus, radial images, using the femoral neck as the axis of rotation, have been recommended as a method for evaluating the femoral head-neck junction over its full circumference, as opposed to just anteriorly as what occurs using the more conventional oblique axial plane method [4, 5, 8, 11, 30]. Radial images are based on a rotating plane such that each image is orthogonal to the femoral surface and visualizes the head-neck junction in profile. A clockface nomenclature can be applied for localization around the femoral head-neck junction

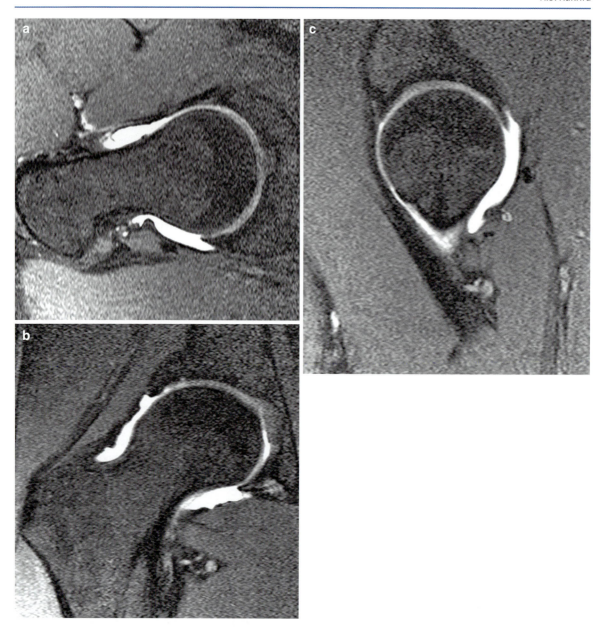

**Fig. 5.1** MR arthrogram of the hip with fat suppressed T1W (**a**) oblique axial, (**b**) oblique coronal and (**c**) oblique sagittal plane images

**Fig. 5.3** Radial Imaging: (**a**) The axis of rotation is the center of the femoral neck (*) as demonstrated on an oblique sagittal image showing the femoral neck in cross-section. (**b**) Localizer image demonstrates superimposed radial reference lines at regular intervals. A clockface nomenclature is implemented with the superior femoral head-neck junction denoted as 12 o'clock. Subsequent rotation of the axis generates images around the circumference of the femoral neck going from superior to anterior, from 12 o'clock in a clockwise direction. (**c**) Sample radial image demonstrating the femoral head-neck contour at the 2 o'clock vector (*)

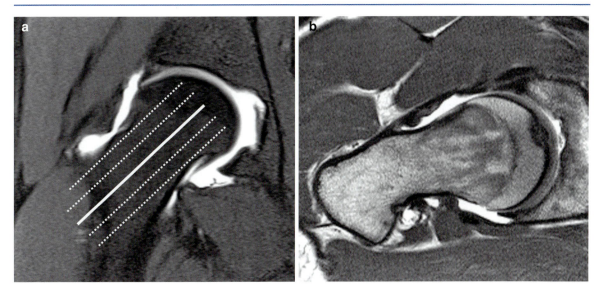

**Fig. 5.2** The oblique axial plane as prescribed from an oblique coronal image (**a**) as being parallel to the long axis of the femoral neck, generating the oblique axial image (**b**) which demonstrates the acetabulum, femoral head, and elongated neck on the same image

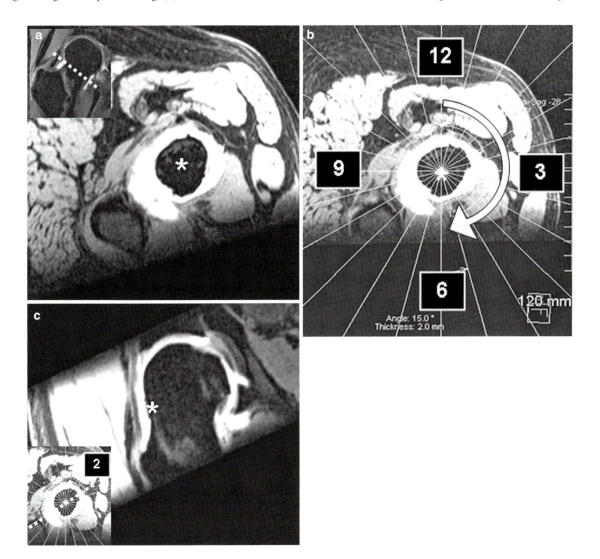

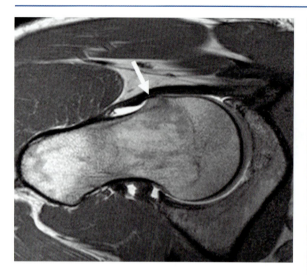

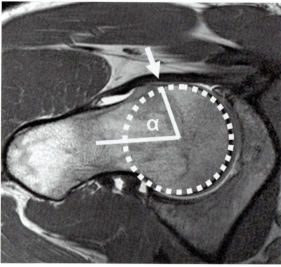

**Fig. 5.4** Oblique axial T1WI demonstrating Cam deformity at the anterior femoral head-neck junction (*white arrow*), resulting in loss of the normal concave contour, and reduced head-neck offset

**Fig. 5.5** Measurement of the alpha angle (α). A best-fit circle is drawn around the perimeter of the femoral head. The alpha angle is formed by the axis of the femoral neck (*1*) and a line (*2*) drawn from the circle center to the point where the femoral head extends beyond the margin of the best-fit circle (*white arrow*)

with the superior and anterior locations designated 12 o'clock and 3 o'clock, respectively.

The alpha angle is a parameter used to quantify the degree of femoral deformity and reflects insufficient offset and femoral head asphericity [9, 10]. Prior MRI studies show that an elevated alpha angle is associated with symptomatic impingement [5, 9–11]. It can be measured on either oblique axial or radial images.

The alpha angle is determined by first drawing a best-fit circle around the perimeter of the femoral head. The first arm of the angle is the long axis of the femoral neck, defined as the line drawn between the center of the femoral neck at its narrowest point and the center of the femoral head. The second arm of the angle is drawn from the center of the femoral head anteriorly to the point where the head extends beyond the margin of the circle [10] (Fig. 5.5).

There is a range of normal values for the alpha angle. In asymptomatic patients, the alpha angle ranges from 39.3° to 48.3° [5, 10, 33]. A recent study measured the alpha angle in a large cohort of 200 asymptomatic subjects [33]. The mean alpha angle using the oblique axial plane on an image through the middle of the femoral neck was 40.8°, ranging from 27.0° to 69.9°. There were significant differences in alpha-angle values at various locations around the femoral head-neck junction. The mean values anteriorly (3:00 clockface position) and anterosuperiorly

(1:30) were 40.8° and 50.1°, respectively. There were significant gender differences with respect to alpha-angle measurements. The mean alpha-angle value in males and females, anteriorly, was reported to be 44.0° and 38.1°, respectively, while anterosuperiorly, it was 54.1° and 47.0°, respectively. Thus, depending on the location around the femoral head-neck junction being evaluated, and on the gender of the patient, the threshold values for the alpha angle considered to be abnormal may have to be varied [33].

In symptomatic cam-type FAI patients, the mean alpha-angle value found in several studies ranges from 66.4° to 74.0° [5, 9, 10, 31].

## Acetabulum

In the pure pincer form of FAI, impingement is the result of overcoverage of the femoral head by the acetabulum. This may be related to acetabular retroversion, coxa profunda, or acetabular protrusio [1, 2, 4].

Acetabular retroversion causes focal overcoverage of the femoral head, while coxa profunda and acetabular protrusio result in more global overcoverage. All result in relative deepening of the acetabular fossa. These dysmorphisms lead to abnormal abutment of the femoral neck against the overcovering acetabulum, resulting in a linear zone of impingement anterosuperiorly [2, 3].

The version of the acetabulum refers to the orientation of the opening of the acetabular fossa relative to the sagittal plane. In the normal hip, the opening of the acetabular fossa is directed anteriorly, or is anteverted. With retroversion the acetabular fossa is oriented posteriorly [3, 23, 34].

Acetabular version is best evaluated on axial plane images [35], whether by MRI or CT. CT, with its better depiction of compact bone, may allow for more accurate delineation of the exact margins of the osseous landmarks. The entire transverse dimension of the osseous pelvis, with both hips in the field of view, is required to correct for any positional tilt of the pelvis.

The normal acetabulum is anteverted by 20–23° [23, 36, 37], with 15–25° generally considered to be within normal limits. On axial images through the retroverted, acetabulum, the anterior acetabular rim sits more lateral than the posterior rim [23].

The orientation of the acetabular version is not fixed at all levels. There is a natural decrease in the degree of anteversion progressing from superior to inferior [23, 35, 38]. It has been suggested that the version of the acetabulum should be evaluated at the level through the mid femoral head, on the image where the diameter of the femoral head is largest [23, 35] or on the image where the head is most congruent with the acetabulum [38] (Fig. 5.6).

## Secondary Abnormalities of FAI

The repetitive mechanical trauma of impingement results in structural changes to various components of the joint, including the labrum, hyaline cartilage, and bone. In cam FAI, injury occurs preferentially in the anterosuperior quadrant of the joint. With pincer FAI, the joint injury can start anterosuperiorly, but later on also posteriorly, with eventual more circumferential, global changes to the joint [1, 2].

## Labrum

There is a spectrum of morphologic labral injury which may be seen with FAI, including degeneration, disruption of the chondrolabral junction, and labral

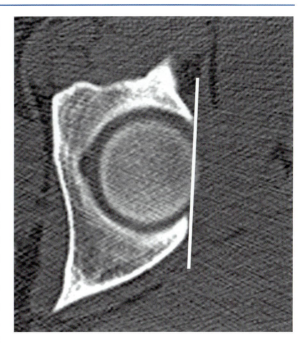

**Fig. 5.6** Acetabular retroversion as measured on axial CT image through the level of the mid femoral head. The acetabular opening is in neutral to minimally retroverted orientation (*white line*) relative to the true sagittal plane. The normal range is 15–25° of anteversion

tears, most commonly occurring in the anterosuperior quadrant. A high prevalence of labral degeneration and tearing in the setting of FAI is known to exist [9].

MRA is the test of choice for evaluation of the acetabular labrum [39–43]. Specifically, it is an excellent investigation for detecting labral tears with recent studies comparing it to arthroscopy reporting sensitivity and accuracy values ranging from 92% to 100% and 93% to 96%, respectively [42–44]. However, recent studies have demonstrated that high-resolution, nonarthrographic MRI is adequate for the evaluation of the labrum and cartilage [8, 29]. With rapidly improving MRI technology, higher field strengths and newer sequences, MRA may become antequated in the future.

Normally, the labrum has a pointed, triangular shape with sharp margins and very low signal intensity across most MRI sequences. There is a firm, continuous attachment of the labrum to the osseous acetabular rim and the acetabular cartilage [45]. This interface between the hyaline cartilage and labrum is referred to as the chondrolabral junction (Fig. 5.7).

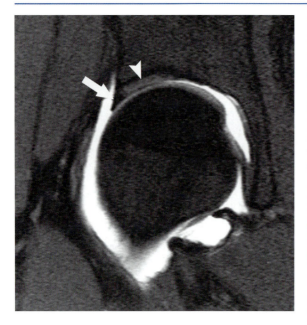

**Fig. 5.7** Normal chondrolabral junction on MRA oblique coronal T1WI with fat suppression. The normal labrum (*white arrow*) is well defined, triangular in configuration and of diffuse low signal. The normal acetabular hyaline cartilage (*arrowhead*) is of intermediate signal compared to the labrum and joint fluid. There is a tight interface between the labrum and cartilage

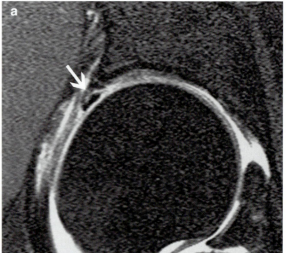

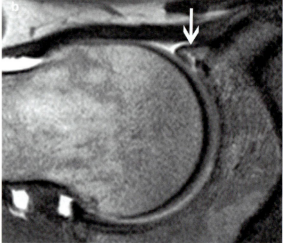

**Fig. 5.8** Labral tears with gadolinium signal extending into substance of labrum (*white arrows*); (**a**) Linear tear of the superior labrum on oblique coronal T1WI with fat suppression, (**b**) Linear tear through degenerate anterior labrum on oblique axial T1WI

The degenerate labrum may manifest on MRI with increased size, globularization, increased intrasubstance signal, and surface irregularity [19]. Labral tears will be demonstrated by contrast solution extending into the substance of the labrum, and are most commonly seen in the anterior-superior quadrant [29, 41, 42, 44, 46] (Fig. 5.8). With labral detachments, the contrast will undermine the base of the labrum at the chondrolabral and acetabular–labral junctions (Fig. 5.9). Paralabral cysts are small fluid-filled cysts which can develop, secondary to labral degeneration, tears and detachments [47] (Fig. 5.10).

Although the aforementioned labral changes in cam and pincer FAI can be similar, there are some features which are more commonly seen in either of the two forms. In cam FAI, the labral injury is initiated at the chondrolabral junction anterosuperiorly where there is repetitive shear trauma [2, 19] resulting in a focal separation of the labrum from the cartilage along the deep, articular margin [1, 8, 48]. This will manifest as imbibition of fluid into the defect at the chondrolabral junction [19] (Fig. 5.11). In pincer FAI, abutment of the anterior acetabular rim onto the femoral neck results in focal impaction on the labrum

[3], most frequently occurring anterosuperiorly [1]. Labral fissuring with prominent intralabral cyst formation is seen more frequently in pincer than cam FAI [2, 3].

Over time, the traumatized labrum can become ossified, leading to increased depth of the rigid component of the acetabular fossa. This in turn will lead to further increased coverage of the femoral head. Ossification of the labrum/acetabular rim can occur in both the cam and pincer forms of FAI, seen most often in the anterosuperior quadrant [11].

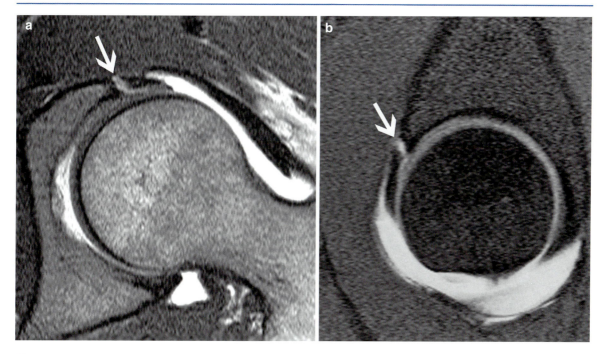

**Fig. 5.9** Labral detachment with gadolinium imbibition between the acetabular rim and the base of the labrum (*white arrows*) on (**a**) oblique axial and (**b**) oblique sagittal, T1W with fat suppression images

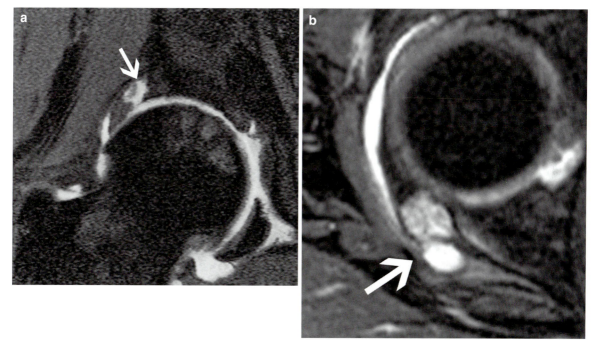

**Fig. 5.10** Paralabral cyst formation secondary to underlying labral tear. (**a**) Globular paralabral cyst (*white arrow*), partially filling with gadolinium, interposed between labrum and acetabular rim on T1W with fat suppression; (**b**) Paralabral cyst with bilobed configuration with greater conspicuity on fluid sensitive, axial proton density with fat suppression image (*white arrow*)

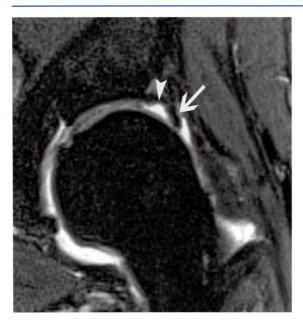

**Fig. 5.11** Disruption of the chondrolabral junction on MRA coronal T1WI with fat suppression. The labrum is globular with irregular surface (*white arrow*). Full thickness chondral defect is present along the lateral margin of the acetabular roof articular surface with gadolinium fluid imbibition into the defect (*arrowhead*)

## Cartilage

Both cam and pincer FAI are known to result in significant cartilage abnormality, with almost all patients demonstrating varying degrees of chondral injury [1, 9, 11]. The chondral morphologic changes may be in the form of surface fraying, fissuring, partial or full thickness loss of cartilage, and delamination. However, the dominant pattern of damage to the cartilage can vary between the cam and pincer forms.

MRI is the optimal radiologic modality for the evaluation of cartilage status [49]. In FAI chondral abnormality can be manifest with signal and morphologic changes. Both routine MRI [8, 29] and MRA [9, 19, 26, 50, 51] can be used to detect chondral defects of the femoral and acetabular articular surfaces. Various MR sequences have been used to evaluate cartilage morphology in the hip. These include proton density, gradient echo, and T1 sequences, with or without fat suppression, and with our without arthrographic technique. Recently, more quantitative techniques such as dGEMRIC, T2 and T1-rho mapping have been introduced in hope of detecting bio-

chemical changes in cartilage before gross, morphologic damage occurs [14]. In situations where MRI is contraindicated, CT arthrography may allow for evaluation of gross cartilage morphology and thickness [25, 26].

The initial chondral insult in cam FAI occurs at chondrolabral junction, anterosuperiorly, with disruption of the normally continuous interface between the two structures. With repetitive impingement of the cam deformity against the acetabulum, the damage extends more medially, into the hyaline cartilage [19]. With cam FAI, chondral injury preferentially occurs along the peripheral margin of the acetabulum, anterosuperiorly, tending to be more focal and deeper than with pincer FAI [1, 11]. The insult may begin as fissuring, thinning, and eventually evolve to full thickness chondral defect (Fig. 5.12).

One form of chondral injury specifically seen in cam FAI is the delamination whereby a focal area of cartilage detaches from the acetabular subchondral compact bone. This debonding manifests as a signal change within the substance of the cartilage, typically focal, linear hypointensity paralleling the articular surface, on various sequences, including gradient echo, proton density, and intermediate weighted images [51, 52]. When the debonding coexists with a full thickness chondral fissure or defect, a flap is created. On MRI a flap is identified by fluid interposition between the cartilage and the subchondral compact bone [51] (Fig. 5.13). The sensitivity, specificity, and accuracy of routine high-resolution MRI for detecting chondral injury in the hip ranges from 86% to 100%, 72% to 82%, and 82% to 88%, respectively [8, 29]. The sensitivity, specificity, and accuracy of MRA for detecting chondral injury in the hip ranges from 58% to 79%, 69% to 100%, and 69% to 81%, respectively [50, 53].

With pincer FAI, repetitive impaction of the anterosuperior acetabular rim on the femoral neck initially results in a narrow band of injury to the acetabular cartilage. The chondral lesions tend to be more diffuse, and shallower than with cam FAI [1, 11]. With chronic pincer impingement, contrecoup chondral lesions may be seen along the posteroinferior acetabular surface (Fig. 5.14). This relates to reduced excursion of the femoral head anteriorly due to the acetabular overcoverage. This leads to a secondary posterior shift of the femoral head with greater pressure against the posterior cartilage [1].

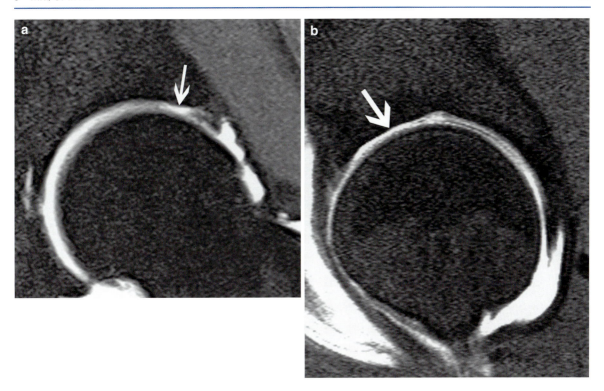

**Fig. 5.12** Cam FAI – Focal full-thickness chondral defect (*white arrows*) along the lateral, anterosuperior acetabular roof on MRA oblique (**a**) coronal and (**b**) sagittal T1WI with fat suppression. Gadolinium fills in the space void of hyaline cartilage

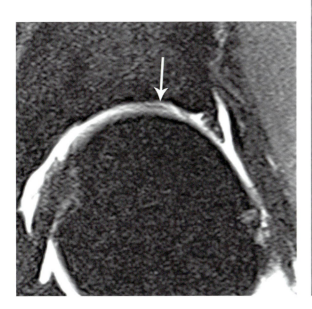

**Fig. 5.13** Cam FAI – Chondral delamination on oblique coronal T1WI with fat suppression. Delamination manifests as fine, linear imbibition of gadolinium between hyaline cartilage and subchondral compact bone (*white arrow*)

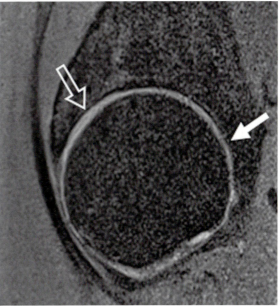

**Fig. 5.14** Pincer FAI – Moderate chondral thinning along the posterior joint space (*white arrow*) compared to normal chondral thickness along the anterosuperior joint (*open white arrow*) on oblique sagittal T1WI with fat suppression

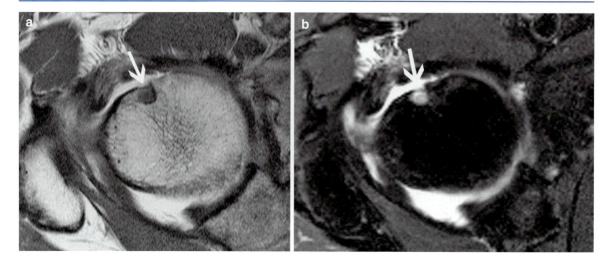

**Fig. 5.15** Fibrocyst along the anterosuperior femoral head-neck junction (*white arrows*) on (**a**) axial T1 and (**b**) axial proton density with fat suppression images

## Bone

Fibrocysts are known to be associated with both cam and pincer FAI [11, 54] and can be demonstrated by both CT [24, 49] and MRI [9, 11, 24, 49, 55]. Although the general population prevalence of fibrocysts has long been presumed to be approximately 5%, a recent CT based study found the prevalence to be 43% [24]. In patients with FAI, using MRI, the reported prevalences range from 4% to 24% [8, 9, 11], and with MR arthrography, 52% [54].

Fibrocysts can vary in size, ranging from 2 to 15 mm [24, 54, 55] and may be unilocular or multilocular [49]. It has been reported that the small fibrocysts may progressively evolve into larger cysts with continuing impingement [56].

On CT, fibrocysts appear as lucent lesions just below the cortex. They are typically well defined with sclerotic margins although the overlying cortex may be thin and irregular. The attenuation value varies from that of fluid to soft tissue, depending of the composition of the internal contents [24].

On MRI, fibrocysts appear as well-defined lesions which peripherally are of low T1 and T2 signals, and centrally of variable T1 and T2 signals, again depending the internal composition [54] (Fig. 5.15).

Although originally referred to as herniation pits, the term fibrocyst has now been adopted, reflecting the differences in the underlying pathophysiology of the two entities. Herniation pits are believed to develop second-ary to mechanical pressure on the anterior femoral neck by the iliofemoral ligament/anterior capsule during extreme hip extension. Herniation pits contain variable amounts of synovium, fluid, fibrous tissue, and metaplastic cartilage [57]. Fibrocysts, on the other hand, develop as result of repetitive mechanical contact between the femur and the acetabular rim during flexion and internal rotation. Histologically, they are composed of varying amounts of fluid and fibrous tissue [54].

A spatial relationship between the location of fibrocysts and site of impingement has been established [54]. They are most commonly seen along the anterosuperior femoral neck, just at the margin of the articular surface [1]. Fibrocysts may be associated with local marrow edema seen on MRI [49]. Fibrocysts have been noted to be associated with higher alpha angles [24]. Given the prevalence, location, and association with higher alpha-angle values, fibrocysts may be a radiologic marker of FAI [54].

Marrow edema may be seen in a subchondral location due to chondropathic changed. Nonsubchondral, or marginal, marrow edema may also develop as a result of focal contact of impingement. The edema can occur on either femoral or acetabular sides of the joint [18].

Impingement leads to increase stress along the anterosuperior acetabular rim. This may lead to focal osseous fracture or fragmentation, or chronic nonfusion of the normal epiphysis in this area, referred to as the os acetabuli [58]. Os acetabuli can be seen with both cam and pincer FAI [9].

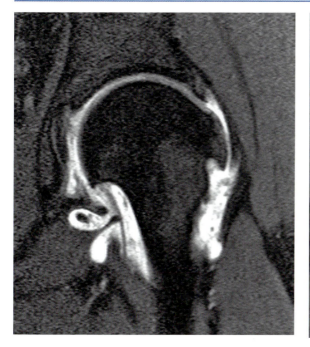

**Fig. 5.16** Synovitis with small focal nodular areas of low signal along the intra-articular capsular lining on MRA oblique coronal T1WI with fat suppression. TIFF

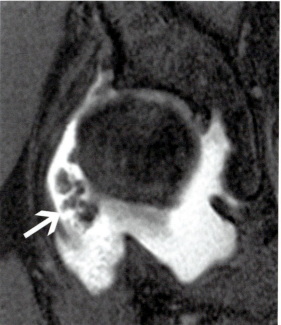

**Fig. 5.17** End stage hip OA with multiple intra-articular bodies (*white arrow*) presenting as irregular shaped low signal foci surrounded by gadolinium fluid

## Joint

In both cam and pincer FAI, the primary morphologic abnormalities of the hip along with secondary derangement of the articular structures, result in altered biomechanics leading to osteoarthritis. The variable constellation of findings including chondral loss, osteophytosis, synovitis, effusion, capsular thickening, and loose bodies, can be demonstrated by MRI Fig. 5.16 and Fig. 5.17. However, it should be noted that these findings are nonspecific and can be seen in a variety of arthritides in the absence of FAI.

## Conclusion

FAI is known to create a predisposition to hip osteoarthritis. The impingement results from anatomic abnormalities, which lead to altered hip biomechanics and joint injury. These dysmorphisms require radiologic investigation in order to be detected and characterized. MRI is the optimal radiologic modality to evaluate the primary anatomic deformities of the joint, as well as to detect the secondary derangements which result from the impingement.

Cam FAI is result of a contour abnormality at the anterosuperior femoral head-neck junction, which can be quantified by the alpha angle. Associated findings include disruption of the chondrolabral junction, focal anterosuperior acetabular chondral lesions, delamination, and labral degeneration and tearing. The MRI triad of elevated alpha angle, anterosuperior labral tear, and anterosuperior chondral lesion may be seen in a large number cam FAI patients [9].

Pincer FAI is characterized by a relatively deep acetabular fossa with overcoverage of the femoral head, either focal or global. Associated abnormalities include more diffuse acetabular chondral damage, both anterosuperiorly and posteriorly, and labral injury including degeneration, tearing, and prominent intralabral cyst formation.

Both forms of FAI may also result in fibrocyst formation, ossification of the labrum, marrow edema, and changes of OA.

MRI and CT provide information that may impact significantly on patient management. Based on the radiologic findings, patients can be stratified into conservative, arthroscopic or open surgical treatment regimes. The images provide a preoperative anatomic road-map localizing, grading, and quantifying the primary and/or secondary abnormalities. They may also be useful in the pre-, intra-, or postoperative settings in combination with computer aided navigation software programs. This may allow for the earlier characterization and diagnosis of, and intervention for, FAI, potentially delaying or preventing the secondary joint derangements which can lead to premature OA.

# References

1. Beck M et al (2005) Hip morphology influences the pattern of damage to the acetabular cartilage: femoroacetabular impingement as a cause of early osteoarthritis of the hip. J Bone Joint Surg Br 87(7):1012–1018
2. Ganz R et al (2008) The etiology of osteoarthritis of the hip: an integrated mechanical concept. Clin Orthop Relat Res 466(2):264–272
3. Ganz R et al (2003) Femoroacetabular impingement: a cause for osteoarthritis of the hip. Clin Orthop Relat Res 417:112–120
4. Ito K et al (2001) Femoroacetabular impingement and the cam-effect. A MRI-based quantitative anatomical study of the femoral head-neck offset. J Bone Joint Surg Br 83(2):171–176
5. Beaule PE et al (2005) Three-dimensional computed tomography of the hip in the assessment of femoroacetabular impingement. J Orthop Res 23(6):1286–1292
6. Meyer DC et al (2006) Comparison of six radiographic projections to assess femoral head/neck asphericity. Clin Orthop Relat Res 445:181–185
7. Tannast M, Siebenrock KA, Anderson SE (2007) Femoroacetabular impingement: radiographic diagnosis – what the radiologist should know. AJR Am J Roentgenol 188(6):1540–1552
8. James SL et al (2006) MRI findings of femoroacetabular impingement. AJR Am J Roentgenol 187(6):1412–1419
9. Kassarjian A et al (2005) Triad of MR arthrographic findings in patients with cam-type femoroacetabular impingement. Radiology 236(2):588–592
10. Notzli HP et al (2002) The contour of the femoral head-neck junction as a predictor for the risk of anterior impingement. J Bone Joint Surg Br 84(4):556–560
11. Pfirrmann CW et al (2006) Cam and pincer femoroacetabular impingement: characteristic MR arthrographic findings in 50 patients. Radiology 240(3):778–785
12. Clohisy JC et al (2009) Radiographic evaluation of the hip has limited reliability. Clin Orthop Relat Res 467(3): 666–675
13. Dudda M et al (2009) Do normal radiographs exclude asphericity of the femoral head-neck junction? Clin Orthop Relat Res 467(3):651–659
14. Mamisch TC et al (2008) Magnetic resonance imaging of the hip at 3 Tesla: clinical value in femoroacetabular impingement of the hip and current concepts. Semin Musculoskelet Radiol 12(3):212–222
15. Petersilge CA (2000) From the RSNA Refresher Courses. Radiological Society of North America. Chronic adult hip pain: MR arthrography of the hip. Radiographics 20(Spec No):S43–S52
16. McCarthy JC, Busconi B (1995) The role of hip arthroscopy in the diagnosis and treatment of hip disease. Orthopedics 18(8):753–756
17. Yamamoto Y et al (2007) Usefulness of radial contrast-enhanced computed tomography for the diagnosis of acetabular labrum injury. Arthroscopy 23(12):1290–1294
18. Bredella MA, Stoller DW (2005) MR imaging of femoroacetabular impingement. Magn Reson Imaging Clin N Am 13(4):653–664
19. Werlen S (2005) Magnetic resonance arthrography of the hip in femoroacetabular impingement. Oper Tech Orthop 15:191–203
20. Kassarjian A (2006) Hip MR arthrography and femoroacetabular impingement. Semin Musculoskelet Radiol 10(3): 208–219
21. Hodler J et al (1995) MR arthrography of the hip: improved imaging of the acetabular labrum with histologic correlation in cadavers. AJR Am J Roentgenol 165(4):887–891
22. Steinbach LS, Palmer WE, Schweitzer ME (2002) Special focus session. MR arthrography. Radiographics 22(5):1223–1246
23. Reynolds D, Lucas J, Klaue K (1999) Retroversion of the acetabulum. A cause of hip pain. J Bone Joint Surg Br 81(2):281–288
24. Panzer S, Augat P, Esch U (2008) CT assessment of herniation pits: prevalence, characteristics, and potential association with morphological predictors of femoroacetabular impingement. Eur Radiol 18(9):1869–1875
25. Nishii T et al (2007) Disorders of acetabular labrum and articular cartilage in hip dysplasia: evaluation using isotropic high-resolutional CT arthrography with sequential radial reformation. Osteoarthritis Cartilage 15(3):251–257
26. Wyler A et al (2009) Comparison of MR-arthrography and CT-arthrography in hyaline cartilage-thickness measurement in radiographically normal cadaver hips with anatomy as gold standard. Osteoarthritis Cartilage 17(1):19–25
27. Ramnath RR (2006) 3 T MR imaging of the musculoskeletal system (part II): clinical applications. Magn Reson Imaging Clin N Am 14(1):41–62
28. Kassarjian A, Brisson M, Palmer WE (2007) Femoroacetabular impingement. Eur J Radiol 63(1):29–35
29. Mintz DN et al (2005) Magnetic resonance imaging of the hip: detection of labral and chondral abnormalities using noncontrast imaging. Arthroscopy 21(4):385–393
30. Siebenrock KA et al (2004) Abnormal extension of the femoral head epiphysis as a cause of cam impingement. Clin Orthop Relat Res 418:54–60
31. Rakhra KS et al (2009) Comparison of MRI alpha angle measurement planes in femoroacetabular impingement. Clin Orthop Relat Res 467(3):660–665
32. Jager M et al (2004) Femoroacetabular impingement caused by a femoral osseous head-neck bump deformity: clinical, radiological, and experimental results. J Orthop Sci 9(3): 256–263
33. Hack K et al. (2010) Prevalence of cam-type femoroacetabular impingement morphology in asymptomatic volunteers. J Bone Joint Surg Am 92(14):2436–2444.
34. Siebenrock KA, Schoeniger R, Ganz R (2003) Anterior femoro-acetabular impingement due to acetabular

retroversion. Treatment with periacetabular osteotomy. J Bone Joint Surg Am 85-A(2):278–286

35. Anda S, Terjesen T, Kvistad KA (1991) Computed tomography measurements of the acetabulum in adult dysplastic hips: which level is appropriate? Skeletal Radiol 20(4): 267–271

36. Stem ES et al (2006) Computed tomography analysis of acetabular anteversion and abduction. Skeletal Radiol 35(6):385–389

37. Murphy SB et al (1990) Acetabular dysplasia in the adolescent and young adult. Clin Orthop Relat Res 261:214–223

38. Tonnis D, Heinecke A (1999) Acetabular and femoral anteversion: relationship with osteoarthritis of the hip. J Bone Joint Surg Am 81(12):1747–1770

39. Czerny C et al (1996) Lesions of the acetabular labrum: accuracy of MR imaging and MR arthrography in detection and staging. Radiology 200(1):225–230

40. Leunig M et al (1997) Evaluation of the acetabular labrum by MR arthrography. J Bone Joint Surg Br 79(2):230–234

41. Czerny C et al (1999) MR arthrography of the adult acetabular capsular-labral complex: correlation with surgery and anatomy. AJR Am J Roentgenol 173(2):345–349

42. Chan YS et al (2005) Evaluating hip labral tears using magnetic resonance arthrography: a prospective study comparing hip arthroscopy and magnetic resonance arthrography diagnosis. Arthroscopy 21(10):1250

43. Toomayan GA et al (2006) Sensitivity of MR arthrography in the evaluation of acetabular labral tears. AJR Am J Roentgenol 186(2):449–453

44. Freedman BA et al (2006) Prognostic value of magnetic resonance arthrography for Czerny stage II and III acetabular labral tears. Arthroscopy 22(7):742–747

45. Ito K, Leunig M, Ganz R (2004) Histopathologic features of the acetabular labrum in femoroacetabular impingement. Clin Orthop Relat Res 429:262–271

46. Blankenbaker DG et al (2007) Classification and localization of acetabular labral tears. Skeletal Radiol 36(5):391–397

47. Magee T, Hinson G (2000) Association of paralabral cysts with acetabular disorders. AJR Am J Roentgenol 174(5): 1381–1384

48. Eijer H, Myers SR, Ganz R (2001) Anterior femoroacetabular impingement after femoral neck fractures. J Orthop Trauma 15(7):475–481

49. James SL et al (2007) Femoroacetabular impingement: bone marrow oedema associated with fibrocystic change of the femoral head and neck junction. Clin Radiol 62(5):472–478

50. Schmid MR et al (2003) Cartilage lesions in the hip: diagnostic effectiveness of MR arthrography. Radiology 226(2): 382–386

51. Beaule PE, Zaragoza E, Copelan N (2004) Magnetic resonance imaging with gadolinium arthrography to assess acetabular cartilage delamination. A report of four cases. J Bone Joint Surg Am 86-A(10):2294–2298

52. Pfirrmann CW et al (2008) MR arthrography of acetabular cartilage delamination in femoroacetabular cam impingement. Radiology 249(1):236–241

53. Knuesel PR et al (2004) MR arthrography of the hip: diagnostic performance of a dedicated water-excitation 3D double-echo steady-state sequence to detect cartilage lesions. AJR Am J Roentgenol 183(6):1729–1735

54. Leunig M et al (2005) Fibrocystic changes at anterosuperior femoral neck: prevalence in hips with femoroacetabular impingement. Radiology 236(1):237–246

55. Nokes SR et al (1989) Herniation pits of the femoral neck: appearance at MR imaging. Radiology 172(1):231–234

56. Gunther KP et al (2007) Large femoral-neck cysts in association with femoroacetabular impingement. A report of three cases. J Bone Joint Surg Am 89(4):863–870

57. Pitt MJ et al (1982) Herniation pit of the femoral neck. AJR Am J Roentgenol 138(6):1115–1121

58. Klaue K, Durnin CW, Ganz R (1991) The acetabular rim syndrome. A clinical presentation of dysplasia of the hip. J Bone Joint Surg Br 73(3):423–429

# Future Strategies for the Assessment of Cartilage and Labral Lesions in Femoroacetabular Impingement

Ara Kassarjian, Luis Cerezal, and Eva Llopis

Over the past few years, interest in the concept of femoroacetabular impingement (FAI) has grown tremendously. As the orthopedic community has begun to show intense interest in the apparent relationship between FAI and early onset of degenerative change, there has been a concomitant increase in the desire for high-quality imaging of the hip. Although traditional imaging modalities have, to date, been sufficient for imaging the extra-articular structures and the osseous structures, imaging of intra-articular structures, specifically the cartilage and labrum, remains challenging.

There is mounting evidence that labral lesions and cartilage lesions are intimately related to degenerative change and that treatment of such lesions at earlier stages may result in better outcomes [1]. With the more widespread use of hip arthroscopy and continual advances in treatment of cartilage and labral lesions, there is ever increasing pressure on radiologists to provide high-resolution accurate imaging of subtle cartilage and labral lesions, lesions that were essentially imperceptible with prior imaging techniques. Specifically, the current challenge is to accurately image damage of morphologically normal cartilage, subtle cartilage flaps, thin partial-thickness cartilage surface lesions, and subtle non-displaced labral tears. Preoperative knowledge of the presence and severity of such lesions is important in treatment planning and patient counseling [2]. This chapter will discuss some emerging techniques and strategies for imaging of subtle yet potentially important lesions of the hip cartilage and acetabular labrum.

## General Principles

Imaging of the acetabular and femoral cartilage and the acetabular labrum presents significant challenges. To begin with, the hip is a deeply seated joint resulting in some imaging artifacts or attenuation of signal from the intra-articular structures. Also, since the hip is a relatively stable and tight joint, there is typically little separation between the intra-articular structures.

The most widely used techniques for imaging the intra-articular structures of the hip are MR, MR arthrography, and CT arthrography. Aside from demonstrating mineralized intra-articular loose bodies, non-arthrographic CT has a very limited role in assessing the intra-articular structures of the hip.

As in most other joints, conventional hip MR provides excellent overall soft tissue contrast. In addition, MR can demonstrate osseous abnormalities such as marrow edema. However, since the hip is covered by large muscle groups and, in some patients, a significant amount of subcutaneous fat, MR coils cannot be placed in very close proximity to the joint. In addition, since there are currently no dedicated hip coils on the

A. Kassarjian (✉)
Department of Radiology, Division of Musculoskeletal Radiology, Massachusetts General Hospital, Boston, MA, USA

Corades, S.L, Madrid, Spain
e-mail: akassarjian@gmail.com

L. Cerezal
Department of Radiology, Clínica Mompía, Instituto Radiológico Cántabro, Cantabria, Spain
e-mail: lcerezal@gmail.com

E. Llopis
Department of Radiology, Hospital de la Ribera, Valencia, Spain

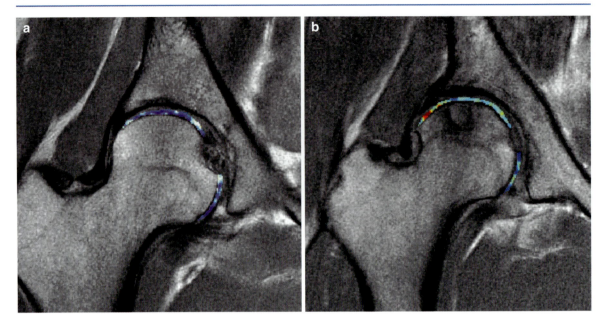

**Fig. 6.1** (**a**) T2 map demonstrates normal cartilage T2 values in the hip. (**b**) T2 map shows degeneration of hip cartilage (Images courtesy of Atsuya Watanabe M.D., Ph.D.)

market, imaging is typically done with some level of improvisation such as using a combination of flex coils, torso coils, or even cardiac coils. Even with adequate signal to noise and reasonable spatial resolution, it is challenging to accurately image the very thin cartilage of the acetabulum and femur and the small acetabular labrum not only due to their small dimensions but also due to the fact that they are very closely opposed to one another. For this reason, although conventional MR can be used to assess the hip cartilage and labrum, its accuracy in assessing intra-articular structures is generally inferior to that of MR arthrography [3]. Two possible exceptions that will subsequently be discussed are the techniques of MR T2 mapping and delayed gadolinium-enhanced MR imaging of cartilage (dGEMRIC).

At MR arthrography or CT arthrography, introduction of contrast into the hip joint results in joint distention and some separation of the intra-articular structures. This aids in assessing the surfaces of these structures. If there is a defect along the articular surface of these structures (e.g., labral tear, cartilage defect), the contrast can flow into the defect and thus make it more conspicuous at imaging. For this reason, when assessing intra-articular lesions of the hip, it is common to choose MR arthrography or CT arthrography over conventional non-arthrographic MR imaging [4].

## Cartilage

### Non-arthrographic Imaging

To date, conventional (non-arthrographic) MR imaging has poor sensitivity and poor to moderate accuracy in assessing hip cartilage [3]. Although higher field strength (e.g., 3T) appears to improve accuracy, published figures are still suboptimal [5].

T2 mapping of hip cartilage has been receiving increasing attention recently. One of the reasons is that advances in MR hardware and software have made it possible to apply this technique to the hip despite the absence of dedicated hip coils. The lack of such a coil is partially overcome by increasing field strengths. With T2 mapping, one can indirectly assess cartilage macromolecular orientation and organization and cartilage water content [6]. The main theoretical advantage of T2 mapping is that it can detect structural abnormalities in grossly morphologically normal cartilage and can do so in a noninvasive manner (Fig. 6.1). This may be a significant prognostic indicator as cartilage treatment procedures evolve. One of the major drawbacks to T2 mapping is that there is no consistent widely agreed-upon definition of what constitutes a "normal" T2 map of acetabular and femoral cartilage. Preliminary studies have demonstrated that there are definite zonal variations in the hip [7]. Studies demonstrating potential normal variations associated with level of activity, intensity or timing of exercise, and surrounding osseous morphology are lacking. With further study and establishment of normal values and patterns of distribution of the T2 characteristics of hip cartilage, T2 mapping has the potential to become a powerful tool for evaluating the structural integrity of morphologically normal cartilage. However, the actual application and clinical utility of such a technique, as well as its potential effect on decision-making and outcomes, is unknown.

dGEMRIC has been widely cited in the evaluation of knee cartilage. Although this is not a new technique, its application in the evaluation of hip cartilage is relatively recent [8, 9]. Briefly, dGEMRIC uses the properties of intravenously injected gadolinium to indirectly assess the biochemical composition of cartilage [10]. Regions of degenerated cartilage theoretically have lower glycosaminoglycan (GAG) concentrations. Due to the negative charge of gadolinium (Gd-DTPA), and the negative charge of GAGs, more gadolinium will theoretically bind to the degenerated (and thus GAG-deficient) regions of cartilage. Using this technique, 1–2 h following the intravenous administration of gadolinium, a conventional MR is performed, and the biochemical nature of cartilage can be inferred based on the amount of T1 shortening of the cartilage. The main advantage of dGEMRIC is that it may demonstrate abnormal biochemical properties of grossly morphologically normal cartilage. However, dGEMRIC does have some disadvantages. First of all, one must wait a significant amount of time between injection and imaging. This can prove to be impractical in a busy clinical setting. Also, reproducibility of the technique may not be as high as widely believed. A recent study looking at dGEMRIC of knee cartilage demonstrated 10–15% test-retest variability [11].

Although diffusion-weighted imaging and tractography have been applied to cartilage imaging (mainly in the knee), their feasibility and utility in hip cartilage imaging are currently not known.

Both T2 mapping and dGEMRIC have the theoretical advantage of detecting cartilage structural and biochemical abnormalities before they are visible at standard imaging or at arthroscopy. Since it appears that outcomes of treatment of FAI may be related to the degree of cartilage damage at the time of surgery, the potential of detecting subtle structural and biochemical lesions may eventually be of use in determining whether surgery would be expected to have good outcomes and, if so, which type of surgery would be best. Perhaps the degree of structural or biomechanical cartilage damage at presentation will determine the best treatment: osteochondroplasty vs. resurfacing vs. hemi- or total arthroplasty vs. other yet to be determined procedures. Currently, these decisions are often based on the degree of *visible* cartilage damage.

## Arthrographic Imaging

Until the true accuracy and utility of non-arthrographic techniques such as T2 mapping and dGEMRIC become evident, currently available and widespread techniques continue to be improved.

For MR arthrography, ever-improving MR hardware and software including the design of better coils and more robust gradients has increased the spatial and contrast resolution that can be achieved within a reasonable scan time. For example, the recent description of very subtle cartilage signal abnormalities at 3T which indicate underlying delaminating cartilage lesions (although the actual lesion is not visible) is an example of better use and understanding of currently available tools [12]. In addition, a recent study has demonstrated that placing traction on the leg at the time of MR imaging can help separate the femoral and acetabular cartilage surfaces and thus enable visualization of subtle surface lesions [13] (Fig. 6.2). Knowledge of the presence of these subtle cartilage lesions is having increasing influence on the timing and type of FAI surgery. Recently, the experimental use of direct MR arthrography and subsequent intra-articular gadolinium-enhanced MR imaging of cartilage (iGEMRIC) of the hip has been described [14]. This has the potential to provide the best of both worlds as the arthrographic component provides morphologic data while the delayed imaging provides biochemical data.

For CT arthrography, advances in gantry design, tube design, and detector configurations have led to exquisite imaging of femoral and acetabular cartilage. The isotropic data sets that are obtained with multi-detector scanners can then be reformatted retrospectively in any desired plane yielding detailed imaging of the areas of interest (Fig. 6.3). Although scientific evidence is sparse, it appears that CT arthrography with modern equipment

**Fig. 6.2** Multiple images
from dGEMRIC study of hip
show low GAG content (*red
areas*) most prominent
adjacent to acetabular
subchondral cyst (*arrow*)
(Reprinted with permission
from Cunningham et al. [8])

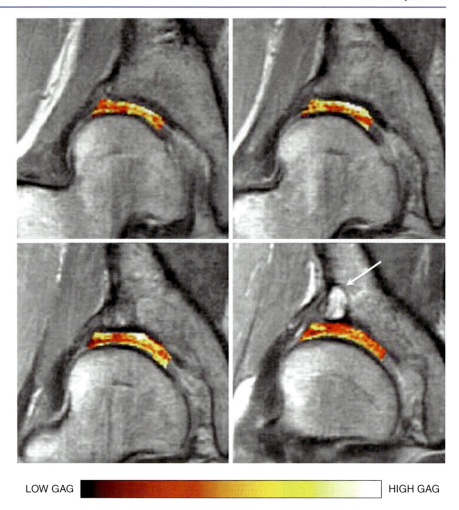

LOW GAG                                                    HIGH GAG

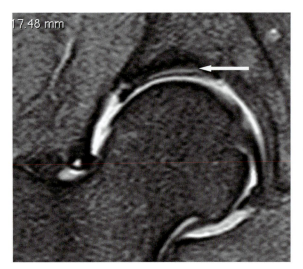

**Fig. 6.3** Hip MR arthrography with traction demonstrates a
delaminating lesion (*arrow*) of the acetabular cartilage

is equal to, if not superior to, MR arthrography in the
detection of hip cartilage lesions [15]. Also, as with MR
arthrography, addition of leg traction may prove beneficial in allowing better visualization of the cartilage
surfaces. However, CT arthrography provides little information regarding cartilage signal and composition, and
detection of delaminating lesions remains difficult
(Fig. 6.4). Finally, since many patients with cam-type
FAI are young, one must always take into account the
gonadal radiation dose from high-resolution hip CT
imaging.

As the indications and prognostic factors of FAI
surgery evolve, the role of the acetabular cartilage at
the time of surgery appears to be a focal point. As a
result, investigations and applications of new and
improved hip cartilage imaging techniques (both mac-
roscopic and structural/biomechanical) should be a
focus of future research.

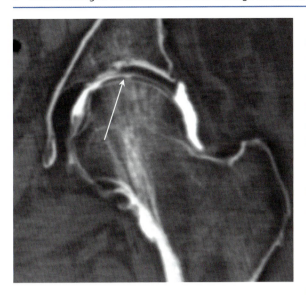

**Fig. 6.4** Hip CT arthrography shows a subtle cartilage lesion (*arrow*)

## Labrum

As with imaging of hip cartilage, most studies demonstrate the superiority of MR and CT arthrography over non-arthrographic studies. In comparing CT arthrography with MR arthrography, results seem to be similar in recent studies [4]. Although CT has the advantage of slightly higher spatial resolution, MR typically provides higher contrast resolution. MR has the advantage of demonstrating other factors such as bone marrow edema and cartilage signal abnormalities that would not be appreciated on CT arthrography. Finally, the superior soft tissue contrast of MR provides the additional advantage of allowing accurate evaluation of extra-articular causes of hip pain.

In 1996, there were two publications concerning the classification of acetabular labral tears which have since served as the most widely used classification systems [16, 17]. Czerny et al. proposed a classification system based on labral morphological abnormalities as seen at MR arthrography. This classification system has similarities to the meniscal tear classification system with the added component of including the presence or absence of enlargement/loss of triangular configuration and presence/absence of a paralabral recess of the labrum. In the same year, Lage et al. published an arthroscopic classification of acetabular labral tears based on the morphology and location of the tear. These included radial

flap tears, radial fibrillated tears, longitudinal peripheral tears, and unstable tears. Clearly, these two classification systems use different criteria and different aspects of tear morphology to classify the tears. Also, the concept of an unstable tear is difficult to apply directly to imaging. Ideally, the classification system used at imaging should be similar to that used at arthroscopy. With this in mind, Blankenbaker et al. compared the Czerny classification system as well as a modified MR arthrographic version of the Lage classification system to arthroscopic Lage classification in 65 patients with arthroscopically proven labral tears [18]. They found that the Czerny classification did not have significant correlations with the arthroscopic Lage classification. In addition, they found only borderline correlation between the modified MR arthrographic Lage classification and the arthroscopic Lage classification. However, MR arthrography and arthroscopy had good agreement regarding the location of the tear (based on a clockface).

As has been done for the shoulder, a consensus classification system needs to be developed to better correlate the findings at MR arthrography (or CT arthrography) and arthroscopy. Most radiologists and orthopedists would agree that the location and extent of a labral tear based on a clockface numbering system are fundamental components of such a classification system. However, agreement must be reached as to which arthrographic and arthroscopic classification system should be used. Having a consistent reproducible classification system will be important as treatment of labral tears continues to evolve with increasing use of labral repair and reattachment procedures.

As both arthroscopic and MR arthrographic experience of labral lesions increases, there is increasing interest in potential normal variants in labral morphology. Although the concept of a normal recess along the posteroinferior labrum is widely accepted, there remains controversy regarding a possible normal recess along the anterosuperior labrum [19]. This is an important region to study as approximately 90% of labral tears involve this region. In addition, there are variants in the shape of the labrum (rounded, hypoplastic, etc.) that have yet to be adequately studied in a scientific manner. As was done with the glenoid labrum, further study is needed into the normal variants that may be encountered in the acetabular labrum and assessment as to whether some of these normal variants are associated with an increased risk of labral tears.

In conclusion, although there have been significant advances in imaging of hip cartilage and labrum, there is much room for improvement. Structural and biomechanical imaging of cartilage as well as better imaging of cartilage flaps and subtle cartilage surface lesions may a have significant impact on the preoperative evaluation and intraoperative treatment of cartilage lesions. Although imaging of the acetabular labrum has become quite accurate, the focus should now shift to better correlation between the findings at imaging and arthrography. A classification system that encompasses and incorporates imaging findings, arthroscopic findings, and potential treatments should be devised. In addition, better understanding of normal variants of the acetabular labrum is needed.

# References

1. Beck M, Kalhor M, Leunig M, Ganz R (2005) Hip morphology influences the pattern of damage to the acetabular cartilage: femoroacetabular impingement as a cause of early osteoarthritis of the hip. J Bone Joint Surg Br 87: 1012–1018
2. Peters CL, Erickson JA (2006) Treatment of femoro-acetabular impingement with surgical dislocation and débridement in young adults. J Bone Joint Surg Am 88:1735–1741
3. Schmid MR, Nötzli HP, Zanetti M, Wyss TF, Hodler J (2003) Cartilage lesions in the hip: diagnostic effectiveness of MR arthrography. Radiology 226(2):382–386
4. Wyler A, Bousson V, Bergot C, Polivka M, Leveque E, Vicaut E, Laredo JD (2009) Comparison of MR-arthrography and CT-arthrography in hyaline cartilage-thickness measurement in radiographically normal cadaver hips with anatomy as gold standard. Osteoarthritis Cartilage 17(1):19–25, Epub Jul 9, 2008
5. Ramnath RR (2006) 3T MR imaging of the musculoskeletal system (part II): clinical applications. Magn Reson Imaging Clin N Am 14(1):41–62
6. Dardzinski BJ, Mosher TJ, Li S, Van Slyke MA, Smith MB (1997) Spatial variation of T2 in human articular cartilage. Radiology 205:546–550
7. Watanabe A, Boesch C, Siebenrock K, Obata T, Anderson SE (2007) T2 mapping of hip articular cartilage in healthy volunteers at 3T: a study of topographic variation. J Magn Reson Imaging 26(1):165–171
8. Cunningham T, Jessel R, Zurakowski D, Millis MB, Kim YJ (2006) Delayed gadolinium-enhanced magnetic resonance imaging of cartilage to predict early failure of Bernese periacetabular osteotomy for hip dysplasia. J Bone Joint Surg Am 88(7):1540–1548
9. Kim YJ, Jaramillo D, Millis MB, Gray ML, Burstein D (2003) Assessment of early osteoarthritis in hip dysplasia with delayed gadolinium-enhanced magnetic resonance imaging of cartilage. J Bone Joint Surg Am 85-A(10):1987–1992
10. Bashir A, Gray ML, Boutin RD, Burstein D (1997) Glycosaminoglycan in articular cartilage: in vivo assessment with delayed Gd(DTPA)(2-)-enhanced MR imaging. Radiology 205(2):551–558
11. Ssakainen J, Multanen J, Rauvala E, Lammentausta E, Ojala R, Kiviranta I, Hakkinen A, Heinonen (2008) Scandinavian Physiological Society's Annual Meeting. Acta Physiologica 193(Suppl 664):p34
12. Pfirrmann CW, Duc SR, Zanetti M, Dora C, Hodler J (2008) MR arthrography of acetabular cartilage delamination in femoroacetabular cam impingement. Radiology 249(1):236–241, Epub Aug 5, 2008
13. Llopis E, Cerezal L, Kassarjian A, Higueras V, Fernandez E (2008) Direct MR arthrography of the hip with leg traction: feasibility for assessing articular cartilage. AJR Am J Roentgenol 190(4):1124–1128
14. Boesen M, Jensen KE, Qvistgaard E, Danneskiold-Samsøe B, Thomsen C, Ostergaard M, Bliddal H (2006) Delayed gadolinium-enhanced magnetic resonance imaging (dGEMRIC) of hip joint cartilage: better cartilage delineation after intra-articular than intravenous gadolinium injection. Acta Radiol 47(4):391–396
15. Nishii T, Tanaka H, Sugano N, Miki H, Takao M, Yoshikawa H (2007) Disorders of acetabular labrum and articular cartilage in hip dysplasia: evaluation using isotropic high-resolutional CT arthrography with sequential radial reformation. Osteoarthritis Cartilage 15(3):251–257, Epub Sep 20, 2006
16. Czerny C, Hofmann S, Neuhold A, Tschauner C, Engel A, Recht MP, Kramer J (1996) Lesions of the acetabular labrum: accuracy of MR imaging and MR arthrography in detection and staging. Radiology 200(1):225–230
17. Lage LA, Patel JV, Villar RN (1996) The acetabular labral tear: an arthroscopic classification. Arthroscopy 12(3):269–272
18. Blankenbaker DG, De Smet AA, Keene JS, Fine JP (2007) Classification and localization of acetabular labral tears. Skeletal Radiol 36(5):391–397, Epub Jan 17, 2007
19. Studler U, Kalberer F, Leunig M, Zanetti M, Hodler J, Dora C, Pfirrmann CW (2008) MR arthrography of the hip: differentiation between an anterior sublabral recess as a normal variant and a labral tear. Radiology 249(3):947–954, Epub Oct 7, 2008

# Part III

# FAI Surgical Treatment

# Evidence-Based Medicine in the Treatment of Femoroacetabular Impingement

**7**

Ricardo Larraínzar Garijo, R. García-Bógalo, and E. Díez-Nicolás

When it comes to providing a medical indication and selecting a certain surgical technique, surgeons make their decision based on their professional experience, previous results, and personal skills. However very few of them can affirm with scientific rigor that their perceptions are real and are not influenced by some type of bias, either voluntary or not. The great challenge that we are confronted with is trying to bring light to the darkness of scientific knowledge with the help of the different works published.

Evidence-based medicine (EBM) is quickly becoming the standard in today's health environment. In 1991, Guyatt [1] published an editorial in the ACP Journal Club in which he defines it as "an attitude of illustrated skepticism regarding the application of diagnostic, therapeutic and prognostic technologies to the daily handling of patients." From that day many physicians, managers, and health-care professionals have incorporated it to their daily practice. However, Guyatt only expressed with words what has been, and it will remain, the very essence of the medical act: finding the best solution to our patients' problem. The main

contribution of this attitude of enlightened skepticism was to systematize [2], and therefore parameterize, the ways in which medical decisions are made [3].

## Methodology

There are more than a 100 published studies at our disposal that we can use as a guide when making our individual decisions. However not all works follow the same methodology, and therefore the conclusions reached by the authors are not always comparable. The main hurdle to research is bias, that is to say, the possibility that the findings are the result of factors other than those postulated by the investigator.

The area of surgery for femoroacetabular impingement (FAI) is rife with methodological errors that lead to biased assumptions:

- Selection errors. Not all patients are equal, and therefore the results obtained in a specific group of patients may not be extrapolated to the general population. There are practically no papers that provide a detailed account of the characteristics of the population studied.
- Errors in measuring the results. In order to compare different studies, it is essential to quantify their results using the same parameters. Although there seems to be uniformity in terms of radiologic assessment (alpha angle), there is wide variation in terms of clinical quantification.
- Nondiscrimination errors. Not all surgeries are done by the same surgeon, and even the same individual may not carry out similar, exactly the same surgery in all cases as this depends on baseline physical and psychological conditions. Moreover, there is an

R.L. Garijo (✉)
Department of Orthopedic and Trauma Surgery,
Infanta Leonor Hospital,
Madrid, Spain

Jefe de Servicio COT,
Madrid, Spain
e-mail: ricardo.larrainzar@salud.madrid.org

R. García-Bógalo • E. Díez-Nicolás
Department of Orthopedic and Trauma Surgery,
Infanta Leonor Hospital,
Madrid, Spain

Ó. Marín-Peña (ed.), *Femoroacetabular Impingement*,
DOI 10.1007/978-3-642-22769-1_7, © Springer-Verlag Berlin Heidelberg 2012

assumption that a surgical technique was uniformly applied to all patients in a series when it is most likely that this was not the case. These two circumstances are probably the major factor that has impaired the methodological quality of surgeons' research work.

All the reasons expounded above should make us resort to prospective randomized studies when seeking the "best current knowledge on a certain topic."

## Searching for the Information

Fortunately, new technologies have emerged that provide us with a fabulous tool that would have delighted classical researchers. Nevertheless, there are so many of them that there is risk that valuable information may be lost as a result of too much "noise." For preparation of this work, we selected the MEDLINE database. As a starting point, we carried out a first search with the sequence: "Femur Neck"[MeSH] AND ("Surgical Procedures, Operative"[MeSH] OR "surgery" [Subheading]) and ("Reproducibility of Results"[MeSH] OR "Treatment Outcome"[MeSH]) without language restrictions. Our search provided us 96 hits containing many diseases unrelated to our object of interest.

In order to eliminate "noise" and select only papers focused exclusively on FAI, we supplemented our initial sequence with:

- ("Femur Neck"[MeSH] AND ("Surgical Procedures, Operative"[MeSH] OR "surgery" [Subheading]) and ("Reproducibility of Results"[MeSH] OR "Treatment Outcome"[MeSH])) and (femoral head (free term) and impingement (free term)). Seven hits were returned.
- ("Femur Neck"[MeSH] AND ("Surgical Procedures, Operative"[MeSH] OR "surgery "[Subheading]) and ("Reproducibility of Results"[MeSH] OR "Treatment Outcome"[MeSH])) and (femoral head (free term) and impingement (free term)). Eight hits were returned.

## Analysis of the Search

Following the established criteria, we came up with a total of 29 articles related to FAI, which were available for evaluation. However, an analysis the methodology followed in them reveals that none of them is a randomized prospective study. Therefore the level of evidence they provide is limited, with none of the publications having enough methodological quality to warrant study or comparative analysis. But there is reason for hope since of the 164 publications on FAI indexed in MEDLINE, 92 (56%) were published in the past 2 years, which reflects the recent interest this disease is attracting and raises the possibility that developmental randomized studies will be published in the near future.

Interestingly, regardless of where the publication was made, the authors' research focused on three areas: surgical technique, radiological diagnosis, and relationship to degenerative process.

## Evidence-Based Treatment of FAI

For the sake of didactics and interest, we shall respond to a few clinical questions and discuss the personal reflections of the authors who only seek to evoke in the reader a systematic reflection of other explanations to the findings analyzed.

## Origin of the Mechanical Conflict

The cause of the conflict generated in a "cam"-type impingement can be traced back to a defect of closing of the growth plate as stated by Siebenrock [4] in a case-control study (level III evidence) involving 30 patients, 15 diagnosed with "cam" type impingement and 15 controls. The author conducted an MRI study that revealed 4.3-mm femoral displacement anterosuperiorly in the FAI group, as compared with 7.6 mm in the control group, which pointed to an anterosuperior extension of the epiphysis of 97% in the FAI group and of 84% in the control group.

In another case-control study (level III evidence), Ito [5] analyzed the effect of the acetabular component on "cam"-type FAI. The author conducted a case-control MRI analysis of 24 patients (12 males and 12 females) diagnosed with FAI, and demonstrated that the symptomatic male patients presented with a significant decrease in neck offset, especially in the anterolateral region, while this occurrence was only found in the anterior region in middle-aged women. All FAI cases had femoral anteversion of 9.7°, as compared with 15.9° in the control group. It would seem clear that this is, in essence, a condition that creates a conflict and a mechanical disturbance in the normal functioning of the hip joint.

## Relationship Between FAI and Hip Arthritis

We assume the existence of a conflict that generates mechanical symptoms, but the question to be answered is whether this is the initial stage of articular degeneration and if by solving the mechanical conflict, we can halt the natural progression of the disease.

Wagner [6] presented a comparative retrospective study (level III evidence) with three groups – FAI (22 patients diagnosed and treated surgically), hip arthritis (14 adult patients who underwent prosthetic hip surgery), and controls (6 autopsy samples with a morphologically normal hip) – and performed an immunohistochemical study.

All samples of the FAI group showed that the hyaline cartilage presented with degenerative signs; using the Makin criteria, such changes were very different from those observed in the control group ($p = 0.007$) but not from those in the arthritic group ($p = 0.014$). These findings suggest that the mechanical conflict could constitute an early sign of the development of hip arthritis further to a biological conflict.

In the same vein, Jager [7] conducted an immunohistochemistry study of 19 patients diagnosed with FAI and demonstrated the recruitment of pluripotent cells in the perilesional zone of the mechanical conflict. There is no evidence to confirm whether the elimination of mechanical conflict can halt the natural progression of the disease.

## Imaging of FAI

Clohisy [8] presented a paper on 56 symptomatic FAI patients and compared them with 24 healthy hips to determine the effectiveness of simple imaging studies. He analyzed various common x-ray views: AP, lateral, and "frog-leg" lateral. By comparing the alpha angle, the asphericity of the femoral head, and head-neck offset, he concluded that all the aforementioned views show similar values but that the "frog-leg" lateral view provided the best appreciation of the magnitude of head neck offset.

Another way to quantify the concavity of the femoral neck is through 3D tomography. Beaulé [9] used this method to determine alpha and beta angles in 30 FAI patients and 12 healthy patients. Both values are higher in the presence of a mechanical conflict (alpha angles: FAI 66.4°, control 43.8°; beta angles: FAI 40.2°, control 43.8°).

FAI is not the only source of pain in the hip of the young adult. Although MRI can be considered the "gold standard" in the diagnosis of this condition, the presence of cysts in the radiographs of the anterosuperior region of the neck is suggestive of FAI as shown by Leuning [10] in a retrospective comparative study (level III evidence) of 117 patients diagnosed with FAI as compared with 132 patients with hip dysplasia. None of the patients in the dysplasia group showed these signs on AP pelvic radiographs.

In symptomatic FAI and hip dysplasia (HD) patients with labral pathology, it could be difficult to establish the most appropriate therapeutic strategy. Leuning published a prospective comparative study (level II evidence) [11] using arthro-MRI as a differentiator. In this study, which comprised a total of 28 patients (FAI 14, dysplasia 14), the author discusses various aspects, such as acetabular index, which is greater in dysplasia (FAI 6°, HD 25°), hypertrophy of the labrum, and the presence of ganglia (characteristic of HD).

Thus arthro-MRI seems to be the imaging "gold standard," especially in the context of developmental abnormalities of the hip. But the introduction of contrast into the joint is not always going to be necessary to reach a diagnosis of labral injury [12]. Arthro-MRI also plays a role in the differentiation of "cam"- and "pincer"-type FAI. Pfirmann [13] published a comparative retrospective study (level III evidence) of 33 patients (cam 33, pincer 17). As expected, the "cam" type had a greater alpha angle than the "pincer" type. Moreover, in "cam"-type FAI, patients' chondral lesions of the femoral neck were located anterosuperiorly, whereas in "pincer"-type FAI, these were to be found in the posterosuperior portion.

The value of calculating the alpha angle in the diagnosis of CFA is undisputed; however, it may prove hard to measure. This is demonstrated by Rakhra [14], who in a study comprising 41 arthro-MRI showed that the value of the alpha angle was underestimated in 54% of patients in the axial oblique views; the author recommended systematic use of radial views.

**Table 7.1** Evidence available

| Author | Year | Evidence level | Series | FAI type | Technique | Outcome | Complication |
|---|---|---|---|---|---|---|---|
| Siebenrock [15] | 2003 | IV | $N=22$ (29 hip)<br>M: 14 / F: 5<br>Mean age: 36 years<br>Follow-up: 56.4 months | Pincer | Periacetabular osteotomy | Improvement in all ROM-related parameters | 3 revisions (10%) |
| Beck [16] | 2004 | IV | $N=19$<br><br>M: 19 / F: 10<br>Mean age: 23 years<br>Follow-up: 30 months | Pincer: 14<br><br>Cam: 14 | | Improvement Merle d'Aubigne grade I | THA: 5 (26.3%)<br>Arthroscopy: 1 (3.4%) |
| Murphy [17] | 2004 | IV | $N=23$<br><br>Mean age: 35.4 years<br>Follow-up: 62.4 months | Pincer: 1<br><br>Cam: 10<br><br>Both: 12 | Surgical dislocation | Improvement Merle d'Aubigne | THA: 7 (30.4%)<br>Arthroscopy: 1 (4.3%) |
| Peters [18] | 2006 | IV | $N=29$ (30 hips)<br>M: 16 / F: 13<br>Mean age: 31 years<br>Follow-up: 32 months | Pincer: 1<br>Cam: 14<br>Both: 15 | Surgical dislocation | Improvement Harris Hip Score (70 preop / 87 post-op) | THA: 4 (13.3%) |
| Beaulé [19] | 2007 | IV | $N=34$ (37 hips)<br>M: 18 / F: 16<br>Mean age: 40.5 years<br>Follow-up: 37.2 months | Cam: 34 | Osteochondroplasty | Improvement WOMAC (61.2 preop / 81.4 post-op) | EMO: 9 (24.3%) |
| Bizzini [20] | 2007 | IV | $N=5$<br>M: 5<br>Mean age: 21.4 years<br>Follow-up: 32.4 months | Cam: 5 | Open decompression | Improvement of ROM. Returned to high-performance sports | – |
| Espinosa [21] | 2007 | III | $N=52$ (60 hips)<br>M: 33 / F: 19<br>Mean age: 30 years | Labral lesion | Fixation vs. no fixation | Better result after labral fixation | – |
| Kim [22] | 2007 | IV | $N=43$<br>M: 18 / F: 25<br>Mean age: 40 years<br>Follow-up: 50 months | – | Arthroscopy | Improvement in all ROM-related parameters | – |
| Krueger [23] | 2007 | IV | $N=16$<br>M: 6 / F: 10<br>Mean age: 33.5 years<br>Follow-up: 25 months | Pincer: 10<br>Cam: 5<br>Both: 3 | Arthroscopy | Improvement Merle d'Aubigne (13 preop / 16 post-op) | – |

**Table 7.1**  (continued)

| Author | Year | Evidence level | Series | FAI type | Technique | Outcome | Complication |
|---|---|---|---|---|---|---|---|
| Philippon [24] | 2007 | IV | N=45<br>M: 42 / F: 3<br>Mean age: 31 years<br>Follow-up: 19 months | Pincer: 3<br>Cam: 22<br><br>Both: 21 | Arthroscopy | 35 (78%) patients returned to high-performance sport | Surgical revision 5 (11%) |
| Pierannunzii [25] | 2007 | IV | N=6<br>M: 6 /F: 2<br>Mean age: 30 years<br>Follow-up: 15 months | Pincer: 4<br>Cam: 1<br>Both: 3 | Osteoplasty anterior approach | Improvement Harris Hip Score (74.4 preop / 85.3 post-op) | – |
| Ribas [26] | 2007 | IV | N=32 (35 hips) | – | Anterior approach | Improvement Merle d'Aubigne(13.8 preop / 16.9 post-op) | Neural damage 6 (17.1%) |
| Byrd [27] | 2009 | IV | N=200 (207 hips)<br>M: 138 / F: 62<br>Mean age: 33 years<br>Follow-up: 16 months | Pincer: 44<br>Cam: 163 | Arthroscopy | Improvement Harris Hip Score (20 points at post-op) | THA: 1 (0.5%) |
| Laude [28] | 2009 | IV | N=97 (100 hips)<br>Mean age: 33.4 years<br>Follow-up: 28.6 months | – | Arthroscopically assisted anterior approach | Improvement NAHS (29.1 points at post-op) | 1 neck fracture (1%) |

## FAI Surgery

The authors' interest has focused on analyzing their results, but there is no direct clinical comparison between the different options. Table 7.1 shows the various published studies and briefly describes the baseline characteristics of patients, surgical techniques, and functional outcomes.

Sussman [29] published a comparative cadaver study ($n=8$) on the implementation of the osteoplasty technique via arthroscopy as compared with an open technique. The study showed no statistical differences between the two options, either in terms of the extent or the depth of the resection. The authors concluded that the arthroscopic approach could be a valid alternative to bone resection in the treatment of isolated "cam"-type FAI.

In a cadaver study ($n=15$) aimed at determining the ideal amount of bone that needs to be resected, Mardones [30] concluded that 30% constitutes the largest resection that is possible without compromising the mechanical strength of the femoral neck. According to a paper by Neumann [31], this resection is achieved by achieving a 43° alpha angle, which can be considered "normal." This conclusion comes from a prospective series (level III evidence) comprising 45 patients subjected to FAI treatment and followed for 1 year.

## The Future of Evidence-Based FAI Surgery

As mentioned above, methodology is becoming an increasingly important factor in trying to bring some order to the effort involved in clinical research. The goal is not to "destroy science" but to help build something useful in the absence of noise, confusion, and bias.

Recently published studies raise questions about the most basic aspects of diagnosis. Physical examination should be systematic and conducted by expert personnel [32]; the frog-leg lateral position radiograph may not be valid for measuring the alpha angle [33], with new CT being introduced [34]. Undoubtedly FAI is a pathology that is attracting the interest of many health-care professionals.

In the field of surgery, the challenge is enormous, so surgeons should strive to achieve excellence in the studies they undertake. Once the methodology is right, the next drawback is bound to be the number of patients enrolled in the studies, so the "sharing of patients" between different centers is likely to become the norm, provided that the follow-up period is at least 5 years. These criteria will make it possible to conduct more rigorous studies with more patients in them, but the downside is that more surgeons will be involved, each with their own level of experience. There is no single solution to this dilemma, but an analysis of the literature reveals that there are a large number of publications that lead to no hard-and-fast conclusions, and the surgical community must work proactively to find the "scientific truth." Authors should focus their efforts on using common evaluation criteria to quantify results and make direct comparisons. Likewise, the major challenge that basic science researchers have ahead of them is to determine whether the resolution of the mechanical conflict can halt the normal development of the FAI.

## Conclusions Based on Current Evidence

- FAI is an originally mechanical conflict which, if left untreated, leads to a biological disease.
- MRI, and specially arthro-MRI, is the "gold standard" in the diagnosis of FAI.
- There is no current evidence to support the superiority of any surgical technique over others. The technique selected often depends on the preferences, abilities, and experience of each surgeon.
- The normalization of the 43° angle alpha requires a 30% resection of the femoral neck and should be the aim of all surgeons, regardless of the operative technique used.

## References

1. Guyatt GH (1991) Evidence-based medicine [editorial]. ACP J Club 112(2):16
2. Evidence-Based Medicine Working Group (1992) Evidence-based medicine. A new approach to teaching the practice of medicine. JAMA 268(17):2420–2425
3. PozoRodríguez F (1999) La medicina basada en la Evidencia. Una perspectiva desde la clínica. Medicina Clínica 112(1): 12–16
4. Siebenrock KA, Wahab KH, Werlen S et al (2004) Abnormal extension of the femoral head epiphysis as a cause of cam impingement. Clin Orthop Relat Res 418:54–60
5. Ito K, Minka MA 2nd, Leunig M et al (2001) Femoroacetabular impingement and the cam-effect. A MRI-based quantitative anatomical study of the femoral head-neck offset. J Bone Joint Surg Br 83(2):171–176
6. Wagner S, Hofstetter W, Chiquet M et al (2003) Early osteoarthritic changes of human femoral head cartilage subsequent to femoro-acetabular impingement. Osteoarthritis Cartilage 11(7):508–518
7. Jager M, Wild A, Westhoff B et al (2004) Femoroacetabular impingement caused by a femoral osseous head-neck bump deformity: clinical, radiological, and experimental results. J Orthop Sci 9(3):256–263
8. Clohisy JC, Nunley RM, Otto RJ et al (2007) The frog-leg lateral radiograph accurately visualized hip cam impingement abnormalities. Clin Orthop Relat Res 462:115–121
9. Beaule PE, Zaragoza E, Motamedi K et al (2005) Three-dimensional computed tomography of the hip in the assessment of femoroacetabular impingement. J Orthop Res 23(6): 1286–1292
10. Leunig M, Beck M, Kalhor M et al (2005) Fibrocystic changes at anterosuperior femoral neck: prevalence in hips with femoroacetabular impingement. Radiology 236(1):237–246
11. Leunig M, Podeszwa D, Beck M et al (2004) Magnetic resonance arthrography of labral disorders in hips with dysplasia and impingement. Clin Orthop Relat Res 418:74–80
12. James SL, Ali K, Malara F et al (2006) MRI findings of femoroacetabular impingement. AJR Am J Roentgenol 187(6):1412–1419
13. Pfirrmann CW, Mengiardi B, Dora C et al (2006) Cam and pincer femoroacetabular impingement: characteristic MR arthrographic findings in 50 patients. Radiology 240(3): 778–785
14. Rakhra KS, Sheikh AM, Allen D et al (2009) Comparison of MRI alpha angle measurement planes in femoroacetabular impingement. Clin Orthop Relat Res 467(3):660–665
15. Siebenrock KA, Schoeniger R, Ganz R (2003) Anterior femoro-acetabular impingement due to acetabular retroversion. Treatment with periacetabular osteotomy. J Bone Joint Surg Am 85-A(2):278–286
16. Beck M, Leunig M, Parvizi J et al (2004) Anterior femoro-acetabular impingement: part II. Midterm results of surgical treatment. Clin Orthop Relat Res 418:67–73
17. Murphy S, Tannast M, Kim YJ et al (2004) Debridement of the adult hip for femoroacetabular impingement: indications

and preliminary clinical results. Clin Orthop Relat Res 429: 178–181

18. Peters CL, Erickson JA (2006) Treatment of femoro-acetabular impingement with surgical dislocation and debridement in young adults. J Bone Joint Surg Am 88(8):1735–1741

19. Beaule PE, Le Duff MJ, Zaragoza E (2007) Quality of life following femoral head-neck osteochondroplasty for femoroacetabular impingement. J Bone Joint Surg Am 89(4): 773–779

20. Bizzini M, Notzli HP, Maffiuletti NA (2007) Femoroacetabular impingement in professional ice hockey players: a case series of 5 athletes after open surgical decompression of the hip. Am J Sports Med 35(11):1955–1959

21. Espinosa N, Beck M, Rothenfluh DA et al (2007) Treatment of femoro-acetabular impingement: preliminary results of labral refixation. Surgical technique. J Bone Joint Surg Am 89(Suppl 2 Pt.1):36–53

22. Kim KC, Hwang DS, Lee CH et al (2007) Influence of femoroacetabular impingement on results of hip arthroscopy in patients with early osteoarthritis. Clin Orthop Relat Res 456:128–132

23. Krueger A, Leunig M, Siebenrock KA et al (2007) Hip arthroscopy after previous surgical hip dislocation for femoroacetabular impingement. Arthroscopy 23(12):1285–1289 e1

24. Philippon M, Schenker M, Briggs K et al (2007) Femoroacetabular impingement in 45 professional athletes: associated pathologies and return to sport following arthroscopic decompression. Knee Surg Sports Traumatol Arthrosc 15(7):908–914

25. Pierannunzii L, d'Imporzano M (2007) Treatment of femoroacetabular impingement: a modified resection osteoplasty technique through an anterior approach. Orthopedics 30(2):96–102

26. Ribas M, Marin-Pena OR, Regenbrecht B et al (2007) Hip osteoplasty by an anterior minimally invasive approach for active patients with femoroacetabular impingement. Hip Int 17(2):91–98

27. Byrd JW, Jones KS (2009) Arthroscopic femoroplasty in the management of cam-type femoroacetabular impingement. Clin Orthop Relat Res 467(3):739–746

28. Laude F, Sariali E, Nogier A (2009) Femoroacetabular impingement treatment using arthroscopy and anterior approach. Clin Orthop Relat Res 467(3):747–752

29. Sussmann PS, Ranawat AS, Lipman J et al (2007) Arthroscopic versus open osteoplasty of the head-neck junction: a cadaveric investigation. Arthroscopy 23(12):1257–1264

30. Mardones RM, Gonzalez C, Chen Q et al (2005) Surgical treatment of femoroacetabular impingement: evaluation of the effect of the size of the resection. J Bone Joint Surg Am 87(2):273–279

31. Neumann M, Cui Q, Siebenrock KA et al (2009) Impingement-free hip motion: the 'normal' angle alpha after osteochondroplasty. Clin Orthop Relat Res 467(3):699–703

32. Martin RL, Kelly BT, Leunig M et al (2010) Reliability of clinical diagnosis in intraarticular hip diseases. Knee Surg Sports Traumatol Arthrosc 18(5):685–690

33. Konan S, Rayan F, Haddad FS (2010) Is the frog lateral plain radiograph a reliable predictor of the alpha angle in femoroacetabular impingement? J Bone Joint Surg Br 92(1):47–50

34. Arbabi E, Chegini S, Boulic R et al (2010) Penetration depth method-novel real-time strategy for evaluating femoroacetabular impingement. J Orthop Res 28(7):880–886

# Bone Resection: First Step for Treatment, How Much Is Too Much?

# 8

Rodrigo Mardones and Fernando Nemtala

## Acetabuloplasty (Fig. 8.1)

### Preoperative Planning

A technically correct AP view of the pelvis is paramount for accurate preoperative planning of arthroscopic treatment of the pincer-type impingement. As a general rule, a distance of 3.2 cm in men (and 4.7 cm in women), from the midportion of the sacrococcygeal joint to the upper border of the pubic symphysis, indicates an adequate radiograph [1].

The Wiberg (center-edge) angle should be calculated. The goal is to eliminate acetabular overcoverage (defined as a Wiberg angle > 39° [2]). In case of acetabular dysplasia (defined as a Wiberg angle < 25°), the decision of performing an acetabuloplasty must be revised due to the risk of instability.

It has been defined that no more than 25% of the femoral head should appear uncovered on an anteroposterior view of the pelvis (head extrusion index) [3]. Although no minimal femoral head extrusion index has been defined, we recommend achieving 15 ± 5% of femoral undercoverage.

The areas of focal acetabular overcoverage as seen in presence of acetabular retroversion [4, 5] must also be noted ("crossover sign") and corrected during the procedure.

A simple way of estimating the magnitude of the resection is that a reduction of 2° of acetabular coverage can be expected for every 1 mm of lateral resection.

An easy way to assess the anterior and posterior walls is to remember that in normal conditions, the anterior wall covers the medial third of the femoral head on an AP view and the posterior wall must cover the two medial thirds of the femoral head.

### Access to the Hip Joint and Exposure of the Acetabulum

Although many arthroscopic portals have been described to access the hip joint, the authors use a two-portal technique in which the anterior and anterolateral portals are used only.

The first access is an anterolateral portal 1 cm proximal and 1 cm anterior to the tip of the greater trochanter. The 70° 4-mm arthroscope is employed to visualize the space between the femoral head, acetabular labrum, and the joint capsule (security triangle) for proper placement of an anterior portal. The second portal is marked 1 cm distal and 2–3 cm lateral to the intersection of a line perpendicular to the femoral axis that originates at the anterolateral portal and a line parallel to the femoral axis passing through the anterior superior iliac spine.

The anterior capsulotomy is performed under arthroscopic vision to a length of 1 or 2 cm. The anterolateral capsulotomy is performed employing a banana scalpel to a length of 2 or 3 cm. On occasion, we have extended the capsulotomy joining both portals.

Once the proximal pole of the acetabulum has been recognized, correction of the acetabular coverage can be performed as planned in Step 1.

R. Mardones (✉) • F. Nemtala
Orthopedic Department, Clínica Las Condes,
Santiago de Chele, Chile
e-mail: rmardones@clc.cl

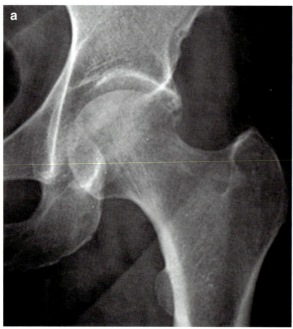
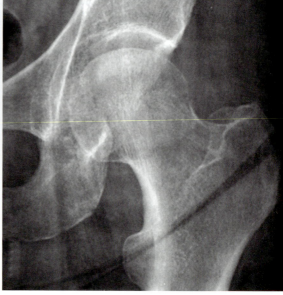

Fig. 8.1 (a) Preoperative radiograph showing pincer-type impingement. Note the acetabular overcoverage of the femoral head. Wiberg angle is 46° and 100% of the femoral head is cov-

ered. (b) Postoperative radiograph showing correction of the acetabular undercoverage. Wiberg angle is 28° and only 80% of the femoral head is covered

If the labrum is to be preserved, it must be detached from the acetabular edge with a banana scalpel. The length of the detachment must be as long as the estimated length of acetabular correction. This area often correlates with the extension of the delaminated cartilage.

If a labrum debridement is decided, it can be performed with the shaver.

In order to gain optimal exposure and perform the subsequent correction, it is very important to adequately visualize the acetabular rim; this can be achieved with the use of the shaver and the radiofrequency instruments.

The trimming can be performed only if there is a perfectly visible bone border.

## Trimming

The trimming is performed with a 5-mm burr. The burr is introduced through the anterior portal for the correction of the anterior wall and through the anterolateral portal for the correction of the posterior wall.

The area of delaminated cartilage is a good landmark for the magnitude of the resection.

Acetabular correction can be monitored with the image intensifier to assess the acetabular coverage and to rule out the presence of the "crossover sign" if acetabular retroversion was diagnosed preoperatively. We also prefer to perform a preoperative template of the amount of resection needed as we normally do in our THR procedures in order to have an idea of how much resection we need to achieve the expected Wiberg angle (30–35°).

It is frequent to observe peripheral chondral defects in the acetabulum; in many cases, these lesions can be resected as a part of the acetabular correction. If they cannot be resected, microfractures can be performed. If applicable, the labrum is reattached.

## Osteoplasty of the Femoral Head–Neck Junction (Fig. 8.2)

### Preoperative Planning

In cam impingement, the goal of the surgical procedure is to restore the anterior femoral neck offset.

The anterior head neck offset is the distance between a line tangential to the femoral head and another line tangential to the femoral neck. Both lines are traced in an axial view of the hip [6].

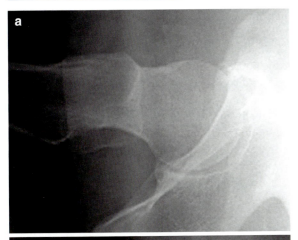

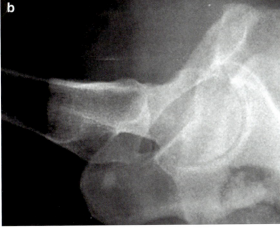

**Fig. 8.2** (**a**) Preoperative radiograph showing cam impingement. Anterior femoral head–neck offset is smaller than posterior offset. (**b**) Postoperative radiograph. Anterior offset has been corrected and mimics posterior offset

Cross-table and Dunn views have been demonstrated to best assess the femoral head–neck asphericity and correlate with MRI [7].

The cross-table lateral view allows measurement of the anterior and posterior femoral neck offset. Normal values for the anterior offset have been described as 11.6 mm ± 0.7 [6].

As described by Notzli et al., the alpha angle depicts the point where an oversized radius appears in the femoral head in an axial view [8]. From that point of view, it can be assumed that the femoral head is ideally spherical under normal conditions. Therefore, the anterior offset should mimic the posterior offset, and thus the anterior/posterior offset ratio should be close to 1.

## The Osteoplasty Itself

The C arm X-ray is positioned to allow an anteroposterior and axial image of the hip, similar to a cross-table view.

Once the traction has been released, the extremity should be flexed 45–50° and abducted 25–30°. The anterolateral head–neck junction is explored, and the extent of the damage is noted as a superficial fibrillar pattern, a notch with an osteophytic margin, or a bump. Articular range of motion is tested, and areas of contact are noted defining the area of resection.

A cross-table view under image intensification is employed to determine the anterior proximal border which matches the curve of the posterior offset of the femoral head. Moving the camera posteriorly and rotating the hip internally, the entrance of the blood vessels to the femoral head may be seen. Regardless to the size of the bump, this must be the posterior limit of the resection to avoid damage to the blood supply.

The femoral osteoplasty is performed with the camera in the anterior portal and the instruments in the anterolateral portal. The extent and shape of the resection are defined by preoperative planning, arthroscopic vision, and fluoroscopic guidance.

The intraoperative cross-table view in neutral rotation (under image intensification) must be comparable to the preoperative view (in conventional radiographs) in which the resection must be calculated initially in order to prevent any bias during the procedure. However, intraoperatively, we perform additional cross-table views in internal and external rotation to make a three dimensional assessment of the deformity based on an overall view (180° minimum) of the femoral head–neck junction.

Since the theoretical normal anterior/posterior offset ratio is 1, this is the ideal goal set for the resection. With the hip in extension, anterior offset is improved using posterior offset as a guideline until ratio between the two appears normal. The anterior and posterior resection areas must be properly assessed by internal, external, and neutral rotation of the extended hip with cross-table views in order to perform an optimal resection. The proximal resection limit can be determined by the AP view, and it usually coincides with the sclerotic line of the physis. When cross-table views in neutral, external, and internal rotations show an anterior offset comparable to the posterior offset in terms of concavity and depth, the surgeon knows that the femoral head–neck

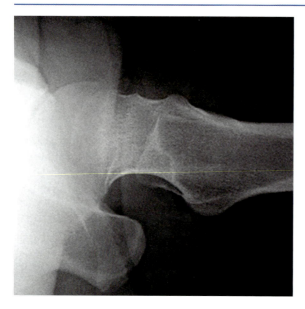

**Fig. 8.3** Postoperative X-ray (cross-table view) after hip arthroscopy

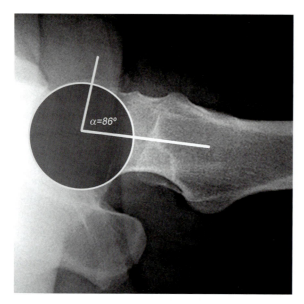

**Fig. 8.4** Undercorrection alpha angle after hip arthroscopy

junction has recovered its asphericity and a normal alpha angle value can be expected (Figs. 8.3 and 8.4).

Mardones et al. published a biomechanical study in which 30% of the femoral head–neck junction diameter was determined as the resection limit beyond which the risk of an iatrogenic fracture increased [9].

Finally, the hip is tested through the complete range of motion, and abnormal contact must be ruled out. Occasionally during flexion, despite the absence of impingement, the resection can be extended distally in order to provide a regular neck margin.

## References

1. Siebenrock KA, Kalbermatten DF, Ganz R (2003) Effect of pelvic inclination on determination of acetabular retroversion: a study on cadaver pelves. Clin Orthop Relat Res 407:241–248
2. Tonnis D, Heinecke A (1999) Acetabular and femoral anteversion: relationship with osteoarthritis of the hip. J Bone Joint Surg Am 81:1747–1770
3. Li PL, Ganz R (2003) Morphologic features of congenital acetabular dysplasia. Clin Orthop Relat Res 416:245–253
4. Siebenrock KA, Schoniger R, Ganz R (2003) Anterior femoroacetabular impingement due to acetabular retroversion and its treatment by periacetabular osteotomy. J Bone Joint Surg Am 85:278–286
5. Reynolds D, Lucac J, Klaue K (1999) Retroversion of the acetabulum: a cause of hip pain. J Bone Joint Surg Br 81:281–288
6. Eijer H, Leunig M, Mahomed N, Ganz R (2001) Cross table lateral radiographs for screening of anterior femoral head-neck offset in patients with femoro-acetabular impingement. Hip Int 11:37–41
7. Meyer DC, Beck M, Ellis T, Ganz R, Leunig M (2006) Comparison of six radiographic projections to assess femoral head-neck asphericity. Clin Orthop Relat Res 445:181–185
8. Notzli H, Wyss T, Stoecklin C, Schmid M, Treiber K, Hodler J (2002) The contour of the femoral head-neck junction as a predictor for the risk of anterior impingement. J Bone Joint Surg Br 84B:556–560
9. Mardones R, Gonzalez C, Chen Q, Zobitz M, Kaufman K, Trousdale R (2005) Surgical treatment of femoroacetabular impingement: evaluation of the effect of the size of the resection. J Bone Joint Surg Am 87:273–279

# Open Surgical Treatment of FAI: Safe Surgical Dislocation of the Femoral Head

**9**

Michael Leunig, Anil Ranawat, Martin Beck, and Reinhold Ganz

## Introduction

Femoroacetabular impingement (FAI) has been proposed as a one of the major causes of osteoarthritis of the hip [2, 10, 11]. Although term such as "head tilt" or "pistol grip" deformities have been introduced previously [5, 14, 28, 31], FAI, as a unique biomechanical process, has only recently been proposed [11]. FAI is a dynamic phenomenon causing chondro-labral damage as a consequence of repetitive hip motion. Impingement results from structural abnormalities including reduced anterolateral femoral head-neck offset, an overcoverage of the anterosuperior acetabular rim or an excessively deep acetabulum. During flexion and internal rotation [8, 11, 29], these abnormalities can produce mechanical impingement of the femoral head against either the acetabular labrum and/or its adjacent cartilage [2, 15, 19, 20, 21, 35, 44]. With time, this repetitive trauma leads to further reduced joint clearance and eventually to early osteoarthritis [3, 10, 24, 30, 42, 43].

M. Leunig (✉)
Orthopädie, Schulthess Klinik,
Zürich, Switzerland
e-mail: michael.leunig@kws.ch

A. Ranawat
Hospital for Special Surgery,
New York, NY, USA

M. Beck
Orthopädie, Kantonsspital Luzern,
Luzern, Switzerland

R. Ganz
Inselspital, University of Bern,
Bern, Switzerland

Based on the osseous deformities present, two distinct types of FAI have been identified, cam and pincer FAI (Fig. 9.1a–d) [11, 16, 17, 18, 37, 38, 39]. These morphological variations are not mutually exclusive. It is common for patients to have combined picture of both cam and pincer FAI [2].

Surgical indications for open treatment of FAI include but are not limited to groin pain and impingement exam findings, impingement osseous abnormalities on imaging, and prearthritic hip disease (Tonnis scale <1). Other indications include large deformities not amenable to arthroscopic treatment and failed arthroscopic treatment. An important factor to consider is the type, magnitude, and location of underlying osseous abnormality. Although arthroscopy is an emerging technique in the treatment of FAI, it is technically challenging and has its limitations. Arthroscopy can easily handle the secondary effects of the morphological abnormality (chondro-labral pathology), while there is as yet no consensus as to how well it can handle the underlying osseous abnormalities [40]. On the other hand, a surgical dislocation provides complete visualization of the acetabular and femoral surfaces, allowing identification of chondral lesions on the labrum surface. In addition, structural morphological changes such as lack of anterior femoral neck offset and acetabular overcoverage can be addressed with relative ease [9, 26, 33, 41]. In addition, failure to address the underlying bony abnormality is likely to lead to continued symptoms, progressive joint degeneration, and poor outcomes [23, 34]. There are relative few contraindications with the open technique such as extensive arthritic changes (Tonnis scale ≥2) and significant acetabular protrusio or dysplasia.

Ó. Marín-Peña (ed.), *Femoroacetabular Impingement*,
DOI 10.1007/978-3-642-22769-1_9, © Springer-Verlag Berlin Heidelberg 2012

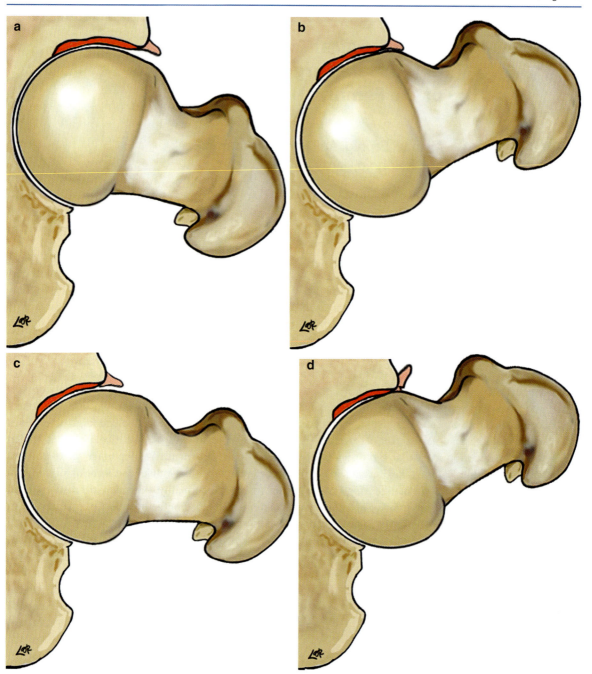

**Fig. 9.1** The two forms of FAI are shown. Cam FAI occurs when the lack of offset on the femoral neck (**a**) leads to mainly anterior damage (*arrow*) through repetitive trauma between the femoral neck and acetabulum during hip flexion (**b**). Pincer FAI occurs secondary to acetabular overcoverage (**c**) causing anterior abutment and subsequent "contrecoup" injury to the cartilage of the posteroinferior acetabulum (*arrows*) during hip flexion (**d**)

## Nonoperative Treatment

The treatment regime should be tailored to the patient. In most cases, conservative treatment is attempted first. These modalities include activity modification, rest, NSAIDs, and most importantly, a physical therapy regimen focusing on abdominal, lower back, and hip flexor strengthening. On occasion, intra-articular injections can be used for both diagnostic and therapeutic purposes. We do not routinely perform intra-articular hip injections, except in selected cases where the origin of a patient's symptoms remains unclear. In many cases, conservative management strategies may only partially alleviate symptoms and often only mask symptoms. Attempts by physical therapists to improve passive range of motion are not often beneficial and may be counterproductive since limitation of internal rotation in FAI is due to abnormal osseous morphology. While some patients can temporarily benefits from these conservative measures, young athletic patients have difficulties to comply with activity modification.

## Background of Surgical Technique

The key to a safe surgical dislocation is an in-depth understanding of the blood supply to the femoral head [12]. Studies dating back more than 40 years [36] as well as a recent cadaveric hips injection study have demonstrated that the medial femoral circumflex artery (MFCA) is the main blood supply to the femoral head [12]. The vessel crosses the obturator externus posteriorly; thereafter, it passes anteriorly to the short external rotators before perforating the joint capsule at the level of superior gemellus. The study also demonstrated that the vessel remained protected even during controlled surgical dislocation, provided that the external rotators and obturator externus remained intact. Unfortunately, the commonly utilized posterior approach requires division of the short external rotators and, doing so, violates the blood supply. As a result of this, a technique allowing a wide operative exposure and a safe surgical dislocation of the femoral head was developed [9]. The general concept of the technique is an anterior dislocation of the femoral head from a postero(lateral) approach. The short external rotators, and thus the MFCA, are left intact, while the joint capsule is exposed anteriorly by a trochanteric flip osteotomy.

## Technique

General or spinal anesthesia is used. The patient is placed in the lateral decubitus positions in well-padded bolsters. Correct orientation is important to allow accurate assessment of acetabular orientation

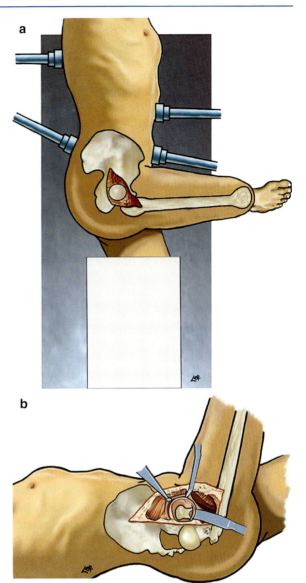

**Fig. 9.2** Lateral decubitus position for surgical hip dislocation (**a**). This technique with exposure of the entire femoral head and acetabulum allows identification and treatment of FAI. In flexion/external rotation, the femoral head can be dislocated allowing nearly circumferential inspection of the entire acetabulum (**b**)

during the procedure. The skin is cleansed with a standard preparation over the trochanteric region. The patient is prepped and draped in standard sterile fashion (Fig. 9.2a) with a free leg sterile bag drape on the opposite side of the operating table to receive the lower leg during hip dislocation (Fig. 9.2b). A second generation cephalosporin antibiotic is given for prophylaxis and continued for 24 h.

A straight lateral incision of approximately 20–25 cm in length is made along the anterior third of the femur which is continued proximal to the trochanteric tip. As a general rule, the more the adipose tissue, the longer the incision required for the trochanteric osteotomy. The fascia lata is incised in line with the incision and extended proximally without any violation of gluteus maximus fibers as described by Gibson [13]. The advantage of this approach is that the gluteus maximus muscle is not split, avoiding damage to the muscle and its anterior neurovascular supply.

The next step is to incise the trochanteric bursa. The innominate tubercle and the border of the vastus lateralis origin are now visible. By careful, superficial exposure of the posterior margin of gluteus medius, the posterocranial tip of the trochanter with the tendinous insertions of the gluteus medius can be seen and palpated. The small trochanteric branch of the MFCA can be identified running anteriorly along the posterior border of the trochanteric crest and should be cauterized. The trochanteric flip osteotomy can now be performed.

Ideally, the osteotomy fragment should provide continuity between the gluteus medius and minimus (specifically the long tendon anteriorly) proximally and the vastus lateralis via the osteotomy fragment distally. Thus, the osteotomy is not a digastric trochanteric osteotomy but actually trigastric in nature [25]. Conversely, the piriformis and short external rotators should remain attached to the nonosteotomized femur (stable trochanter). If done properly, the osteotomy should undercut the tendinous origin of vastus lateralis distally and leave a few remaining gluteus medius fibers proximally at the trochanter. This will increase the certainty that most of the underlying piriformis muscle tendon will remain on the stable trochanter. More recently, a step osteotomy has been used which improves reduction and primary stability of the trochanteric osteotomy.

To expose the posterior border of gluteus medius and trochanter, the limb should be internally rotated 20–30°. The osteotomy is performed with an oscillating saw roughly at an angle parallel to the internally rotated lower extremity. The osteotomy should run from the posterosuperior border of the greater trochanter distally toward the posterior border of the vastus lateralis muscle and remain parallel with the long axis of the femoral shaft. Although the osteotomy was originally described as a single plane cut, we would now recommend the use of a "triplanar" osteotomy to increase the mechanical stability of the osteotomy fragment, especially in older patients who may have compromised bone. The osteotomy consists of two broad chevron-type cuts leaving a step of 5 mm between them. Moreover, the osteotomy should not perforate the anterior cortex of the trochanteric crest, but rather leave it incomplete until an osteotome is used to lever the fragment forward for a controlled fracture. The advantage of this triplanar osteotomy is its increased stability on multiple planes and the relative ease to refix the fragment anatomically at the end of the procedure.

The osteotomy fragment is then mobilized. An 18-mm Hohmann retractor is placed in the osteotomy site, and the fragment is retracted and mobilized anteriorly. The mobile osteotomy fragment is in continuity with the gluteus medius and vastus lateralis. The fibers of the vastus lateralis origin at the posterior femur are gradually released to mid height of the gluteus maximus tendon. The mobile fragment can now be tilted more anteriorly, especially after the anterolateral part of vastus lateralis has been released subperiosteally from the femur with the hip in external rotation, flexion, and abduction. Proximally, the residual tendon insertions of the gluteus medius, still attached to the stable part of the trochanter, are cut. After releasing these fibers, the piriformis tendon becomes visible. Ideally, a portion of the piriformis tendon should be attached to the mobile osteotomy fragment. These residual piriformis fibers on the mobile fragment are then released to further mobilize the osteotomy fragment.

The next step is to develop and expose the hip capsule between the interval of gluteus minimus and the piriformis. The limb is placed in extension and internal rotation. The interval between the gluteus minimus and the posterior capsule is carefully dissected posteriorly down to the acetabular rim. This interval offers the greatest certainty that the blood supply to the femoral head will be preserved. Furthermore, the constant anastomosis between the inferior gluteal artery and the deep branch of the medial circumflex artery is optimally protected. It runs along the lower margin of the piriformis tendon and is of fundamental importance because it alone can guarantee vascularization of the femoral head if there is injury to the deep branch [12]. Finally, the limb is placed in abduction, flexion, and external rotation again; the anterosuperior capsular insertions of the gluteus minimus muscle are then released while preserving the attachment of the long tendon to the mobile fragment. After gradual release of the posterior, superior, and anterior insertions of gluteus minimus from the capsule, the hip capsule is

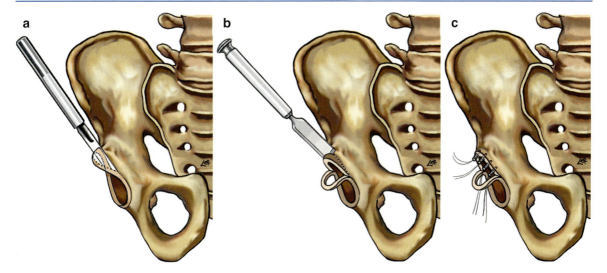

**Fig. 9.3** Resection of excessive anterior rim (**a**) in acetabular retroversion with a curved osteotome (**b**) can be performed after labral detachment as part of the approach to the acetabular rim. After sufficient rim resection, (**c**) labral refixation is performed with bone anchors

completely exposed; however, the short external rotators must always remain protected and attached to the stable trochanter.

With the hip capsule completely exposed, a z-shaped capsulotomy (right hip) is performed. This begins with a linear incision along the line of the femoral neck close to the superior border of the stable trochanter. The capsulotomy then runs posterosuperiorly along the acetabular rim inside out in a proximal direction to avoid injury to the retinaculum, cartilage, and labrum. Finally, an inferomedial extension of the capsulotomy is performed over the front of the anterior capsule in the direction of the lesser trochanter. The labrum and chondral surfaces are also best preserved by an "inside-out" arthrotomy which allows for adequate visualization at all times.

The next critical step is careful dislocation of the femoral head and appropriate positioning of the retractors to visualize the pathology. First, an 8-mm Hohmann hook is hammered into the bone below the capsular margin but above the labrum and holds the soft tissues back at the 12 o'clock position. A Langenbeck hook may also be adequate for this purpose. A bone hook is then placed around the femoral calcar, and hip is gently subluxed with traction, flexion, and external rotation as the limb is prepared to be placed into the sterile leg bag. The ligamentum teres, which is preventing complete dislocation, is then cut with parametrium scissors taking care not to damage the chondral surfaces of the acetabulum or femoral head. On rare occasions, the hip is only subluxed, and all operative work is done in this position. The lower extremity is then dislocated anteriorly and placed in the sterile leg bag. Two additional retractors are placed: one at the anterior acetabular rim and the other inferiorly by the transverse acetabular ligament. A 360° view is now possible of the entire acetabulum. Posterior retractors can also be placed if necessary. Finally, a bump is placed on the femur (slight abduction), and a posterior force is applied to the femur by an assistant for further acetabular visualization.

The hip can now be inspected for evidence of injury secondary to femoroacetabular impingement. Open inspection initially begins with capsulotomy when the amount of synovial effusion and the degree of synovitis are documented. Next, attention turns to the acetabular chondro-labral surfaces. As soon as the cartilage is exposed, it should be protected from drying out with a constant trickle of saline solution. Damage to the acetabular cartilage and labrum is documented. A blunt probe can be used to examine the labrum for detachments or tears; the cartilage must be assessed for softening or delamination. By altering the position of the leg in flexion, all articular surfaces can be visualized and any chondro-labral injuries in both the anterosuperior and posterosuperior regions documented. If labral tears are irreparable, then the labrum is debrided. Likewise, grade four contained chondral lesions are often microfractured.

If pincer impingement is noted preoperatively and confirmed intraoperatively, then acetabular rim trimming is performed (Fig. 9.3). First, the labrum must be

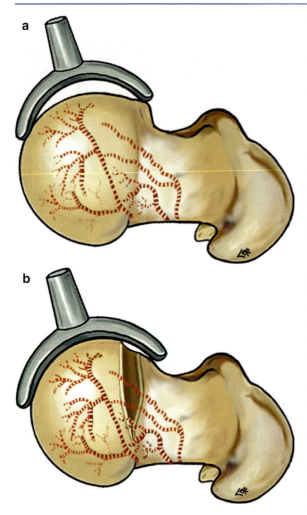

**Fig. 9.4** Resection osteoplasty of the femoral head/neck junction can be used to recreate the normal concave contour of the femoral neck. (**a**) Transparent templates are used to determine femoral head sphericity. (**b**) Femoral osteochondroplasty is performed to repair the insufficient offset

detached from the acetabular rim by sharp dissection. If there is a full-thickness chondral defect, then a microfracture is performed. Since the typical location for acetabular rim lesions is the anterosuperior margin, the excess rim segment can be removed with a curved osteotome. The amount of rim resected depends on the location of the cross-over sign and the value of the lateral center-edge angle seen on the preoperative plain film. Additionally, intraoperative impingement tests are performed to assess the degree of overcoverage causing impingement. Rim excision is performed until no impingement exists but not at the expense of creating instability or dysplasia. Following rim resection, the labrum is reattached by driving two to four small mini

G2 suture anchors (Mitek Surgical Products, Westwood, MA) into a bed of bleeding cancellous bone approximately 5–10 mm apart [6]. At this moment, the sutures are only placed through the labrum; tightening is postponed until the femoral head is repositioned into the socket. This allows a more homogeneous expansion of the labrum over the head contour.

Next, attention turns to the femoral side. The retractors are gently removed, and the knee is lowered; the femoral head can be elevated out of the wound so that there is excellent visualization of the proximal femur. First, the posterosuperior retinaculum and vessels are identified and protected. Next, the sphericity of the femoral head can now be assessed after two blunt retractors are placed under the femoral neck. Nonsphericity is tested using appropriately sized transparent spherical templates. With these templates, a safe resection is predictable and the risk of femoral neck fracture is minimized [22]. The commonest location for this pathology is the anterosuperior head/neck junction, with the abnormal cartilage having a slightly hypervascular, pink appearance. The presence of a cyst near the peripheral border of the non-spherical segment is sometimes noted, which indicates the point of maximum impingement.

The abnormal bone can be removed carefully using curved chisels until a normal head/neck offset is recreated, taking great care not to injure the terminal branches of the MFCA in the posterosuperior retinaculum (Fig. 9.4a). Unfortunately, this area may also be non-spherical, in which case, the debridement should start proximally on the neck and reach the point where the vessels enter their intraosseous course. A periosteal elevator may also be used to strip a portion of the retinaculum off the bone as well. Femoral resection should be done cautiously with regular reassessment using the spherical templates to avoid overresection, which would not only increase the risk of femoral neck fracture (with excessive resection) but also endanger the loss of the labrum's suction seal effect with the femoral head.

Prior to relocation, the ligamentum teres is debrided. Perfusion should be confirmed by bleeding from the fovea and a raw cancellous surface created following neck debridement. Bone wax can be applied to the debrided surface prior to relocation. Hip relocation can be achieved with simple traction and controlled internal rotation, with care not to avulse the labral sutures. Following relocation, the sutures are tightened, and the range of movement is assessed to look for any residual impingement prior to closure.

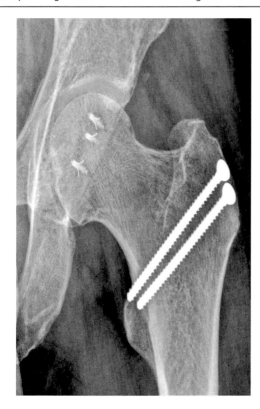

**Fig. 9.5** Postoperative radiograph showing surgical dislocation through a transtrochanteric approach with acetabular rim trimming, labral refixation, and femoral offset correction

Capsular closure is done without excessive tension to avoid compression of the retinacular vessels. The trochanteric fragment is reduced anatomically according to the triplanar osteotomy cuts and reattached using 3.5- or 4.5-mm screws. With the triplanar trochanteric osteotomy, 3.5-mm screws are sufficient. On the other hand, 4.5-mm screws are much easier to remove if they become symptomatic. The fascia lata, fat, and cutaneous layers are carefully closed in a layered fashion. Drains are rarely indicated.

## Postoperative Management and Rehabilitation

A postoperative radiograph is obtained in the recovery room (Fig. 9.5). The patient is usually immobilized postoperatively on crutches with toe-touch weight-bearing for a total 6–8 weeks. The patient is prohibited from hip flexion >70° and from actively abducting the extremity to allow proper healing of the osteotomy site. Continuous passive motion (with flexion limited to 70°) is started on postoperative day number one until discharge in order to prevent formation of intra-articular adhesions. If a microfracture was performed, then continuous passive motion use must be prolonged a total of 6–8 weeks. The patient is usually discharged after 5–7 days. All patients receive low-molecular-weight heparin until full mobilization occurs.

If after 8 weeks, radiographs show evidence of healing of the osteotomy site, then weight-bearing and motion restrictions are lifted. If there is any doubt, then therapy should be postponed for another 3–4 weeks. Full activities are allowed once the patient has regained full motion and strength, which usually requires 3 months.

## Results

A review of the literature and results of open impingement surgery is presented in Table 9.1. To date, there have been approximately eight series with approximately 200 patients [1, 3, 4, 7, 23, 27, 32]. Prognosis generally depends on the extent of articular damage [1, 3, 4, 7, 23, 27, 32]. In other words, the extent of preoperative arthritis is an important predictor of outcome. In addition, labral refixation appears to yield better clinical and radiographic results, while cases with combined impingement and instability have had poorer results.

## Complications

General complications such as infection, blood loss, and venous thrombosis are quite rare. Specific complications to this procedure include iatrogenic osteonecrosis, osteotomy nonunion, symptomatic hardware, under/over correction, and femoral neck fracture.

Although the risk of osteonecrosis exists, in numerous series, no instances have been reported [1, 3, 4, 7, 23, 27, 32]. A thorough understanding of the course of the medial femoral circumflex artery helps prevent this potential complication. Similarly, all these reports mention minimal trochanter fixation problems. If trochanter pseudoarthrosis does develop, then repeat stable osteosynthesis is recommended. With the new triplane osteotomy, trochanter nonunions have been almost eliminated. On the other hand, symptomatic hardware is not infrequent. If present, it takes a small outpatient procedure to

**Table 9.1** Open clinical results of surgical dislocation for FAI

| Paper | Hips | F/U | Impingement type | Other | Complications | Results |
|---|---|---|---|---|---|---|
| Beaule et al. [1] | 37 | | Cam | | No revisions or AVN, 9 ROH | Improvement in WOMAC, UCLA, and SF-12. 6/34 dissatisfied |
| Bizzini et al. [4] | 5 | 2.7 years | Combined | Professional hockey players | None | All retuned to hockey |
| May et al. [23] | 5 | 16.3 months | Cam | After arthroscopic labral debridement | None | Good |
| Peters and Erickson [32] | 30 | 2 years | Combined | Worse results with worse pre-op arthritis | None | 8 hips had progressive DJD. 4 got THA. 2 had staged PAOs |
| Espinosa et al. [7] | 60 | 2 years | Combined | Labral refixation had less arthrosis | None | 80% of labral refixation vs. 28% of labral resection had good/excellent |
| Beck et al. [3] | 19 | 4.7 | Combined | Worse results with worse pre-op arthritis | No AVN | 5 patients THA, while 13 hips rated good/excellent |
| Murphy et al. [27] | 23 | 2–12 years | Combined | Worse results with pre-op arthritis and combined impingement and instability | None | 7 went on to THA, 1 had arthroscopic labral debridement |
| Tanzer et al. [45] | 10 | 26 months | Cam | Technique was not with surgical dislocation but cheilectomy | None reported | HHS improved to 90, no reoperations |

remove the hardware with minimal disability associated with it. Finally, under/over correction are also rare problems that can be eliminated with proper preoperative radiographic assessment in conjunction with carefully performed intraoperative impingement testing. Likewise, femoral neck fractures can be avoided with the use of templates to avoid excessive resections [22].

## Conclusion

Open treatment of femoroacetabular impingement with surgical dislocation provides the surgeon with numerous advantages. First, it is a safe and extensile exposure of the hip joint. Second, a surgical dislocation provides the surgeon with the ability to evaluate all of the pathology under direct visualization. Finally, a surgical dislocation is a versatile procedure since it enables the surgeon to perform numerous impingement procedures from one exposure. Elimination of femoroacetabular impingement significantly improves patients' symptoms, and with further study, chondral disease may be delayed or prevented. At present, the best results are seen in patients with early chondral disease.

## References

1. Le Beaule PE, Duff MJ, Zaragoza E (2007) Quality of life following femoral head-neck osteochondroplasty for femoroacetabular impingement. J Bone Joint Surg Am 89(4): 773–779
2. Beck M, Kalhor M, Leunig M, Ganz R (2005) Hip morphology influences the pattern of damage to the acetabular cartilage: femoroacetabular impingement as a cause of early osteoarthritis of the hip. J Bone Joint Surg Br 87(7): 1012–1018
3. Beck M, Leunig M, Parvizi J, Boutier V, Wyss D, Ganz R (2004) Anterior femoroacetabular impingement: part II.

Midterm results of surgical treatment. Clin Orthop Relat Res (418):67–73

4. Bizzini M, Notzli HP, Maffiuletti NA (2007) Femoroacetabular impingement in professional ice hockey players: a case series of 5 athletes after open surgical decompression of the hip. Am J Sports Med 35(11):1955–1959

5. Eijer H, Myers SR, Ganz R (2001) Anterior femoroacetabular impingement after femoral neck fractures. J Orthop Trauma 15(7):475–481

6. Espinosa N, Beck M, Rothenfluh DA, Ganz R, Leunig M (2007) Treatment of femoro-acetabular impingement: preliminary results of labral refixation. Surgical technique. J Bone Joint Surg Am 89(Suppl 2 Pt.1):36–53

7. Espinosa N, Rothenfluh DA, Beck M, Ganz R, Leunig M (2006) Treatment of femoro-acetabular impingement: preliminary results of labral refixation. J Bone Joint Surg Am 88(5):925–935

8. Ganz R, Bamert P, Hausner P, Isler B, Vrevc F (1991) Cervico-acetabular impingement after femoral neck fracture. Unfallchirurg 94(4):172–175

9. Ganz R, Gill TJ, Gautier E, Ganz K, Krugel N, Berlemann U (2001) Surgical dislocation of the adult hip a technique with full access to the femoral head and acetabulum without the risk of avascular necrosis. J Bone Joint Surg Br 83B(8):1119–1124

10. Ganz R, Leunig M, Leunig-Ganz K, Harris WH (2008) The etiology of osteoarthritis of the hip: an integrated mechanical concept. Clin Orthop Relat Res 466(2):264–272

11. Ganz R, Parvizi J, Beck M, Leunig M, Notzli H, Siebenrock KA (2003) Femoroacetabular impingement: a cause for osteoarthritis of the hip. Clin Orthop Relat Res (417):112–120

12. Gautier E, Ganz K, Krugel N, Gill T, Ganz R (2000) Anatomy of the medial femoral circumflex artery and its surgical implications. J Bone Joint Surg Br 82(5):679–683

13. Gibson A (1950) Posterior exposure of the Hip joint. J Bone Joint Surg Br 32B:183–186

14. Guevara CJ, Pietrobon R, Carothers JT, Olson SA, Vail TP (2006) Comprehensive morphologic evaluation of the hip in patients with symptomatic labral tear. Clin Orthop Relat Res 453:277–285

15. Ito K, Leunig M, Ganz R (2004) Histopathologic features of the acetabular labrum in femoroacetabular impingement. Clin Orthop (429):262–271

16. Ito K, Minka MA 2nd, Leunig M, Werlen S, Ganz R (2001) Femoroacetabular impingement and the cam-effect. A MRI-based quantitative anatomical study of the femoral head-neck offset. J Bone Joint Surg Br 83(2):171–176

17. Kalberer F, Sierra R, Madan S, Ganz R, Leunig M (2008) Ischial spine projection into the pelvis. In: Clin Orthop Relat Res 466(3):677–683

18. Lavigne M, Parvizi J, Beck M, Siebenrock KA, Ganz R, Leunig M (2004) Anterior femoroacetabular impingement: part I. Techniques of joint preserving surgery. Clin Orthop (418):61–66

19. Leunig M, Fraitzl CR, Ganz R (2002) Early damage to the acetabular cartilage in slipped capital femoral epiphysis. Therapeutic consequences. Orthopade 31(9):894–899

20. Leunig M, Podeszwa D, Beck M, Werlen S, Ganz R (2004) Magnetic resonance arthrography of labral disorders in hips with dysplasia and impingement. Clin Orthop Relat Res (418):74–80

21. Locher S, Werlen S, Leunig M, Ganz R (2002) MR-arthrography with radial sequences for visualization of early hip pathology not visible on plain radiographs. Z Orthop Ihre Grenzgeb 140(1):52–57

22. Mardones RM, Gonzalez C, Chen Q, Zobitz M, Kaufman KR, Trousdale RT (2005) Surgical treatment of femoroacetabular impingement: evaluation of the effect of the size of the resection. J Bone Joint Surg Am 87(2):273–279

23. May O, Matar WY, Beaule PE (2007) Treatment of failed arthroscopic acetabular labral debridement by femoral chondro-osteoplasty: a case series of five patients. J Bone Joint Surg Br 89(5):595–598

24. McCarthy JC, Noble PC, Schuck MR, Wright J, Lee J (2001) The Otto E. Aufranc award: the role of labral lesions to development of early degenerative hip disease. Clin Orthop 393:25–37

25. Mercati E, Guary A, Myquel C, Bourgeon A (1972) A postero-external approach to the hip joint. Value of the formation of a digastric muscle. J Chir (Paris) 103(5):499–504

26. Meyer DC, Beck M, Ellis T, Ganz R, Leunig M (2006) Comparison of six radiographic projections to assess femoral head/neck asphericity. Clin Orthop Relat Res 445:181–185

27. Murphy S, Tannast M, Kim Y-J, Buly R, Millis M (2004) Debridement of the adult Hip for femoroacetabular impingement. Clin Orthop Relat Res 429:178–181

28. Murray RO (1965) The aetiology of primary osteoarthritis of the hip. Br J Radiol 38(455):810–824

29. Notzli HP, Wyss TF, Stoecklin CH, Schmid MR, Treiber K, Hodler J (2002) The contour of the femoral head-neck junction as a predictor for the risk of anterior impingement. J Bone Joint Surg Br 84(4):556–560

30. Parvizi J, Leunig M, Ganz R (2007) Femoroacetabular impingement. J Am Acad Orthop Surg 15(9):561–570

31. Pauwels F (1976) Biomechanics of the normal and diseased hip: theoretical foundation, technique and results of treatment. An atlas. Springer, Berlin

32. Peters CL, Erickson JA (2006) Treatment of femoro-acetabular impingement with surgical dislocation and debridement in young adults. J Bone Joint Surg Am 88(8):1735–1741

33. Reynolds D, Lucas J, Klaue K (1999) Retroversion of the acetabulum. A cause of hip pain. J Bone Joint Surg Br 81(2):281–288

34. Robertson WJ, Kadrmas WR, Kelly BT (2007) Arthroscopic management of labral tears in the hip: a systematic review of the literature. Clin Orthop Relat Res 455:88–92

35. Seldes RM, Tan V, Hunt J, Katz M, Winiarsky R, Fitzgerald RH Jr (2001) Anatomy, histologic features, and vascularity of the adult acetabular labrum. Clin Orthop (382): 232–240

36. Sevitt S, Thompson RG (1965) The distribution and anastomoses of arteries supplying the head and neck of the femur. J Bone Joint Surg Br 47:560–573

37. Siebenrock KA, Kalbermatten DF, Ganz R (2003) Effect of pelvic tilt on acetabular retroversion: a study of pelves from cadavers. Clin Orthop Relat Res (407): 241–248

38. Siebenrock KA, Schoeniger R, Ganz R (2003) Anterior femoro-acetabular impingement due to acetabular retroversion. Treatment with periacetabular osteotomy. J Bone Joint Surg Am 85-A(2):278–286

39. Siebenrock KA, Wahab KH, Werlen S, Kalhor M, Leunig M, Ganz R (2004) Abnormal extension of the femoral head epiphysis as a cause of cam impingement. Clin Orthop (418): 54–60

40. Sussmann PS, Ranawat AS, Lipman J, Lorich DG, Padgett DE, Kelly BT (2007) Arthroscopic versus open osteoplasty of the head-neck junction: a cadaveric investigation. Arthroscopy 23(12):1257–1264

41. Tannast M, Siebenrock KA, Anderson SE (2007) Femoroacetabular impingement: radiographic diagnosis – what the radiologist should know. AJR Am J Roentgenol 188(6):1540–1552

42. Tonnis D, Heinecke A (1999) Acetabular and femoral ante-version: relationship with osteoarthritis of the hip. J Bone Joint Surg Am 81(12):1747–1770

43. Wagner S, Hofstetter W, Chiquet M, Mainil-Varlet P, Stauffer E, Ganz R, Siebenrock KA (2003) Early osteoarthritic changes of human femoral head cartilage subsequent to femoro-acetabular impingement. Osteoarthritis Cartilage 11(7):508–518

44. Wenger DE, Kendell KR, Miner MR, Trousdale RT (2004) Acetabular labral tears rarely occur in the absence of bony abnormalities. Clin Orthop Relat Res (426): 145–150

45. Tanzer M , Noiseux N  (2004) Osseous abnormalities and early osteoarthritis: the role of hip impingement. Clin Orthop Relat Res (429):170–177

# Mini-Anterior Approach

Manuel Ribas and Óliver Marín-Peña

Femoroacetabular osteoplasty or osteochondroplasty comprises in the removal of the anatomical abnormalities causing femoroacetabular impingement (FAI) and the repair of labral and retrolabral chondral lesions. Since the beginning of the twenty-first century, different techniques have been proposed to address this condition, which can be classified as follows:

1. Purely arthroscopic technique [1–5]
2. Safe surgical dislocation of the femoral head [6–8]
3. Combined techniques using an anterior approach [9–15]

In the year 2003, we developed a technique for the treatment of patients with symptoms of FAI, with the following characteristics:

1. Intermuscular approach to the hip with full protection of muscular structures.
2. Extensive access to the central and the peripheral compartments.
3. Enhanced accuracy in femoroacetabular reshaping based on preoperative planning.
4. Preservation of blood supply to the femoral head.
5. Interligamentous arthrotomy. The degree of ligament repair will depend on the patient's preoperative status.

6. All of the femoral head–neck junction can be approached by managing extension, flexion, and distraction of the hip. (We shall discuss appropriate management of these maneuvers to optimize hip exposure).
7. It is not necessary to perform a trochanterotomy or a dislocation. As a last resort, a safe dislocation can be obtained by applying traction, hyperextension, and external rotation. Biomechanical function of ligamentum teres is not currently well known; this step is best avoided.
8. The use of an arthroscope can be used if necessary.
9. The postoperative protocol is identical to that used for arthroscopic treatment of FAI.

In our institution, surgical treatment of FAI is performed according a specified protocol, which is expounded in Table 10.1.

## Surgical Technique

This technique is divided into different stages:

## Preoperative Assessment

1. Clinical examination: This includes tests to detect general and specific pathology such as the impingement test, the apprehension test, the log roll test, the Faber test, and the adductor test. Instead of repeating the impingement test upon intraarticular injection of local anesthetic, 2 years ago we decided to introduce the Ribas compression-decompression test, which provides 100% sensitivity of symptomatic FAI patients and 94% specificity of FAI-related

M. Ribas (✉)
Department for Orthopedic Surgery and Traumatology,
USP – Dexeus University Hospital,
Barcelona, Spain
e-mail: mribas.icatme@idexeus.es

Ó. Marín-Peña
Department of Orthopedic and Traumatology,
University Hospital Infanta Leonor (Madrid-Spain),
e-mail: olivermarin@yahoo.es

Ó. Marín-Peña (ed.), *Femoroacetabular Impingement*,
DOI 10.1007/978-3-642-22769-1_10, © Springer-Verlag Berlin Heidelberg 2012

**Table 10.1** Osteoplasty techniques used at the Dexeus University Institute (Barcelona)

| | Alpha angle | FAI type | Bump site | Specific pathology | Sex | BMI |
|---|---|---|---|---|---|---|
| Arthroscopy | <70° | Moderate pincer Cam (bump<6 mm) | Anterior | Overcoverage<5 mm | Indifferent (preferably women) | Better if<25 |
| Anterior MIS | Indifferent often>70° | Indifferent Severe pincer Cam (large bump) | Anterior, anterolateral, posterior (moderate) | Overcoverage≥5 mm Coxa retroversa (associated to dysplasia) | Indifferent (preferably men) | Indifferent |
| Safe dislocation | Indifferent | Indifferent Severe pincer Cam (large bump) | Anterior, anterolateral, posterior (severe) | Coxa profunda Coxa protrusa Posterior labral cysts Sequelae: epiphysiolysis | Indifferent (preferably men) | Indifferent |

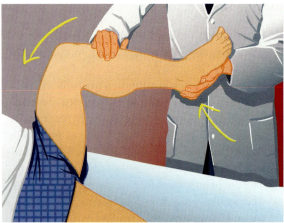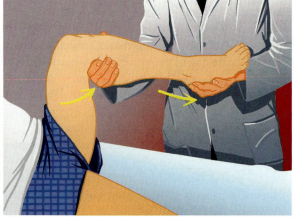

**Fig. 10.1** Compression-decompression test (Ribas test). *Left*: the femoral condyles are compressed as the hip flexed, adduced, and externally rotated to the position where pain is elicited. *Right*: immediate pain relief when the explorer's forearm is placed behind the patient's knee and femoral traction is induced, which induces decompression of the affected hip

labral lesions in the 88 patients we operated on in 2008 (Fig. 10.1).

2. Anteroposterior weight-bearing hip joint views with the feet in a neutral position with 30° external rotation, heels side by side [16–18].
3. Weight-bearing Dunn (45° flexion – 20° abduction – 10° external rotation) and cross-table views (Fig. 10.2) [19]. In pincer-type FAI patients, it is also advisable to carry out a weight-bearing Lequesne-Seze false profile film. With the results of these x-ray examinations, it is possible to classify patients according to the Tönnis scale [20].
4. Gadolinium-enhanced arthro-MRi with radial, coronal, oblique-axial, and sagittal views are useful to identify labral lesions, retrolabral injuries, and areas of damaged cartilage [18, 21, 22]. Cam-type FAI is characterized by a "typical radiological triad": an increased alpha angle

(above 50°), cartilage injury, and injury to the labrum in the anterosuperior acetabulum [23].

5. Measurement of the alpha angle and preoperative consideration of the amount of bone that needs to be resected (in millimeters) based on the above-mentioned radiographic views. This x-ray planning can be compared to the intraoperative arthroscopic findings to enhance correction of any deformities [24, 25].
6. A helical 3D CT-scan is carried out in complex deformities, e.g., posttraumatic injury.

In standard analog x-rays, we use a dedicated template that provides information as to how much bone must be removed and from what areas in order for femoroacetabular reshaping to be successful [26]. These measurements can also be performed with digital radiographs if the appropriate software is available.

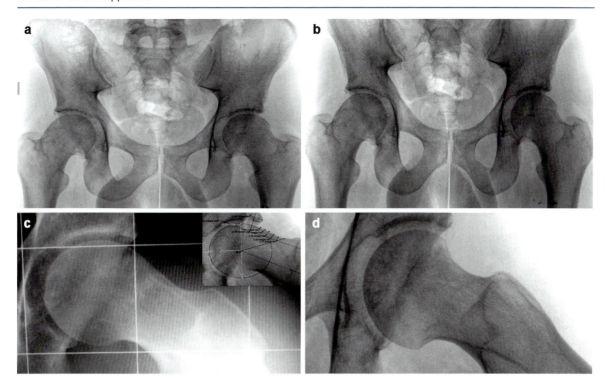

**Fig. 10.2** Superior views: neutral AP view that does not show a head/neck bump (**a**) and 30° external rotation view 1 year post-osteoplasty (**b**). Note that at 30° external rotation, the femoral bump becomes apparent on the right hip; the bump was not vis-ible on the *upper left* view (**b**) following osteoplasty. The lower images are Dunn axial views of the same patient preoperatively (**c**) and 1 year after arthroplasty (**d**)

We use always AP, 30° external rotation, and Dunn's axial views (Fig. 10.2).

## Anesthesia and Positioning

The patient is placed in the supine position on the operating table (Fig. 10.3). Epidural anesthesia is administered with a catheter, which will be left in place during the first 2 days post-op to assist with early mobilization of the hip. We recommend using a multi-mobile traction table to hyperextend the hip and apply capsular distraction. Anyway, it is of paramount importance to move the hip in the three planes of space during the whole procedure (Fig. 10.3).

## Surgical Approach

A 6–8-cm skin incision is performed, starting 1 cm distal and lateral to the anterosuperior iliac spine and directed distally toward the peroneal head (Fig. 10.4).

A fascial incision 1–2 cm behind the first fibers of the tensor fascia latae is recommended to prevent injury to the posterior branch of lateral femorocutaneous nerve.

The fascia is then opened, and the fat interval between the sartorius and tensor fascia lata muscles can easily be palpated. At this point, the surgeon may optionally flex the hip to 30°. The lateral circumflex artery lies medially at the inferior edge of the incision. Sometimes ligation or coagulation of the artery is necessary. Following blunt dissection, detachment of the reflected portion of rectus femoris muscle is performed to allow a wide exposure of the hip capsule. Subsequently, two retroverted curved blunt Hohmann retractors are introduced (Fig. 10.4), one over the upper part of the capsule and one around iliac wing. After careful dissection, an additional Hohmann retractor for large fragments is placed under the femoral neck to extend hip exposure until the iliofemoral muscle. An "I" shaped capsulotomy is performed from distal to cranial through the interval between both iliofemoral ligaments. At this point, it is advisable to place a pair of curved dissection forceps to pull up the capsule crani-

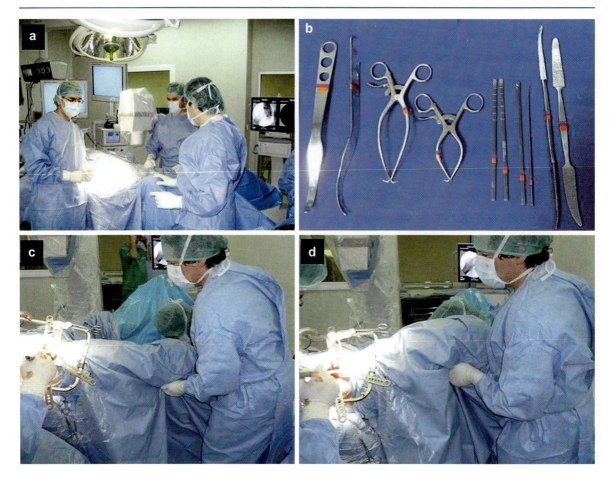

**Fig. 10.3** The patient must be positioned on an extension table that affords full control of hip movement, in accordance with the "rules of space"

ally while it is being incised to avoid any labral damage. Reference sutures are placed at both sides of the capsule. At this point, the curved blunt curved Hohmann retractors can be intraarticularly repositioned on both sides of the femoral neck.

## FAI Inspection

We recommend starting with the acetabular side and then inspect the femoral side (Figs. 10.5 and 10.6). At this stage, an additional light source can be used or even fixed to one of the retroverted Hohmann retractors. Chondral and labral acetabular lesions are inspected as the FAI-inducing movement is recreated. Application of traction in a mini-anterior procedure produces a good joint space that allows accurate assessment of acetabular deformity. This is normally easier with a 30° scope, although a 70°

one could also be used. On the femoral side, lesions were easily identified as the pathologic cartilage that covers the bone bump had a darker appearance than the normal cartilage due to inflammatory changes. At this point, the mechanism causing the impingement can be clearly tested because of the free hip motion provided by this approach (Figs. 10.6 and 10.7).

## The "Rule of Spaces" in Femoroacetabular Osteoplasty

Our principle, called the "rule of spaces," is applicable not only to mini-open procedures but also to arthroscopic management (Fig. 10.7). It provides a comprehensive approach to the femoral head–neck junction and to the anterior and posterior acetabular rim, which is especially useful in cases of coxa pro-

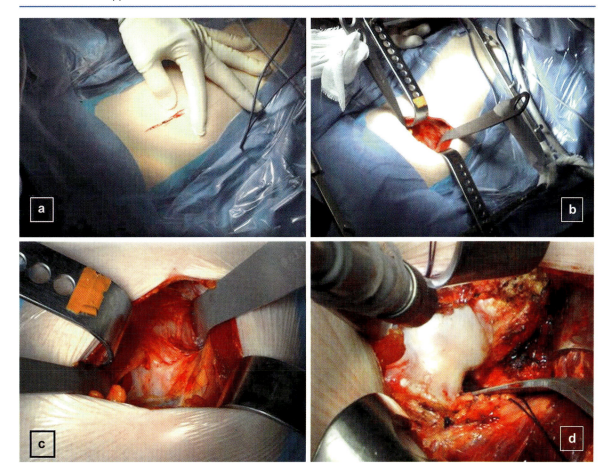

**Fig. 10.4** The incision begins 1 cm inferiorly and laterally to the ASIS and extends 6–8 cm distally and 2 cm more laterally than the medial-most fibers of the tensor fascia latae. This makes it possible to avoid the posterior branch of the femorocutaneous nerve. The lower figures demonstrate capsuloligamentous exposure and direct view of the femoroacetabular impingement through an open capsule

funda. To gain adequate access to the posterior rim or the posterosuperior head–neck junction, the hip needs to be approached firstly by detaching the capsule posteriorly and secondly by applying hyperextension, adduction, and internal rotation of the hip. Once this space has been addressed and reshaped, sufficient clearance of the hip is achieved to apply gradual flexion-abduction and external rotation to allow good visualization of the central area of the bump and reach the posterointerior area of the head–neck junction or even the inferior acetabular wall.

This principle is of paramount importance to perform the osteoplasties by means of this approach and even through arthroscopy. If this rule is not strictly followed, many femoral (generally anterolateral) prominences and cases of FAI-inducing coxa profunda cannot completely be reshaped.

## Osteoplasty

Taking into account the "rule of spaces" above, a fluoroscope is used to take AP and Dunn views of the hip (Figs. 10.5–10.7). Intraoperative landmarks are identified according to the preoperative measurements. Calibrated osteotomes are introduced into the bone under fluoroscopic guidance until the templated depth reached both on the femoral and the acetabular side. In cam-type impingement, the femoral bump is excised with ultra-sharp curved osteotomes, and round burrs were used counterclockwise to avoid excessive bone penetration. In pincer-type impingement, the labrum is detached partially at 45° inclination, according to the preoperative plan and intraarticular findings. Once acetabular trimming is completed, the labrum is reattached with 3.1-mm resorbable anchors fixed to the

**Fig. 10.5** (**a**) Arthroscopic examination following hip traction. (**b**) Classical delamination. (**c**) Classical outside-in reshaping. (**d**, **e**) Microfractures according to Steadman's technique. (**f–h**) Labral reattachment with bioresorbable suture anchors placed at a distance of 1 cm from one another

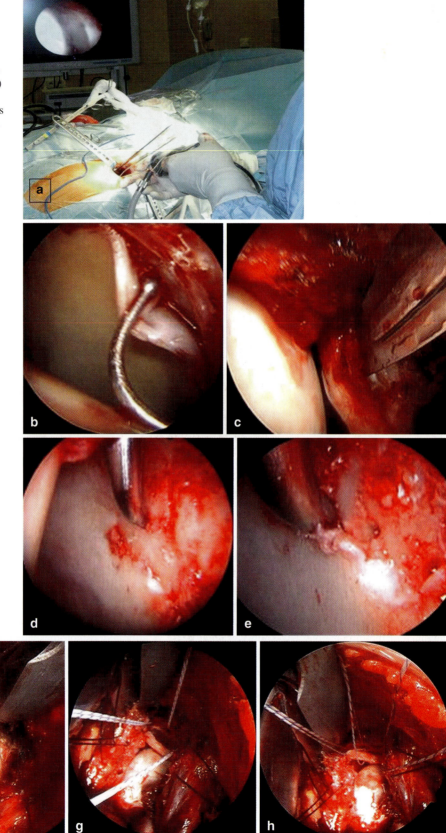

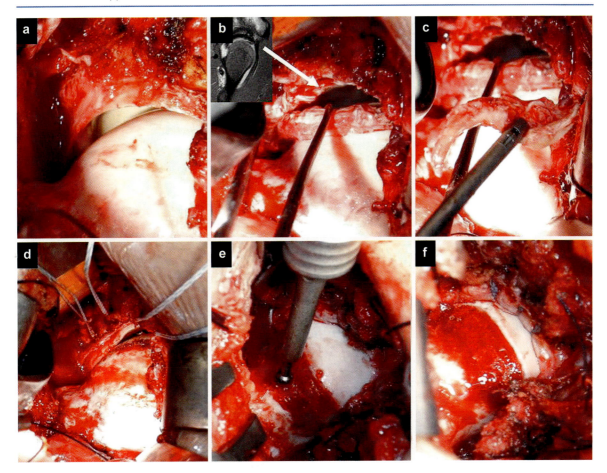

**Fig. 10.6** (**a–d**) Chondrolabral delamination with resection of the injured fragment. (**e, f**) Prior labral reattachment and release of traction. Osteoplastic remodeling

acetabular rim (Figs. 10.5 and 10.6). Pulse lavage is used during all procedures to avoid heterotopic ossification. A final fluoroscopic view is performed after bone resection is completed. Subsequently, femoroacetabular clearance is checked. The procedure normally results in increased range of motion, especially in terms of flexion and internal rotation (Fig. 10.8). Finally, a diamond burr is used over the femoral osteoplasty to obtain hemostasis. Autologous fibrin spray is applied to seal the interface. We do not recommend use of bone wax due to it could induce osteomyelitis or granuloma.

## Closure

We only leave a drain in place when the reshaped head–neck junction bleeds excessively. Soft tissue planes are sutured in full extension of the hip to avoid capsular retraction. At this point, reference sutures are very useful. Special care is taken not to impinge on the posterior branch of lateral femorocutaneous nerve branches during fascial closure. Resorbable 4/0 intradermal suture is used for skin.

## Postoperative Care

An indomethacin protocol is used to prevent heterotopic ossification. Gastroprotective drugs and tlow-molecular-weight heparin are also administrated according to the hip surgery protocol. Drains (if used) and the epidural catheter are removed the first day post-op, immediately after the patient has completed his/her first day of rehabilitation. Later on, patients are trained to walk with crutches with a non-weight-bearing

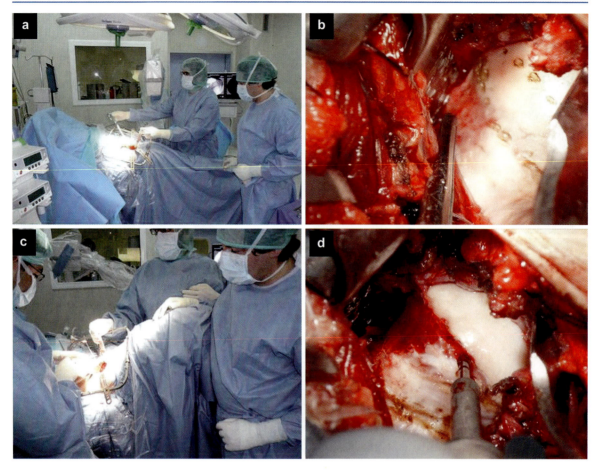

**Fig. 10.7** Rule of the spaces. (**a**, **b**) The posterosuperior space of the head-neck junction and the posterior acetabular rim are approached by application of hyperextension, adduction and internal rotation. Note the synovial flap that contains the reti-nacular vessels. (**c**, **d**) Following posterosuperior reshaping, progressive flexion-abduction-external rotation is applied in order to address the central area and the posteroinferior space of the femoral head-neck junction

restriction for 10 days. When microfractures are performed (for severe chondral lesions), crutches must be used for at least 4 weeks.

## Rehabilitation Program

Immediate passive motion is indicated without any rotational restriction. Active motion is introduced according to patient's tolerance, but in cases of labral reattachment, hip flexion restriction of 90° is recommended for 6 weeks to protect the sutures and the cancellous reshaping osteoplasty. Quadriceps and gluteus isometric exercises and electrostimulation are performed from post-op day one. Closed-chain exercises, including cycling and crawl swimming, are gradually introduced after 3 weeks. Patients are allowed to

resume low-impact sports after 8 weeks, depending on the result as seen on Dunn's views. At this time, a clearly defined line at the new head–neck junction can be observed as sign of corticalization. High-impact sports are only allowed after 12 weeks (see chapter 25 of postoperative rehabilitation in arthroscopic FAI treatment).

**Technical Remarks**
1. If the preoperative impingement test is positive at 90°, a distal bump prevails, whereas if it is positive at 40–50° of flexion, combined FAI, a larger bump, or even both situations may be suspected.

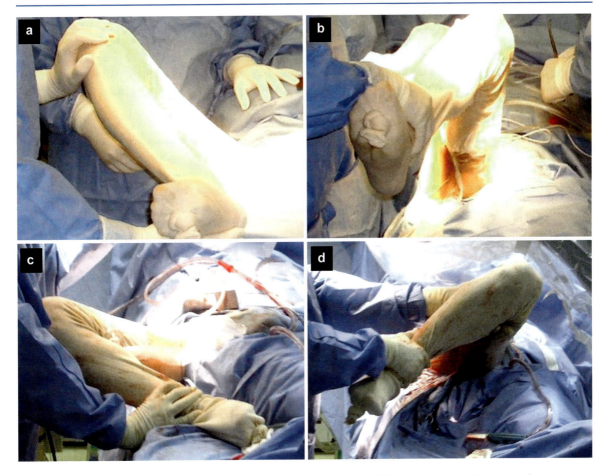

**Fig. 10.8** (**a**, **b**) Preoperative rotational range of motion. (**c**, **d**) Range of motion following femoroacetabular osteoplasty

2. The most common error, especially in arthroscopy, is not to promote the required remodeling in the distal portion of the femoral head–neck interface. This induces undercorrection and leaves a bump deformity above the posterosuperior retinacular vessels. This can be addressed by the mini-invasive technique presented here, with or without arthroscopy.

3. After 30 s of burr-induced remodeling, we recommend use of burrs, pulse lavage, and aspiration to avoid leaving remnants of bone chips in the surgical field. On the other hand, it is advisable not to encroach on the intermuscular aponeurosis during dissection. These surgical details have decreased heterotopic ossification rate below 1% in our series.

From 2003 to the present, more than 400 patients have undergone femoroacetabular osteoplasty in our institution by means of a mini-anterior procedure. The mean follow-up of this series was 3.7 years (3–6, 5 years). Eighty-seven hips corresponded to male patients (ten of them were bilateral), and 28 to females. The average age of patients was 37.1 years (range: 14–57 years). Twenty-four hips were pincer type, 36 cam type, and 57 combined. Injuries in 76 patients (64.9%) were related to sports, either recreational or competitive. The remaining patients (35.1%) only performed occasional physical activity. However, in the latter group, all of those occasional activities required prolonged sitting. Mean operating time was 116 min (range: 65–195). In cases where drainage was used, mean drained blood was 157 cm$^3$ (range: 55–320 cm$^3$), mean hospital stay was 2.6 days (range: 2–4 days), and mean rehabilitation time was 5.4 weeks (range 3–11 weeks). Since 2007, we have sealed the femoral osteoplasty surface by means of autologous fibrine spray so that no drainage is necessary locally. In 12 cases, additional surgical techniques were associated such as percutaneous adductor tenotomies (12 cases) and iliotibial band z-plasties at the level of greater trochanter to address concomitant coxa saltans (three cases). Fifty-nine labra were reanchored, seven partially were remodeled, and four calcified labra were resected. We nowadays use labrum grafts for these cases. In two cases, an additional periacetabular osteotomy was performed.

Radiologically, a well-defined radiodense line was observed in all cases at the femoral head–neck junction between 3 and 6 months post-op on an axial view, indicative of new cortical bone formation (Fig. 10.2).

Complications: There were two cases of hematoma, one of them was punctured, the other one requiring surgical debridement. In 37 cases (31.2%), the surgical scar was hypertrophic. It is important for female patients to be informed about the risk of hematoma preoperatively. In 12 cases (10.2%), patients had local dysesthesias in the area of the lateral femorocutaneous nerve, which disappeared within the first year. The dysesthesias could be attributed to application of lateral distraction on both sides by the bone retractors attached to a square frame. In this series, there was no instance of either necrosis or bone infection. In one case, a small Brooker type I calcification was seen at the anterosuperior portion of the head–neck junction, which did not correlate with any unsatisfactory result. The Merle D'Aubigne (MDA) score improved from 15.8 before surgery to 17.5 one year post-op ($p < 0.001$).

## Conclusions

It seems clear that after 3 years, the majority of patients improved in terms of their symptoms and clinical-functional results. Special mention should be made of prearthritic patients, that is to say, patients with Tonnis grades 0 and 1. Therefore, this study reinforces the findings of other published studies with fewer cases [27]. This applies specifically to patients with incipient stages of degeneration (Tönnis grades 0 and 1). Thus, we can say that osteoplasty is effective to address hip osteoarthritis only if mild radiological changes are present [28].

For this reason, we need to establish a model to detect symptomatic FAI patients, first by providing guidance to other healthcare professionals like general practitioners, rheumatologists, sport physicians, physiotherapists, and secondly by including the impingement test in our regular medical examinations.

In terms of technique, Sadri et al. published a comparative study of patients treated by arthroscopic and open surgery. In this study, neither of the two groups showed any significant differences in terms of their clinical-functional outcomes on the HSS and WOMAC scoring systems after 2 years' follow-up [29].

Another factor that needs consideration when safe dislocation is used is not only the potential morbidity associated with trochanterotomy but also the current lack of knowledge about the real role of the ligamentum teres in hip biomechanics.

In addition, we have stated that in terms of postoperative evolution, there is not much difference between patients treated with a mini-anterior approach and those treated with arthroscopy in our institution. Although patients in the mini-anterior group had more severe lesions, they were operated with open surgery to comply with the surgical protocol (see Table 10.1).

On the other hand, we might wonder whether patients with radiological signs compatible with asymptomatic FAI should be operated prophylactically. To date, there are no studies in the literature providing evidence that all patients with characteristic signs of FAI will suffer from clinical symptoms. Therefore, the data available so far do not warrant performance of preventive surgery. However, the authors do believe that in light of their results, it is advisable to treat symptomatic patients surgically [28].

Actually, we don't know how long can we delay hip osteoarthritis with the arthroscopic osteoplasty, safe dislocation or a mini-anterior approach. We do believe that surgeons who only treat FAI patients arthroscopically should be trained in technical aspects of the mini-anterior approach. In our opinion, it is necessary for the surgeon to know how to approach a hip in a mini-invasive intermuscular way, which will not change postoperative management. In addition, with arthroscopic osteoplasty, it is sometimes impossible to determine whether the bump deformity was fully resected. In addition, other pitfalls need to be considered such as hardware breakage inside the hip. In all these cases, a mini-anterior approach technique is extremely helpful.

# References

1. Philippon MJ, Schenker ML (2006) Arthroscopy for the treatment of femoroacetabular impingement in the athlete. Clin Sports Med 25:299–308
2. Sampson TG (2006) Arthroscopic treatment of femoroacetabular impingement: a proposed technique with clinical experience. Instr Course Lect 55:337–346
3. Sampson T (2005) Arthroscopic treatment of femoroacetabular impingement. Tech Orthop 20:56–62
4. Byrd JW (2006) Hip arthroscopy: surgical indications. Arthroscopy 22(12):1257–1259
5. Crawford JR, Villar RN (2005) Current concepts in the management of femoroacetabular impingement. J Bone Joint Surg Br 87(11):1459–1462 Review
6. Ganz R, Gill TJ, Gautier E, Ganz K, Krügel N, Berlemann U (2001) Surgical dislocation of the adult hip: a technique with full access to femoral head and acetabulum without the risk of avascular necrosis. J Bone Joint Surg Br 83:1119–1124
7. Lavigne M, Parvizi J, Beck M, Siebenrock KA, Ganz R (2004) Anterior femoroacetabular impingement. Part I. Techniques of joint preserving surgery. Clin Orthop 418:61–66
8. Murphy S, Tannast M, Kim YJ, Buly R, Millis MB (2004) Debridement of the adult hip for femoroacetabular impingement: indications and preliminary clinical results. Clin Orthop Relat Res (429):178–181
9. Ribas M, Vilarrubias JM, Ginebreda I, Silberberg J, Leal J (2005) Atrapamiento o choque femoroacetabular. Rev Ortop Traumatol 49:390–403
10. Ribas M, Marín-Peña O, Regenbrecht B, De la Torre B, Vilarrubias JM (2007) Femoroacetabular osteochondroplasty by means of an anterior minimally invasive approach. Hip Int 2:91–98
11. Ribas M, Regenbrecht B, Vilarrubias JM, Wenda K (2006) Femurazetabuläres Impingement: Konzept und chirurgische Behandlung durch ein minimalinvasives Verfahren. Orthop Prax 42(7):484–490
12. Ribas M, Mercede M, Vilarrubias JM, Sadile F (2006) Impingement femoro-acetabolare: concetto e trattamento con nuova tecnica chirurgica mini-invasiva. G Ital Ortop Traum 32:168–173
13. Parvizi J, Leunig M, Ganz R (2007) Femoroacetabular impingement. J Am Acad Orthop Surg 15(9):561–570
14. Clohissy JC, MacClure JT (2005) Treatment of anterior femoroacetabular impingement with combined hip arthroscopy and limited anterior decompression. Iowa Orthop J 25:164
15. Laude F, Boyer T, Nogier A (2007) Anterior femoroacetabular impingement. Joint Bone Spine 74(2):127–132
16. Reynolds D, Lucas J, Klaue K (1999) Retroversion of the acetabulum: a cause of hip pain. J Bone Joint Surg Br 81:281–288
17. Siebenrock KA, Kalbermatten DF, Ganz R (2003) Effect of pelvic inclination on determination of acetabular retroversion. A study on cadaver pelves. Clin Orthop 407:241–248
18. Beall DP, Sweet CF, Martin HD et al (2005) Imaging findings of femoroacetabular impingement syndrome. Skeletal Radiol 34:691–701
19. Harris WH (1986) Etiology of osteoarthritis of the hip. Clin Orthop 213:20–33
20. Tönnis D (1976) Normal values of the hip joint for the evaluation of x-rays in children and adults. Clin Orthop 119:39–47
21. Ito K, Minka MA, Leunig M, Werlen S, Ganz R (2001) Femoroacetabular impingement and the cam-effect: a MRI-based quantitative anatomical study of the femoral head-neck offset. J Bone Joint Surg Br 83:171–176
22. Leunig M, Podeszwa D, Beck M, Werlen S, Ganz R (2004) Magnetic resonance arthrography of labral disorders in hips with dysplasia and impingement. Clin Orthop 418:74–80
23. Kassarjian A (2005) Triad of MR arthrographic findings in patients with cam-type femoroacetabular impingement. Radiology 236(2):588–592
24. Meyer DC, Beck M, Ellis T, Ganz R, Leunig M (2006) Comparison of six radiographic projections to assess femoral head/neck asphericity. Clin Orthop Rel Res 445:181–185
25. Notzli HP, Wyss TF, Stoecklin CH, Schmid MR, Treiber K, Hodler J (2002) The contour of the femoral head-neck junction as a predictor for the risk of anterior impingement. J Bone Joint Surg Br 84:556–560
26. Marin-Peña O, Ribas-Fernandez M, Valles-Purroy A, Gomez-Martin A (2007) Metodo de valoración intraoperatoria de la resección ósea en el choque femoroacetabular. Rev Ortop Traumatol 51(Suppl 2):57
27. Beaulé PE, Le Duff MJ, Zaragoza E (2007) Quality of life following femoral head-neck osteochondroplasty for femoroacetabular impingement. J Bone Joint Surg Am 89:773–779
28. Ribas-Fernández M, Marin-Peña O, Ledesma R, Vilarrubias JM (2007) Estudio de los primeros 100 casos mediante abordaje mini-anterior. Rev Ortop Traumatol 51(Suppl 2):57
29. Graus E, Sadri H, Menetrey J, Hoffmeyer P (2008) Therapie des femoroazetabulären Impingements: Artroskopische Technik versus Chirurgische Luxation. Vortrag Nr. 52 bei der 56. Jahrestagung der Vereinigung Süddeutscher Orthopäden. e.V. 1 bis 4 Mai 2008 in Baden – Baden. Aceptado para su publicación en JBJS-Br

# Arthroscopic Treatment of FAI: Position, Portals, and Instrumentation

**11**

Victor M. Ilizaliturri

## Introduction

The anatomical conditions of the hip joint and the technical complexity of hip arthroscopy contribute to a steep learning curve and make for a time-consuming procedure. The late 1990s and the present decade have witnessed the development of most of the significant technical advances that have contributed to making hip arthroscopy a safe and reproducible procedure [1–3].

The most important part of hip arthroscopy after adequate patient selection is access. Access in hip arthroscopy is determined by patient positioning and portal placement. Both conditions are fundamental and must be clearly understood and adequately performed [4].

The treatment of femoroacetabular impingement (FAI) was introduced to the world of hip arthroscopy by Thomas Sampson [5], who adapted technical steps from the open decompression technique for cam-type deformities [6] to hip arthroscopy techniques. The arthroscopic technique for management of pincer-type deformities was introduced by Marc Philippon [7].

Today there is some difference between authors as regards patient positioning and the placement of arthroscopic portals for the treatment of FAI. Common features of the surgical techniques used for arthroscopic management of FAI include the use of traction to access the central compartment of the hip, where pincer-type deformities and intra-articular pathology are treated; traction release and flexion of the hip to access the hip periphery (essential for the treatment of cam-type deformities); and a combination of anterior hip capsulotomy and capsulectomy to expose both the pincer- and cam-type FAI deformities [8].

In what follows, we present some key aspects of the technique we use for patient positioning and portal placement in the arthroscopic treatment of FAI.

## Patient Positioning

Patient positioning is the first step to success in hip arthroscopy. Poor patient positioning will result in inadequate distraction with poor access to the central compartment or inadequate hip mobilization limiting access to the hip periphery [9]. Accessing the hip periphery is fundamental in the treatment of femoroacetabular impingement deformities.

In general, there are two different positioning methods for hip arthroscopy: supine and lateral. There is slight variation between authors regarding these two methods.

Modern hip arthroscopy requires dynamic patient positioning. The surgeon must be capable of applying and releasing traction intraoperatively and mobilizing the hip joint to different degrees of flexion and rotation.

V.M. Ilizaliturri
Department of Adult Hip and Knee Reconstruction,
Universidad Nacional Autónoma de México,
National Rehabilitation Institute of Mexico,
Mexico City, Mexico
e-mail: vichip2002@yahoo.com.mx

Ó. Marín-Peña (ed.), *Femoroacetabular Impingement*,
DOI 10.1007/978-3-642-22769-1_11, © Springer-Verlag Berlin Heidelberg 2012

**Fig. 11.1** This photograph demonstrates supine positioning for hip arthroscopy. A model is resting supine on a fracture table. Both feet are fixed to holding devices to stabilize the pelvis. In this case, the "operative side" is the right hip; an oversized extra-padded perineal post has been installed medially to the right thigh. This provides lateralization of the tensile force, which results in traction being exerted more in the direction of the femoral neck than in the direction of the femoral shaft. The C-arm is positioned distally between the legs and placed over the right hip providing an anteroposterior view

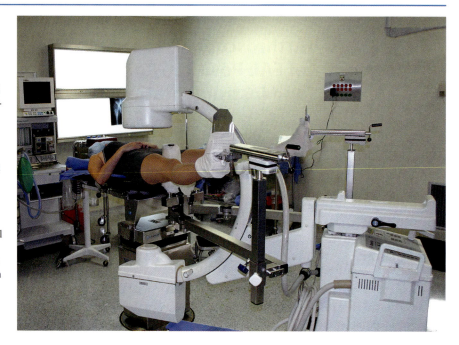

## The Supine Position

Even though dedicated distractors for hip arthroscopy in the supine position exist, fracture tables are more popular because they are within the reach of most hospitals. Thomas Byrd has developed modern supine positioning techniques for hip arthroscopy [10].

In the case of the supine position, both feet are fixed to holding devices to avoid pelvic tilt when traction is applied to the operative side. An oversized extra-padded perineal post (minimum 10 cm in diameter) is vertically attached to the fracture table and rests against the groin of the operative side providing a lateralizing vector to the traction force. The resulting direction of the traction is not applied following the femur shaft but closer to the direction of the femoral neck. The image intensifier is placed between the legs, with the C-arm in a vertical position aiming at the operative side, thereby providing an anteroposterior view of the hip (Fig. 11.1).

## The Lateral Position

The lateral position for hip arthroscopy was originally introduced by Glick and Sampson [11]. The main difference with the supine position is that the patient is positioned in lateral decubitus on the operating table with the operative side upward. Only the foot of the operative side is fixed to the traction device, and pelvic tilt is avoided by the patient's body weight, the length of the nonoperative side leg lying freely on the operating table. A horizontal extra-padded oversized perineal post is positioned on the operative side groin. The post provides lateralization of the tensile forces, which results in traction that is more in line with the femoral neck, as is the case with the supine position. The C-arm is positioned horizontally under the operating table to provide an anteroposterior view of the hip (operative side). In large patients, the arch of the C-arm may not be big enough to reach the area of the hip joint from under the table; if that is the case, the C-arm can be positioned over the table focusing on the area of the hip joint with the arch tilted over the patient's head. Special operating table accessories are required to position a patient in lateral decubitus for hip arthroscopy on a fracture table (Fig. 11.2). As these accessories are often unavailable, the lateral approach has lost favor to the supine approach. More recently dedicated distractors for lateral approach hip arthroscopy have been developed (McCarthy-type distractor, Inomed, GA; Smith and Nephew lateral distractor, Smith and Nephew Endoscopy, Andover, MA). These may contribute to making the lateral position more accessible to surgeons especially to those working in OR set-up in the classical way.

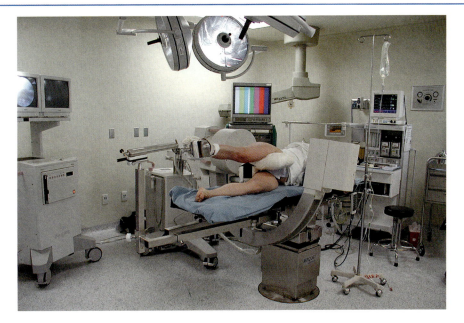

**Fig. 11.2** This photograph demonstrates the lateral decubitus position for hip arthroscopy on a fracture table. The right hip is the operative side. The patient is lying on her left side; only the right foot is fixed to the traction device. An oversized extra-padded perineal post is positioned horizontally against the medial thigh. Raising the perineal post (*black arrow*) provides a lateralization vector for the traction force as is the case of the supine position. The C-arm is positioned horizontally under the operating table to provide an anteroposterior image of the operative hip. The screens are behind the patient because the surgeon stands in the front. The arthroscopy monitor is positioned as far as possible on the head end of the room to allow the assistant standing in front of the surgeon an appropriate view. The fluoroscopy screens are positioned far to the feet end of the room for the same reason

Both surgical positions have been successfully used in the arthroscopic treatment of femoroacetabular impingement [5, 7, 12–14]. The choice of the surgical position depends on the surgeon's preference and experience.

Because our experience is based on the lateral position, the latter is used as an example for the present chapter. The same techniques can be performed using supine patient positioning.

We position the patient laterally, resting on the non-operative side on a fracture table either with special accessories or on a dedicated hip distractor. A perineal post of at least 10 cm in diameter is attached to the table in a horizontal configuration. The perineal post is positioned laterally on the medial thigh and is elevated to provide a lateralization vector to the traction force. The lateralization also distances the post from the pudendal nerve preventing direct compression during surgery. The operative side foot is fixed to the traction device. The nonoperative lower limb rests free on the table. Before traction is applied, the patient's genitalia should be inspected to verify that they are free from compression.

The hip is positioned at 20° flexion to relax the anterior hip capsule. Flexion of more than 20° does not improve distraction of the hip joint and increases the possibility of injury to the sciatic nerve. Abduction is kept neutral to maximize separation of the iliofemoral joint. Neutral rotation is preferred while establishing arthroscopic portals to maximize the distance between the posterior edge of the greater trochanter and the sciatic nerve [15] (Fig. 11.3a, b).

The C-arm is positioned horizontally under the table to provide an anteroposterior fluoroscopic view of the hip. A traction test is always performed before preparing and draping the patient to confirm effective separation of the femoral head from the acetabulum at the image intensifier. This separation should be of at least 10 mm [16]. When separation does not occur, foot fixation should be verified. Inadequate foot fixation to the traction device is the most common cause of ineffective traction. The foot must be firmly fixed to the traction device and well padded to avoid compression injuries. There are different options available for foot fixation to the traction device. A "ski boot" design was introduced by McCarthy and is very effective in

**Fig. 11.3** (**a**) A patient is positioned for arthroscopy of the left hip in lateral decubitus using a portable lateral hip distractor (Smith and Nephew, Andover, MA). The horizontal perineal post is fixed to the surgical table on both lateral rails. Elevation of the post is obtained by increasing the angle between the support bars of the perineal post and the lateral rails. The traction device is attached to the center of the perineal post. A C-arm is positioned horizontally under the table providing an anteroposterior view of the operative hip. The orange lever at the end of the traction bar releases a ball joint at the attachment with the perineal post, facilitating movement between the perineal post and the traction bar. This is used to flex, extend, adduct, or abduct the hip if necessary. (**b**) The same patient as in **a**. The photograph was taken from the front. The foot fixation with adequate padding to the traction device is clearly visible (bootie with Velcro straps). Traction is obtained by sliding the foot train on the traction bar and fine-tuned using a crank. The screens are at the back of the patient because the surgeon stands in the front

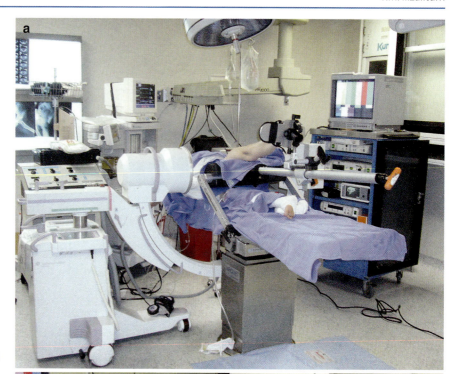

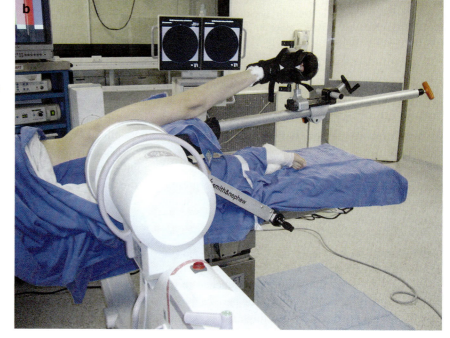

providing foot fixation to the traction device. Most fracture tables have "booties" that fix the foot using Velcro straps or belt buckles.

After a successful traction test is completed, the hip is taken through a full range of motion. Flexion of at least 40° is important to relax the anterior hip capsule and access the hip periphery. Flexion of 90° or more, internal and external rotation, and hip abduction and adduction may be necessary to ascertain adequate decompression of impinging deformities during the procedure (Fig. 11.4). It is important to perform this test before draping the patient because the table accessories

**Fig. 11.4** This photo demonstrates dynamic patient positioning to facilitate access to the hip periphery. A patient is positioned on a lateral distractor for arthroscopy of the left hip. The foot train is slid toward the perineal post flexing the hip and knee; the traction bar was moved to provide abduction and more flexion of the hip. This results in hip flexion of almost 90° and slight abduction. Also, the foot plate was externally rotated. Notice that the hip remains in the field of view of the image intensifier

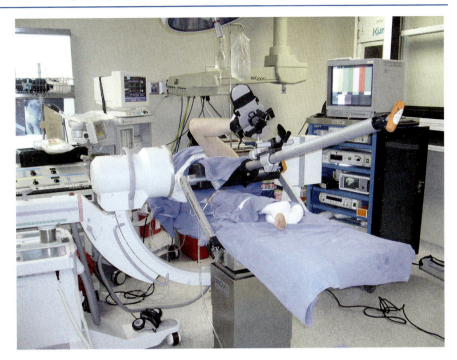

will be manipulated by the unscrubbed operating room staff; they need to be familiar with manipulation of the traction device. In our experience, a dedicated lateral hip distractor is easier to handle by the operating room staff because it is easier to manipulate under the drapes (Fig. 11.5).

## Preparing and Draping the Patient for Hip Arthroscopy

The hip is brought back to the starting position without traction (flexion 20°, abduction 0°, neutral rotations) and the surgical area prepared for surgery.

When applying sterile drapes, we first start by covering both ends of the C-arm using sterile bags. Then waterproof adhesive sterile drapes are placed in a standard fashion. The surgeon should be careful not to cover portal sites with the drapes. The medial drape should be slightly medial to the anterior superior iliac spine. The posterior drape should be behind the posterior edge of the greater trochanter. The superior drape should be level with the anterior superior iliac spine, and the distal drape should be 10–15 cm below the tip of the greater trochanter. After drapes are in position, a sterile gauze is placed over the area where the portals will be established and an adhesive transparent surgical

drape is placed over the surgical area (including the gauze) (Fig. 11.6). The gauze is removed with the adhesive tape on it leaving the area of the portals uncovered by the adhesive drape. This will prevent adhesive material from being brought into the portals by needles and instruments creating a waterproof seal preventing fluid from leaking through the drapes to the patient when the procedure starts (Fig. 11.7).

After cables and tubes for arthroscopy are ready, traction is applied (traction starting time should be recorded to monitor its duration). With the traction established, landmarks are identified and marked on the skin with a skin marker (we prefer to mark the skin after traction is applied to avoid migration of the marks).

## Surgical Technique and Instruments for Arthroscopic Treatment of Femoroacetabular Impingement

### Landmarks and Topographic Anatomy of the Hip Joint

Surface landmarks around the hip joint and their relationship to anatomic structures are the road map of hip arthroscopy. Understanding portal placement in relation to these landmarks and the anatomic structures around

**Fig. 11.5** A patient is positioned and prepared for arthroscopy of the left hip on a lateral hip distractor. The distractor is covered by the drapes. It is important for the operating room staff to know the distractor to position the hip as required by the surgeon

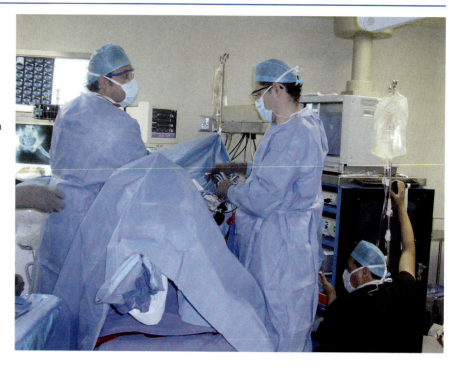

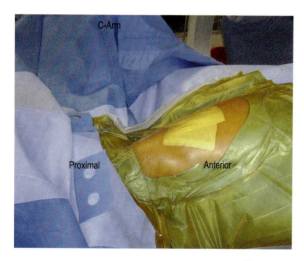

**Fig. 11.6** A patient is positioned and prepared for arthroscopy of the left hip on a lateral hip distractor. Drapes are positioned without covering the surgical area. A transparent adhesive drape is placed over the surgical area and over a sterile gauze that covers the portal sites

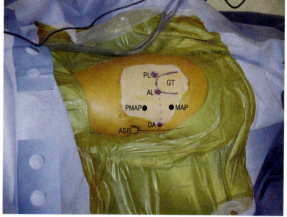

**Fig. 11.7** Clinical photograph demonstrating portal sites on a left hip. The gauze that covered the portals has been removed; the surgical area is limited by the transparent adhesive drape, creating a waterproof seal for the patient. The anterior superior iliac spine (*ASIS*) and the greater trochanter (*GT*) were delineated. The anterolateral portal (*AL*) is at the superior anterior corner of the greater trochanter; the posterolateral (*PL*) portal is at the posterior superior corner of the greater trochanter. The direct anterior (*DA*) portal is located 1 cm lateral to the intersection of a vertical line descending from the anterior superior iliac spine with a horizontal line directed anteriorly from the tip of the greater trochanter. The midanterior portal (*MAP*) and proximal midanterior portal (*PMAP*) are also indicated

the portal path in every anatomic layer is paramount in the performance of safe and successful hip arthroscopy.

The most important and apparent skin landmarks around the hip joint are the greater trochanter and the anterior superior iliac spine. When hip arthroscopy is performed, the greater trochanter and the anterior superior iliac spine should be marked before the case is started.

Byrd performed an anatomic cadaveric study and described the relation of the classic central compartment portals, the skin landmarks, and the anatomic structures around the hip joint [17]. According to Byrd, the anterolateral portal is situated at the anterosuperior corner of the greater trochanter, the posterolateral portal is situated at the posterosuperior corner of the greater trochanter, and the direct anterior portal is at the intersection of a horizontal line running anteriorly from the tip of the greater trochanter with a vertical line running down from the anterior superior iliac spine. The sciatic nerve lies about 1.5 cm behind the posterior aspect of the greater trochanter. The femoral neurovascular bundle lies medial to the vertical line running down from the anterior superior iliac spine. Two or three branches of the lateral femorocutaneous nerve lie at the site of the direct anterior portal (the lateral femorocutaneous nerve is the structure which is at the highest risk of injury by puncture when portals are established). Because the anterolateral portal lies most centrally in the safe zone (between the posterior aspect of the greater trochanter and a vertical line running down from the anterior superior iliac spine), it is always the first to be established. The anterolateral portal penetrates the gluteus medius before entering the lateral aspect of the hip capsule at its anterior margin; the superior gluteal nerve is on average 4.4 cm proximal to the anterolateral portal. The posterolateral portal penetrates the gluteus medius and minimus muscles before entering the lateral hip capsule at its posterior margin. The course of the posterolateral portal is anterior and superior to the piriformis tendon; it lies at a mean 2.9 cm from the sciatic nerve and draws closer to it at the level of the hip capsule. The superior gluteal nerve is at a mean 4.4 cm proximal to the posterolateral portal. The direct anterior portal penetrates the muscle belly of the sartorius and rectus femoris before entering through the anterior hip capsule. Some surgeons prefer to position the direct anterior portal 1 cm lateral to a vertical line descending from the anterior superior iliac spine to avoid penetrating the rectus femoris tendon, thus steering clear from the branches of the lateral femorocutaneous nerve that lie at the site of the direct anterior portal [17].

Gradually, variations of the original portals and other accessory portals have been introduced to access the hip joint. Kelly [18] studied the anatomic relationships of 8 different skin incisions (including the traditional anterolateral, posterolateral, and direct anterior portals) with 11 different portal trajectories used for arthroscopy of both the hip joint and the pertrochanteric space by different authors using a study design similar to Byrd's [17]. In the study by Kelly, the direct anterior portal was positioned 1 cm lateral to the intersection of the vertical line running down from the anterior superior iliac spine and a horizontal line running from the tip of the greater trochanter. It then penetrated the muscle belly of the tensor fasciae latae and passed through the interval between gluteus minimus and rectus femoris before entering the joint through the anterior hip capsule. Branches of the lateral femorocutaneous nerve were found at a mean 1.54 cm form the trajectory of the direct anterior portal. The midanterior portal was positioned using the anterolateral and direct anterior portals as vertices; a third point was marked distally so that all three would form an equilateral triangle. The tip of this triangle was the site of the midanterior portal. The midanterior portal for both the central and peripheral compartment penetrated the tensor fasciae latae before passing through the interval between the gluteus minimus and rectus femoris and entering the anterior hip capsule. The closest neurovascular structure was the lateral femorocutaneous nerve, 1.92 cm away on average. The same equilateral triangle was performed this time with the tip directed proximally; this marked the site of the proximal midanterior portal. The proximal midanterior portal was found to run through the gluteus medius and minimus muscle bellies on its way to the anterior hip capsule with an average distance of 5 cm to the superior gluteal nerve (Fig. 11.7).

## Equipment for Portal Establishment and Surgical Technique

The anatomical situation of the hip joint makes it difficult to access arthroscopically as compared to other joints. A hip arthroscopy-dedicated set of instruments is mandatory when attempting arthroscopic access to the hip joint. The use of standard nondedicated hip arthroscopy equipment for access to the hip joint will result in increased risk of iatrogenic damage to structures inside and around the hip joint [3].

**Fig. 11.8** (**a**) The photograph demonstrates a hip arthroscopy needle (spinal needle) and a nitinol guidewire. The stylus has been removed from the needle and rests beside it. The nitinol guidewire is inside the needle. (**b**) Fluoroscopy photograph of a right hip. There is separation between the femoral head and the acetabulum as a result of traction. A nitinol guidewire is in position inside the hip joint and is used as a monorail to guide a cannulated switching stick into the joint

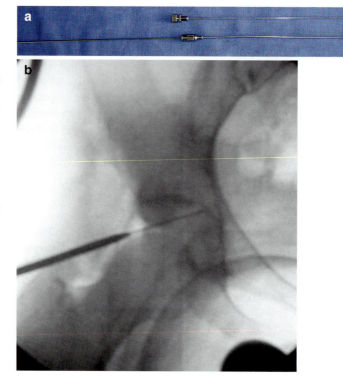

Cannulated instruments are the workhorse of hip arthroscopy and are common to every commercially available hip arthroscopy instrument set. Cannulated instruments are used in combination with a spinal needle guidewire technique (Fig. 11.8a, b).

The most popular technique to access the hip joint arthroscopically is to start by establishing traction and entering the central compartment first. Michael Dienst [19] described an alternative method whereby the hip periphery is accessed first without traction, the anterolateral labrum is identified, traction is applied under direct arthroscopic vision to observe the separation between the femoral head and the acetabulum in vivo, and the spinal needle is positioned between the head and the acetabulum by direct arthroscopic visualization.

As mentioned before, the most common technique is to start at the central compartment with traction. The anterolateral portal is typically the first portal established because it is at the center of the safety zone between the posterior edge of the greater trochanter and a vertical line descending from the anterior superior iliac spine. The sciatic nerve is typically 1.5 cm behind the posterior margin of the greater trochanter and the femoral neurovascular bundle lies medial to a vertical line descending from the anterior superior iliac spine. The anterolateral portal is typically located at the anterior superior corner of the landmark for the greater trochanter [17]. Some authors prefer to establish a single lateral portal more in line with the middle of the tip of the greater trochanter [7]. A spinal needle is introduced at the selected portal site and is navigated by fluoroscopy into the hip joint between the separated acetabulum and the femoral head. Because this first portal is performed blindly, only with the guidance of fluoroscopy, it is the most dangerous one for intra-articular structures. These structures may be damaged by inadequate passage of the needle or the rest of the instruments. A safe technique is to introduce the needle as close as possible to the femoral head, away from the free margin of the lateral labrum with the tip of the needle pointing away from the femoral head. The intra-articular position of the needle should be inferred by the feel of penetrating the hip capsule and not by landing the needle at the medial acetabular wall, which may result in puncture damage to the cartilage. If confirmation of the intra-articular position of the needle is required, this may be obtained with the blunt guidewire, by taking the stylus from the needle and passing the guidewire through it, then palpating the medial acetabulum with the blunt tip of the guidewire. Once the intra-articular position of the needle is confirmed, the guidewire is removed from the needle and 40 cc of

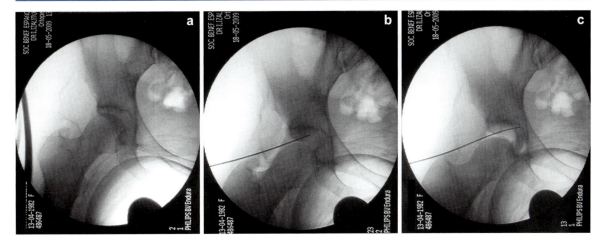

**Fig. 11.9** Fluoroscopy photographic sequence on establishment of the anterolateral portal in a right hip. (**a**) Traction-free fluoroscopic image. (**b**) Fluoroscopic image showing separation of the femoral head from the acetabulum (the hip is with traction). A needle is in position, closer to the head to avoid piercing the labrum. The tip of the needle is turned away from the head to prevent damaging it. The needle is not introduced all the way until reaching the medial acetabular wall to prevent cartilage injury by the tip. (**c**) The joint has been distended with fluid; the separation between the head and the acetabulum has widened from distension, not from increased traction force. The medial acetabular wall is probed with the blunt end of the nitinol guidewire

saline solution is injected into the hip. This will cause the hip joint to distend, and separation between the acetabulum and the femoral head will increase [15]. After distention, the needle must stay closer to the femoral head; if the position of the needle at fluoroscopy is closer to the acetabular rim, the surgeon must suspect that the needle is piercing the labrum and must reposition it closer to the femoral head to avoid further damage to the labrum.

Once the needle is in its final position, the nitinol guidewire is reinserted, the needle removed, and the skin incision performed over the guidewire, then cannulated instruments are used to establish the portals (Fig. 11.9). Our preference is to use a cannulated switching stick mounted on a special handle, which uses the nitinol guidewire as a monorail to follow it into the hip joint. Nitinol guidewires are preferred because they are more flexible than standard K-wires and are more tolerant of bending before kinking and breaking. Once the switching stick is in its intra-articular position, the handle is removed and the standard arthroscopy cannula introduced over the guidewire. A 70° 4-mm arthroscope is positioned in the arthroscopic cannula after removing the switching stick. The rest of the portals are established under direct arthroscopic view. Most surgeons establish the direct anterior portal or one of its variants. The classical direct anterior portal is located at the intersection of the vertical line running down from the anterior superior iliac spine and

a horizontal line directed anteriorly from the tip of the greater trochanter. A spinal needle is introduced at the site of the direct anterior portal and triangulated to the tip of the arthroscope inside the hip joint. The needle should be observed entering the joint at the anterior safety triangle limited superiorly by the free margin of the anterolateral labrum, inferiorly by the femoral head, and laterally by the limit of the arthroscopic field of view. The stylus is removed from the needle and a nitinol guidewire introduced through the needle. The needle is removed and the skin incision performed. The guidewire is used as a monorail to introduce cannulated instruments to establish a working portal. Two alternative techniques may be used to establish a working portal: (1) A modular cannula system (Fig. 11.10) – a cannulated obturator is used to introduce modular cannulas into the hip joint. The cannulated obturator and modular cannula assembly are introduced into the portal using the nitinol guidewire as a monorail. Modular cannulas are available in different diameters and have a proximal attachment for a modular fluid management bridge that serves the purpose of locking the arthroscope inside the cannula, both if the portal is used as a working portal or as a purely arthroscopic one. The system is based in the philosophy of positioning different cannulas in each portal. The arthroscope can be interchanged between these cannulas to access different parts of the joint as needed allowing the free cannulas to act as working cannulas. (2) Slotted

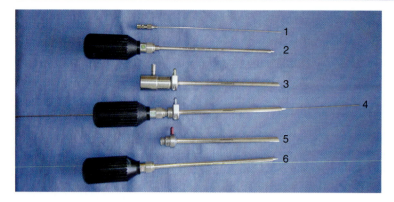

**Fig. 11.10** Photograph of a modular cannula system (Arthrogarde hip arthroscopy cannulas, Smith and Nephew, Andover, MA). (*1*) Hip arthroscopy needle (spinal needle). (*2*) Cannulated obturator for the 4.5-mm modular cannula (*green color* coded for the 4.5-mm obturator–cannula assembly). (*3*) 4.5-mm modular hip arthroscopy cannula. Note a single inflow irrigation extender is attached to the modular end of the cannula. The irrigation extender has an attachment for the arthroscope (Dyonics 4.0-mm 30° or 70° arthroscope, Smith and Nephew, Andover, MA). (*4*) Cannulated obturator–5.0-mm modular cannula assembly. A nitinol guidewire is inside the cannulated obturator (*blue color* coded for the 5.0-mm obturator–cannula assembly). (*5*) 5.5-mm modular cannula. (*6*) 5.5-mm cannulated obturator (*red color* coded for the 5.5-mm obturator–cannula assembly)

**Fig. 11.11** Photograph of a slotted cannula system for hip arthroscopy. (*1*) Hip arthroscopy needle (spinal needle). (*2*) Standard nonmodular arthroscopy cannula with a double valve rotating system for 4.0-mm 30° and 70° arthroscopes (Dyonics, Smith and Nephew, Andover, MA). (*3*) Cannulated T-handle for a cannulated switching stick and dilator. (*4*) Cannulated switching stick with T-handle attachment. (*5*) Dilator with T-handle attachment (instruments *3*, *4*, and *5* are part of the hip access system, Smith and Nephew, Andover, MA). (*6*) Arthrogarde hip arthroscopy slotted cannula with pistol grip (Smith and Nephew, Andover, MA)

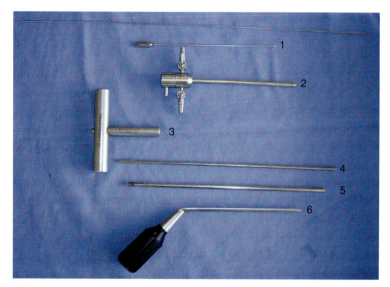

**Fig. 11.12** This photograph demonstrates the T-handle – cannulated switching stick – dilator assembly over a nitinol guidewire. The photograph demonstrates how a slotted cannula is slid using the referred assembly as a guide

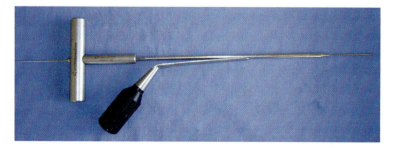

cannula system (Fig. 11.11) [20] – a switching stick is typically positioned over the nitinol guidewire into the joint and the slotted cannula is slid around the switching stick to enter the hip joint (Fig. 11.12). With the slotted cannula inside the hip joint, the switching stick is exchanged for an arthroscopic instrument and the slotted cannula can be removed (Fig. 11.13a, b). After the selected instrument has been used, it serves as a guide to reinsert the slotted cannula preparing the portal for the introduction of a different instrument or for portal exchange. Portal exchange with a slotted cannula is slightly more complicated than with a closed cannula system; a switching stick is introduced into the joint using the slotted cannula which is then removed to be reinserted over the arthroscopy cannula (where the scope is positioned) and confirmed inside the joint with the arthroscope. The arthroscopy cannula arthroscope assembly is removed from the slotted cannula, leaving the latter in position inside the portal. The arthroscope is removed from the arthroscopy cannula which is then introduced at the other portal over the switching stick. The switching stick is removed and the arthroscope positioned inside the arthroscopy cannula.

When working portals are established using either the modular cannula or the slotted cannula method, instruments are brought into the joint under direct arthroscopic vision to prevent iatrogenic damage.

Once the portals are established, a hip capsulotomy is typically performed to increase instrument mobility within the joint and for adequate exposure of impingement deformities. The capsulotomy is typically performed using an arthroscopic banana scalpel. Other instruments such as radiofrequency devices of different shapes may also be used to perform the capsulotomy. An effective technique for a capsulotomy is to connect the anterolateral and direct anterior portals inside the hip joint. This will produce a capsulotomy that is parallel to the anterior acetabular rim (Fig. 11.14). With this exposure, it is very easy to identify the free margin and the capsular side of the labrum providing access to the labral insertion on the acetabular rim. Visualization can be improved by combining the technique with a limited capsulectomy. With the area exposed, the surgeon may proceed to remodel the pincer deformity and treat labral pathology.

Cam-type impingement is treated at the hip periphery (Fig. 11.15). Access to the hip periphery is better without traction and with hip flexion to relax the

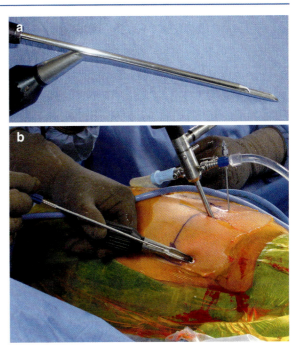

**Fig. 11.13** (**a**) The photograph demonstrates a 45° microfracture awl (Linvatec, Largo, FL) slid through an Arthrogarde slotted cannula (Smith and Nephew, Andover, MA). (**b**) Surgical photograph during hip arthroscopy of a right hip. The patient is in the lateral position. The arthroscope is in the anterolateral portal, and a spinal needle is used for outflow at the posterolateral portal. An Arthrogarde slotted cannula (Smith and Nephew, Andover, MA) is in position at the direct anterior portal. A probe is being introduced using the slotted cannula

anterior hip capsule. A number of accessory portals have been described to access the hip periphery [18]; they can be established with the aid of fluoroscopy and using the cannulated instruments with the same technique as described for the central compartment.

## Conclusion

Hip arthroscopy is a technically demanding procedure with a steep learning curve. The surgeon must understand the anatomy and the effects of traction, capsular distension, and traction-free range of motion on the capsule and its ligaments, as well as the effect these factors have on the working space of hip arthroscopy. Effective patient positioning is based on adequate management of the arthroscopic working space within the hip joint. It is also important to effectively protect areas of compression from distraction devices.

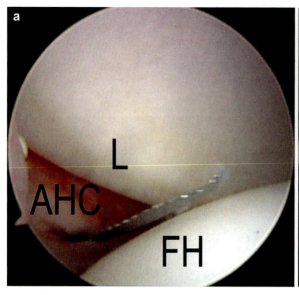 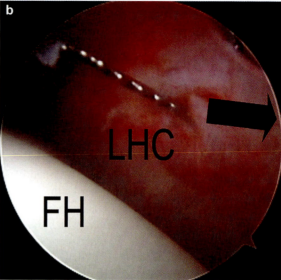

**Fig. 11.14** Arthroscopic photograph inside a left hip. (**a**) The arthroscope is at the anterolateral portal looking at the anterior hip capsule (*AHC*). The anterior labrum (*L*) is at the top and the femoral head (*FH*) at the bottom of the photograph. A serrated banana arthroscopic knife (Erichsen knife system, Stryker, Kalamazoo, MI) is used to perform a capsulotomy. (**b**) The arthroscope has been switched to the direct anterior portal and the capsulotomy of the lateral hip capsule (*LHC*) started. The capsulotomy of the anterolateral portal is performed in the direction of the *black arrow* until it connects to the first capsulotomy performed at direct anterior portal. The femoral head (*FH*) is at the bottom of the photograph

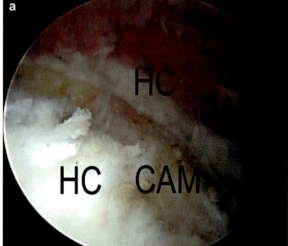 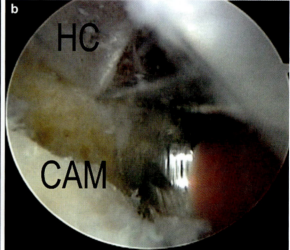

**Fig. 11.15** Arthroscopic photograph of a right hip. The patient is without traction and slight hip flexion. A 4-mm, 30° arthroscope is at the proximal midanterior portal looking anteriorly. (**a**) The margins of the hip capsule (*HC*) after capsulotomy are observed. A cam impingement (*CAM*) deformity is exposed through the capsulotomy. (**b**) A 5.5-mm spherical burr (Smith and Nephew, Andover, MA) is introduced through the direct anterior portal and is used to reshape the cam impingement (*CAM*) deformity

Most of the complications of hip arthroscopy result from inadequate patient positioning, which may lead to suboptimal access conditions for arthroscopic instruments, increasing the possibility of iatrogenic damage to articular structures or insufficient exposure, which will result in inadequate remodeling of deformities, especially in cases of FAI.

Excessive traction time may result in neurological injuries, and inadequate protection of compression points may also produce neurologic or pressure damage to soft tissues.

In-depth knowledge of the topographic anatomy of the hip will facilitate the surgeon's three-dimensional orientation within and around the hip joint. Finally, the surgeon must understand that it is impossible to perform hip arthroscopy safely and effectively without dedicated hip instruments.

# References

1. McCarthy JC (1995) Hip arthroscopy: applications and technique. J Am Acad Orthop Surg 3:115–122
2. Byrd JWT (2006) Hip arthroscopy. J Am Acad Orthop Surg 14:433–444
3. Ilizaliturri VM Jr, Chaidez PA, Aguilera JM, Camacho-Galindo J (2005) Special instruments and techniques for hip arthroscopy. Tech Orthop 20:9–16
4. Ilizaliturri VM Jr, Mangino G, Valero FS, Camacho-Galindo J (2005) Hip arthroscopy of the central and peripheral compartment by the lateral approach. Tech Orthop 20:32–36
5. Sampson TG (2005) Arthroscopic treatment of femoroacetabular impingement. Tech Orthop 20:56–62
6. Leunig M, Beck M, Dora C, Ganz R (2005) Fomoroacetabular impingement: etiology and surgical concept. Oper Tech Orthop 15:247–255
7. Philippon MJ, Stubbs AJ, Shenker ML, Maxwell RB, Ganz R, Leunig M (2007) Arthroscopic management of femoroacetabular impingement: osteoplasty technique and literature review. Am J Sports Med 35:1571–1580
8. Ilizaliturri VM Jr (2009) Complications of arthroscopic femoroacetabular impingement treatment. Clin Orthop Relat Res 467:760–768
9. Dienst M, Godde S, Seil R, Hammer D, Kohn D (2001) Hip arthroscopy without traction: in vivo anatomy of the peripheral joint cavity. Arthroscopy 17:924–931
10. Byrd JW (2001) Hip arthroscopy: the supine position. Clin Sports Med 20:703–731
11. Glick JM, Sampson TG, Gordon RB, Behr JT, Schmidt E (1987) Hip arthroscopy by the lateral approach. Arthroscopy 3:4–12
12. Ilizaliturri VM Jr, Nossa-Barrera JM, Acosta-Rodriguez E, Camacho-Galindo J (2009) Arthroscopic treatment of femoroacetabular impingement secondary to pediatric hip disease. J Bone Joint Surg Br 89:1025–1030
13. Ilizaliturri VM Jr, Orozco-Rodriguez L, Acosta-Rodriquez E, Camacho-Galindo J (2008) Arthroscopic treatment of femoroacetabular impingement. J Arthroplasty 23:226–234
14. Byrd JW, Jones KS (2009) Arthroscopic management of femoroacetabular impingement. Instr Course Lect 58:231–239
15. Dienst M, Seil R, Godde S (2002) Effects of traction, distension and joint position on distraction of the hip joint: an experimental study in cadavers. Arthroscopy 18(8):865–871
16. McCarthy JC, Day B, Busconi B (1993) Hip arthroscopy: applications and technique. J Am Acad Orthop Surg 3(3):115–122
17. Byrd JWT, Pappas JN, Pedley MJ (1995) Hip arthroscopy: an anatomic study of portal placement and relationship to the extraarticular structures. Arthroscopy 11(4):418–423
18. Robertson WJ, Kelly BT (2008) The safe zone for hip arthroscopy: a cadaveric assessment of central, peripheral and lateral compartment portal placement. Arthroscopy 24:1019–1026
19. Dienst M, Seil R, Kohn DM (2005) Safe arthroscopic access to the central compartment of the hip. Arthroscopy 21:1510–1514
20. Ilizaliturri VM Jr, Acosta-Rodriguez E, Camacho-Galindo J (2007) A minimalist approach to hip arthroscopy: the slotted cannula. Arthroscopy 23:560.e1–3

# Normal and Pathological Arthroscopic View in Hip Arthroscopy

**12**

Damian Griffin and Shanmugam Karthikeyan

## Normal Anatomy

Arthroscopy of the hip involves examination of two areas of the joint, often called the central and peripheral compartments. The central compartment is the potential space between the articular cartilage of the femoral head, and that of the acetabulum, and is bounded by the acetabular labrum. The peripheral compartment is the intra-capsular space lateral to the labrum and surrounding the femoral neck.

## Central Compartment

Arthroscopy of the central compartment is performed with traction, typically achieving distraction between the femoral head and acetabulum of about 10 mm. A variety of portal positions have been described. Many surgeons use para-trochanteric portals and an anterior portal, but a thorough examination is possible with just two portals in a relatively posterior postero-lateral position and an antero-inferior position. Portals should be well spaced to avoid interference between instruments and converging by at least 60° to allow optimum triangulation (Fig. 12.1).

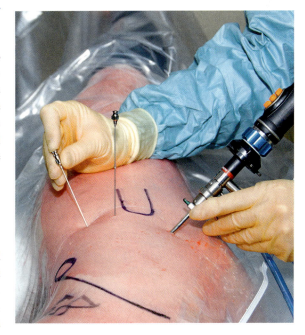

**Fig. 12.1** Spacing of portals for central compartment arthroscopy of a right hip in the lateral position

Most of the central compartment can be well seen from a postero-lateral portal. The medial, posterior, superior and anterior surfaces of the femoral head can be seen and probed. The articular cartilage is white, smooth and glistening in a normal hip. It can be slightly indented with a probe but immediately rebounds. A 70° arthroscope makes it easier to see the medial surface of the femoral head and to look further inferior on the posterior and anterior aspects. During most operations, the inferior aspect of the femoral head is not examined, but when required, this area can be seen with an additional antero-inferior portal.

D. Griffin (✉) • S. Karthikeyan
Warwick Medical School,
University of Warwick,
Coventry, UK
e-mail: Damian.Griffin@warwick.ac.uk;
karthikshanmugam@hotmail.com

Ó. Marín-Peña (ed.), *Femoroacetabular Impingement*,
DOI 10.1007/978-3-642-22769-1_12, © Springer-Verlag Berlin Heidelberg 2012

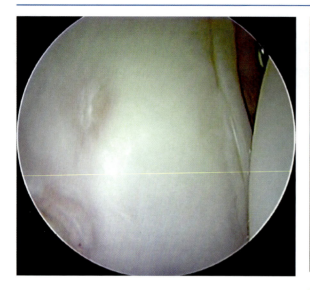

**Fig. 12.2** Antero-superior aspect of the lunate surface and labrum

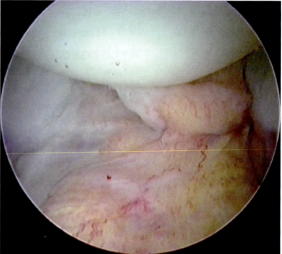

**Fig. 12.4** Ligamentum teres and fat pad in the cotyloid fossa

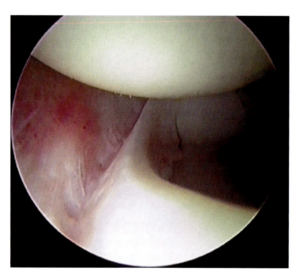

**Fig. 12.3** Perilabral sulcus between the labrum and capsule

The acetabulum forms a roughly hemispherical surface. It is lined by a horseshoe-shaped area of articular cartilage, which curves from the postero-inferior aspect, over the top of the hip to the antero-inferior aspect. This articular cartilage-covered area is often called the lunate surface and makes up about two thirds of the acetabulum (Fig. 12.2). Within the arms of the horseshoe, in the centre of the acetabulum and extending to its inferior margin, is the cotyloid fossa. This fossa is filled with a fat pad. The edge of the acetabulum is made up of the acetabular labrum. This is a fibro-cartilage projection of

the bony margin of the acetabular fossa, roughly triangular in cross-section, and continuous on its inner surface with the articular cartilage of the lunate surface. In the most inferior aspect of the hip, the transverse ligament crosses the gap between the two limbs of the horseshoe-shaped lunate surface. Although the transverse ligament is not supported by underlying bone, there is no apparent difference between it and the labrum so that there is a continuous, circumferential, fibro-cartilaginous rim to the acetabulum. Between the labrum and the adjacent capsule of the hip, there is a potential space, or perilabral sulcus (Fig. 12.3). This sulcus can be easily seen adjacent to the anterior and posterior labrum. On traction, to examine the central compartment, the superior perilabral sulcus tends to be diminished by the forces on the superior capsule.

The ligamentum teres connects the femoral head to the acetabulum (Fig. 12.4). It is a substantial strap-shaped structure, flattened and slightly broader at the base, and usually covered with synovial membrane. The smaller femoral attachment is to a pit, or fovea, in the centre of the femoral head, whilst the broader acetabular attachment is to the base of the cotyloid fossa, close to the posterior attachment of the transverse ligament.

The whole of the acetabulum and the labrum can be seen using the portals described above. A better view of the superior aspect of the acetabulum and of the antero-inferior labrum can be obtained by placing the arthroscope in an anterior portal, but most of the acetabulum can be very well seen from the postero-lateral portal.

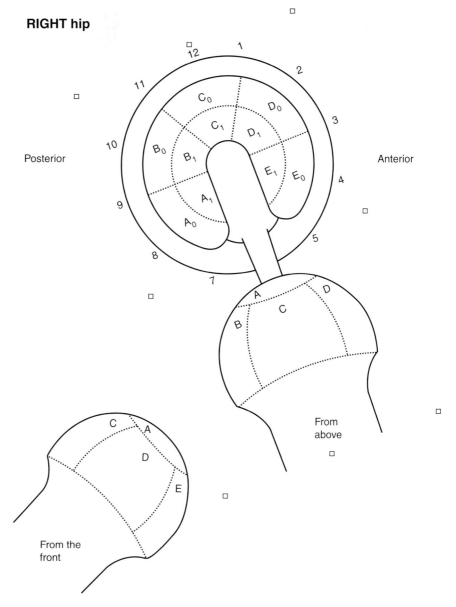

**Fig. 12.5** Hip map dividing the articular surface of the acetabulum into ten zones and the femoral head into five

A 70° arthroscope is ideal for most areas including the ligamentum teres and transverse ligament. A 30° arthroscope provides an excellent view of the depths of the acetabulum and cotyloid fossa.

In order to describe findings at arthroscopy of the central compartment, many surgeons have used some form of map. As in other joints, these maps have usually divided the hip articular cartilage into zones. Since the periphery of the acetabular is continuous and circular, it can be easily described using a clock face nomenclature. Figure 12.5 demonstrates one such scheme. The femoral head is divided into five zones: a central

zone centred on the fovea about 3 cm in diameter and then the posterior, superior, anterior and inferior zones. A clock face is projected onto the labrum, with 6 o'clock defined as the most inferior aspect of the hip, the midpoint of the transverse ligament. The anterior aspect of the hip is defined as 3 o'clock, whether it is a right or left hip. Thus, superior is 12 o'clock and posterior is 9 o'clock. The lunate surface is divided first by radial lines extending from a centre point in the middle of the cotyloid fossa. Lines from this centre radiate toward 3 o'clock and 9 o'clock to separate the upper half from the lower half. The upper half is then divided

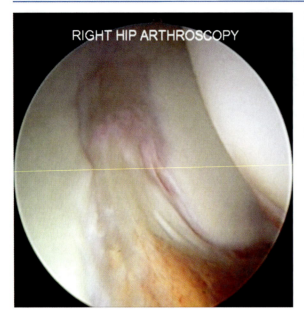

Fig. 12.6 Stellate crease – a normal variant

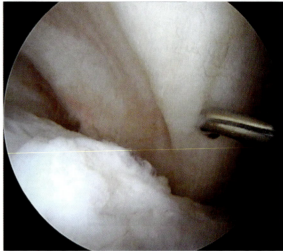

Fig. 12.7 Anterior aspect of the peripheral compartment showing the zona orbicularis and the femoral head to the left

by radial lines projected toward 1 o'clock and 11 o'clock. These five radial segments are each divided into an inner and outer zone by a circle concentric to the rim, which runs halfway between the labro-chondral junction and the edge of the cotyloid fossa.

There are many variations in the intra-articular anatomy of the normal hip. Among these, and most relevant to femoro-acetabular impingement, are variations in the anatomy of the labrum and the articular cartilage of the lunate surface. The cross-sectional shape of the labrum varies considerably around the circumference of the hip and between individuals. It tends to be narrower and more sharply triangular anteriorly, whereas the labrum is less prominent and more rounded in the posterior aspect of the hip. The labro-chondral junction, between the inner aspect of the labrum and the articular cartilage of the lunate surface, is usually continuous and imperceptible anteriorly and superiorly. Posteriorly, there is usually a shallow groove, which can easily be misinterpreted as a labral tear. Sometimes this labral groove continues to the anterior aspect of the hip, and may be normal rather than a sign of pathology. A common variant is the stellate crease, which extends peripherally onto the lunate surface from the antero-superior aspect of the cotyloid fossa (Fig. 12.6). This area of thin or missing articular cartilage is variable in size and sometimes includes a round- or star-shaped defect in the articular cartilage at its tip. A separate linear defect in the articular

cartilage sometimes extends across the anterior limb of the horseshoe-shaped lunate surface, inferior to the stellate crease, at about 3 or 4 o'clock. This probably represents a scar from the fusion of the pubo-iliac component of the tri-radiate cartilage. Occasionally, a similar scar is seen on the posterior limb of the articular surface.

## Peripheral Compartment

The peripheral compartment of the hip is examined without traction. Flexing the hip to about 30° relaxes the capsule and allows the potential space around the femoral neck to be inflated. As in the central compartment, a variety of portals have been described. Most often, antero-superior and antero-inferior portals are used, with a combination of 30° and 70° arthroscopes.

The anterior surface of the femoral neck is an obvious feature, usually covered by shiny periosteum. More medially, the neck widens to form the femoral head, covered with the familiar articular cartilage. Off traction, only a small portion of the articular surface of the head can be seen, although external rotation and adduction exposes more.

Laterally, the anterior capsule is attached to the intertrochanteric line and balloons away from the femoral neck with inflation. The zona orbicularis constricts the capsule around the mid-portion of the neck, and then the capsule is distended again into the perilabral recess (Fig. 12.7). From the peripheral compartment, it is easy to see the outer surface of the anterior labrum and to appreciate its intimate relationship with the reflection of the capsule. The inferior recess of the capsule lies under the femoral neck and is very capacious. The capsule is noticeably thinner here than elsewhere. Antero-superiorly the capsule is thickened by the iliofemoral ligament and is much more closely applied to the femoral neck. In loose and flexible hips, it is sometimes possible to pass the arthroscope between this thickened capsule and the superior femoral neck to observe the much more restricted posterior aspect of the peripheral compartment: In many patients this will require a small capsulotomy.

On the inferior aspect of the femoral neck is a constant feature, the medial synovial fold (sometimes called Weibrecht's ligament). It extends from the edge of the articular surface of the femoral head to the lateral capsular reflection of the inferior recess. The medial synovial fold is quite variable in appearance: It may be a thickening of the periosteum or may bridge across the inferior curve of the femoral neck. This fold, and the zona orbicularis running perpendicular to it, provide excellent orientation landmarks within the peripheral compartment.

On the superior aspect of the neck, a lateral synovial fold is sometimes seen. This is much less obvious than the medial synovial fold, usually just being an area of spongier periosteum and synovium than on the more anterior neck. However, it is important, as it covers the terminal vessels of the ascending branch of the medial femoral circumflex artery as they pass along the neck to enter and supply the femoral head.

Since the hip is not on traction, it is easy to move the joint while examining the peripheral compartment. This can facilitate a better view, especially when looking into the inferior recess or over the top of the neck into the posterior aspect of the compartment. It also allows dynamic assessment of the hip to assess the possibility of femoro-acetabular impingement.

## Pathological Anatomy

Femoro-acetabular impingement can usefully be divided into two types: cam and pincer. They are often present together in a patient, but the arthroscopic appearances associated with each type of impingement are quite different. These differences may help to decide whether one form of impingement is predominant and help to plan treatment.

## Cam-Type Femoro-acetabular Impingement

Often, the most obvious feature of cam-type femoro-acetabular impingement is the damage done to the articular cartilage of the acetabulum, seen during arthroscopy of the central compartment. This is usually in the outer part of the antero-superior aspect of the joint, or zone $D_o$ in Fig. 12.2. Several different pathological features have been observed and described, and the temporal relationship between these is not certain. However, a consensus is beginning to develop which at least provides a framework in which to consider the pathoanatomy associated with cam-type femoro-acetabular impingement. Partial-thickness articular damage is best described by the ICRS classification. Full-thickness damage seems to be specific to this pathology (Fig. 12.8) and may be classified as follows:

- *Bubble.* The most minor damage can be described as a bubble. This is a palpable bulkiness to the articular cartilage at the periphery. If a smooth blunt probe is pushed across the surface of the cartilage, the cartilage rocks up in front of it – a "wave sign". This lesion probably represents delamination of the articular cartilage, either within its substance or at the attachment to the subchondral bone. It seems likely that repeated shearing forces cause this damage.
- *Labro-chondral separation.* Shearing forces can also cause labro-chondral separation. This is a tear of the normal smooth junction between the antero-superior labrum and the adjacent articular cartilage.
- *Pocket.* When the delamination of a bubble connects to a labro-chondral separation tear, a pocket is formed. Here, a probe can be inserted through the opening of the labro-chondral separation tear and into a space between the articular cartilage and the subchondral bone of the lunate surface. This pocket can be quite large, typically 1–2 cm², but it is stable and contained, offering the opportunity for conservative treatments such as gluing of the articular cartilage.
- *Flap.* Once the pocket becomes unstable, usually because of further tears in the articular cartilage, a flap is formed. This flap is the commonest finding in arthroscopy of cam-type femoro-acetabular impingement. It may be extensive, representing several square centimetres of the articular cartilage of the acetabulum.

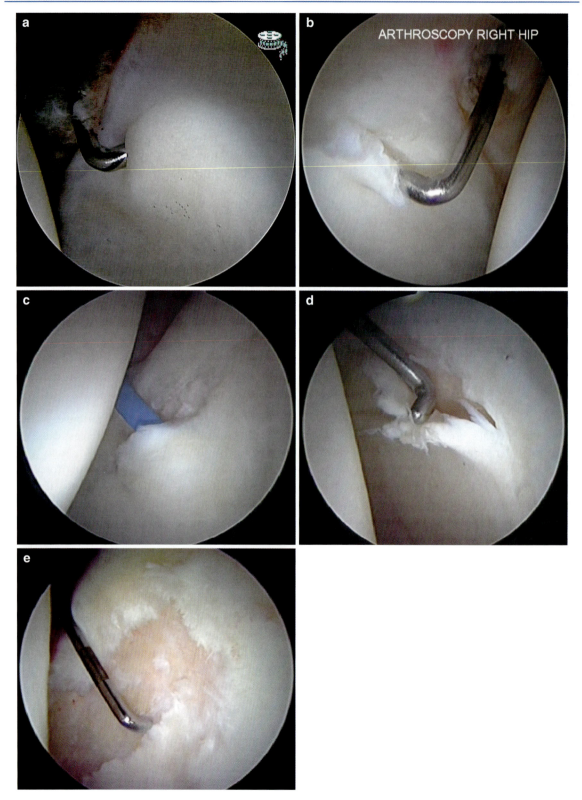

**Fig. 12.8** Acetabular articular cartilage damage in cam-type FAI: (**a**) Bubble; (**b**) Labro-chondral separation; (**c**) Pocket; (**d**) Flap; (**e**) Defect

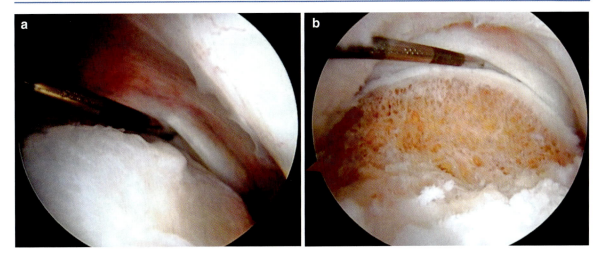

**Fig. 12.9** Peripheral compartment view in cam-type FAI: (**a**) Prominent bone on the femoral head-neck junction; (**b**) After bone reshaping

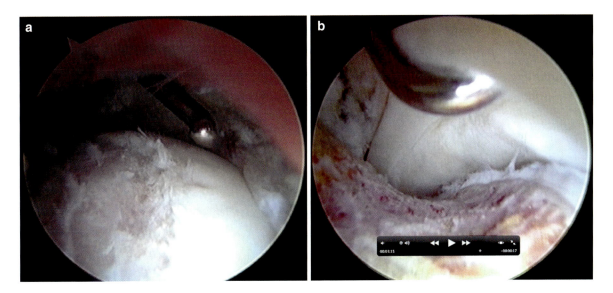

**Fig. 12.10** Profile view in cam-type FAI: (**a**) Prominent bone on the femoral head-neck junction; (**b**) Dynamic assessment after bone reshaping

- *Defect.* The final step is loss of the flap by disintegration or detachment. This leaves a full-thickness articular cartilage defect.

In the peripheral compartment, the bulge of bone causing impingement is often easy to see. Sometimes this is just a fullness of the normal recess at the head neck traction; in other patients, there is prominent bone and secondary osteophyte formation (Fig. 12.9). Dynamic assessment allows the surgeon to identify those areas that are most likely to be responsible for impingement. The prominent bone is usually covered

with articular cartilage, but this may have an abnormal appearance. It is often rough and may be pinkish or bluish compared to the glistening white of normal cartilage. On probing, it is thin and fibrous.

The sphericity of the femoral head can be most easily assessed by making a small capsulotomy during central compartment arthroscopy on traction. With a 70° arthroscope, this allows a profile view of the head and neck junction (Fig. 12.10a), similar to the radiological assessment used to measure alpha angle. Once traction is released, the arthroscope can be allowed to slide into the peripheral compartment to perform a dynamic assessment after a bone resection (Fig. 12.10b).

A variety of techniques have been developed to facilitate arthroscopic head-neck reshaping in cam-type femoro-acetabular impingement. These are relatively straightforward when the abnormal head-neck junction is anterior or antero-superior. They become more complex as the surgeon tries to work on the posterior and inferior aspects of the femoral neck because the arthroscopic view and instrument access is more difficult to achieve.

## Pincer-Type Femoro-acetabular Impingement

Dynamic assessment of the peripheral compartment in pincer-type impingement can demonstrate the crushing of the acetabular labrum against the femoral neck. Often there is a smooth or indented area of the neck, sometimes surrounded by osteophytes. The prominent acetabular rim may be assessed in the perilabral sulcus, and ossification of the labrum is easily appreciated.

In the central compartment, the most obvious feature is the degeneration of the labrum caused by repeated crushing. The labrum may be enlarged, cystic, torn, ossified or completely absent. There is often extensive inflammation of the remnants of the labrum and of the adjacent structures. There may be extensive synovitis filling the perilabral sulcus. If the labrum is relatively undamaged, then it may be detached, the acetabular rim trimmed and then the labrum reattached (Fig. 12.11).

In some cases, there is a defect of the articular cartilage on the postero-inferior aspect of the lunar surface. This is sometimes called a "contre-coup" lesion and is thought to reflect increased pressure on this part of the acetabulum caused by leverage of the femoral neck on the prominent antero-superior acetabular rim.

## Developing Osteoarthrosis

As degeneration due to femoro-acetabular impingement becomes more extensive, the appearances blur

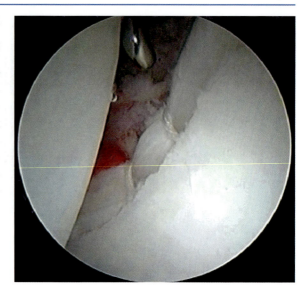

**Fig. 12.11** Reattachment of acetabular labrum after resection of prominent acetabular rim in pincer-type FAI

with generalised osteoarthrosis. Articular cartilage damage becomes more widespread in the acetabulum and then extends onto the femoral head. Increasing amounts of cartilage debris are found floating in the joint at initial arthroscopy. Degeneration and ossification of the labrum worsens, and osteophytes develop on the femoral neck and acetabular rim (Fig. 12.12). In the central compartment, osteophytes form on the margin of the cotyloid fossa (Fig. 12.13) and around the fovea on the femoral head. These may abrade the ligamentum teres, leading to degenerative partial or complete tears. Proliferating synovium fills the perilabral sulcus, and fronds of inflamed synovium make it increasingly difficult to navigate the peripheral compartment.

In a more extensively damaged hip, the surgeon may start to think in terms of established osteoarthrosis. There is no clear dividing line between the early (possibly reversible) pathology associated with femoro-acetabular impingement and osteoarthrosis. The variation in articular damage is probably best considered to be continuous. Factors such as the patient's age, activity level and expectations and the surgeon's capability are probably at least as important as arthroscopic findings in deciding whether to attempt joint-preserving surgery or to recommend arthroplasty for irreversible arthropathy.

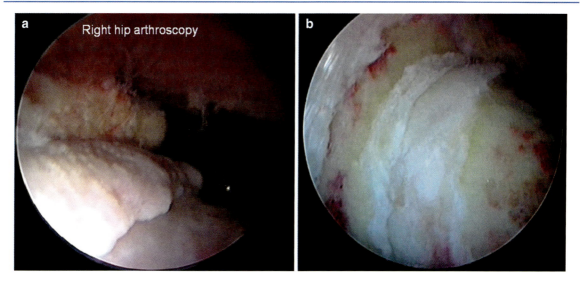

**Fig. 12.12** Combined cam- and pincer-type FAI with secondary osteophytes during arthroscopic joint-preserving surgery: (**a**) Before resection; (**b**) After resection

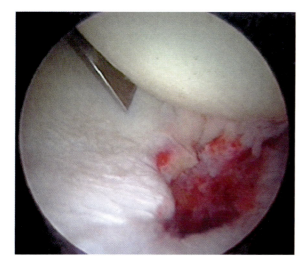

**Fig. 12.13** Osteophytes around the cotyloid fossa

## Bibliography

Beck M (2009) Groin pain after open FAI surgery: the role of intraarticular adhesions. Clin Orthop Relat Res 467:769–774

Bushnell BD, Anz AW, Bert JM (2008) Venous thromboembolism in lower extremity arthroscopy. Arthroscopy 24(5): 604–611

Byrd JW (1994) Hip arthroscopy utilizing the supine position. Arthroscopy 10(3):275–280

Byrd JTW (ed) (1998) Operative hip arthroscopy. Thieme, New York

Byrd JTW, Jones SJ (2000) Prospective analysis of hip arthroscopy with 2-year follow-up. Arthroscopy 16(6):578–587

Clarke MT, Arora A, Villar RN (2003) Hip arthroscopy: complications in 1054 cases. Clin Orthop Relat Res 406:84–88

Dienst M, Godde S, Seil R, Hammer D, Kohn D (2001) Hip arthroscopy without traction: in vivo anatomy of the peripheral joint cavity. Arthroscopy 17:924–931

Dorfman H, Boyer T (1999) Arthroscopy of the hip: 12 years of experience. Arthroscopy 15(1):67–72

Eriksson E, Arvidsson I, Arvidsson H (1986) Diagnostic and operative arthroscopy of the hip. Orthopedics 9(2):169–176

Ganz R, Parvizi J, Beck M, Leunig M, Notzli H, Siebenrock KA (2003) Femoroacetabular impingement: a cause for osteoarthritis of the hip. Clin Orthop Relat Res 417:112–120

Gautier E, Ganz K, Krugel N, Gill T, Ganz R (2000) Anatomy of the medial femoral circumflex artery and its surgical implications. J Bone Joint Surg Br 82B(5):679–683

Glick JM, Sampson TG, Gordon RB, Behr JT, Schmidt E (1987) Hip arthroscopy by the lateral approach. Arthroscopy 3(1):4–12

Griffin DR, Villar RN (1999) Complications of arthroscopy of the hip. J Bone Joint Surg Br 81(4):604–606

Heyworth BE, Shindle MK, Voos JE, Rudzki JR, Kelly BT (2007) Radiologic and intraoperative findings in revision hip arthroscopy. Arthroscopy 23(12):1295–1302

Kim SJ, Choi NH, Kim HJ (1998) Operative hip arthroscopy. Clin Orthop Relat Res 353:156–165

Krueger A, Leunig M, Siebenrock KA, Beck M (2007) Hip arthroscopy after previous surgical hip dislocation for femoroacetabular impingement. Arthroscopy 23(12):1285–1289

Mardones RM, Gonzalez C, Chen Q, Zobitz M, Kaufman KR, Trusdale RT (2005) Surgical treatment of femoroacetabular impingement: evaluation of the size of the resection. J Bone Joint Surg Am 87:273–279

Mardones R, Lara J, Donndorff A, Barnes S, Stuart MJ, Glick J, Trousdale R (2009) Surgical correction of "cam-type" femoroacetabular impingement: a cadaveric comparison of open versus arthroscopic debridement. Arthroscopy 25(2):175–182

Philippon MJ, Schenker ML, Briggs KK, Maxwell RB (2008) Can microfracture produce repair tissue in acetabular chondral defects? Arthroscopy 24(1):46–50

Shetty VD, Villar RN (2007) Hip arthroscopy: current concepts and review of the literature. Br J Sports Med 41(2):64–68

Smart LR, Oetgen M, Noonan B, Medvecky M (2007) Beginning hip arthroscopy: indications, positioning, portals, basic technique, and complications. Arthroscopy 23(12):1348–1353

Villar RN (1994) Arthroscopy. BMJ 308(6920):51–53

# What Goes on During the Learning Curve?

# 13

Luís Perez-Carro and Marc Tey

## Introduction

The recent development of the concept of femoroacetabular impingement (FAI) and the surgical options associated with it have opened an exciting new area of inquiry in hip surgery. Hip arthroscopy has gained popularity as its indications have greatly increased. There is no doubt of the relevance of the new arthroscopic techniques to orthopedics. Out of the five instructional courses offered every year by the Spanish Arthroscopy Association, two were on hip arthroscopy in 2008, one in 2007, and none in 2006.

Hip arthroscopy has a steep learning curve, which greatly depends on the surgeon's previous experience. In our courses, we found that half of the surgeons were not really interested in performing hip arthroscopy and just wanted to be briefly acquainted with it, and the other half were really interested in performing hip arthroscopy. Most of these colleagues come from the field of arthroscopy, but others are experienced hip surgeons. The learning curve will vary widely in these two groups.

It is not easy to determine the exact length of the learning curve or when a surgeon can be considered to have completed it. Is it the number of surgeries we need to achieve the result we planned for? Is it the number of surgeries needed to perform the technique as we had planned it? Is it related to completing the procedure in a reasonable length of time? It may be useful to consider that the learning curve is the number of surgeries we need to achieve our surgical goal with a reasonable number of complications. But few articles in the literature provide reports on complications in hip arthroscopy. This is probably due to the fact that the technique was uncommon until recently and to the fact that surgeons are not inclined to talk about their mistakes.

In a panel of experts in hip arthroscopy held during the 2nd international Hip Meeting at Homburg/Saar in 2006, it was suggested that a minimum of 30 surgeries per year was needed to complete an optimal learning curve. We should probably consider the difficulties the surgeon is likely to encounter as he progresses along his learning curve and how he can best overcome them.

Far from being an easy, hip arthroscopy poses serious challenges to the surgeon: Small hips are difficult to scope, and the problems accessing the hip joint with arthroscopic surgical instruments are just an example. In a seminal paper, Villar published that in 18% of the 194 hips included in his study, access was considered difficult, in (2.8%) the joint was inaccessible, and two patients required an arthrotomy (0.2%), one to remove a loose body and the other for debridement where access was not possible [1].

L. Perez-Carro (✉)
Hospital Universitario Marqués de Valdecilla,
Clinica Mompia Santander,
Santander, Spain
e-mail: lpcarro@gmail.com

M. Tey
Department of Orthopedic Surgery and Traumatology,
USP – University Hospital Dexeus,
Barcelona, Spain

Clínica Quirúrgica Onyar de Girona,
Girona, Spain
e-mail: mtey.icatme@idexeus.es

Ó. Marín-Peña (ed.), *Femoroacetabular Impingement*,
DOI 10.1007/978-3-642-22769-1_13, © Springer-Verlag Berlin Heidelberg 2012

# Mistakes, Complications, and Other Pitfalls During the Learning Curve

Mistakes, complications, and pitfalls during the learning curve can be divided into three categories:
1. Preoperative
   Related to indication
   Related to positioning and traction
2. Intraoperative
   Related to portal creation
   Related to instrument introduction
   Procedure specific
   General arthroscopic complications
3. Postoperative
   Related to rehabilitation program

A meta-analysis of the literature analyzing the complications following 2,049 hip arthroscopies revealed a complication rate of 2.2% [2–8], with most of these complications being minor without residual morbidity. These percentages are probably an underestimation as surgeons are usually reluctant to admit their failures and definitely show no enthusiasm about publishing them.

## Preoperative

### Related to Indication

A good indication is the first step leading to a good result in any technique. During the learning curve, it is mandatory to select not only good indications but especially "easy" indications. Some cases of osteoarthritis can be a good indication (release of loose bodies, locked hips due to everted cartilage, or labral tears, etc.) for hip arthroscopy, but may not be ideal during the learning curve. Synovitis and poor joint distraction can make arthroscopy difficult as such procedures increase the risk of cartilage and labral damage and take demand long surgical time, which augments the risk of traction-induced neuroapraxia.

### Recommendation

Initial cases should ideally be thin women, who are more elastic and have narrower joint spaces, presenting with no degenerative changes as this decreases the risk of iatrogeny. Women with hip dysplasia who require a periacetabular osteotomy can be a good choice; it is essential to assess their labrum and cartilage status.

## Related to Positioning and Traction

Access to the hip joint is difficult because of the resistance to distraction resulting from the large muscular sheath, the strength of the iliofemoral ligament, and the negative intra-articular pressure. To access and visualize the central compartment, traction must be applied to the joint, whereas the peripheral compartment is better examined without traction [9]. When performing arthroscopy of the central compartment, it must be remembered that there is a risk of neuropraxia to the perineal region or distal part of the leg, caused by compression of certain neurological structures due to insufficient protection, excessive traction, or increased traction time. There is practically no risk of neuropraxia during arthroscopy of the peripheral compartment. Most of the injuries reported in the literature consisted of a transient neuropraxia that resolved within a few days. The pudendal nerve was the most common site for neuropraxia, but transient neurapraxia of the femoral, sciatic, lateral femoral cutaneous, and peroneal nerves has been described. Eriksson and colleagues [4] also reported on a case of pressure necrosis of the scrotum, and Rodeo described a case of pressure necrosis in the foot [8].

During our learning curve, 15 of our initial cases developed transient pudendal anesthesia because of neuroapraxia. They resolved when counterpost padding of at least 20 cm was used.

### Recommendations

1. The surgeon should be accustomed to performing the technique both with and without traction and should learn to apply the right amount of traction, neither too much nor too little.
2. The patient must be correctly positioned and padded.
3. The distraction force should be minimal; just enough force should be used to provide sufficient space to manipulate the surgical instruments. The traction time should be as short as possible. Intermittent traction (traction for 45 min and release for 10 min) is superior to continuous traction. There is little clarity as to the length of traction although most surgeons suggest that it should not exceed 2 h.
4. Use of an oversized, heavily padded perineal post.
5. General anesthesia should be used in preference to other anesthetic techniques as it enables adequate articular distraction with less traction than is required with other types of anesthesia.

**Fig. 13.1** Limited instrumental motion due to soft tissue thickness

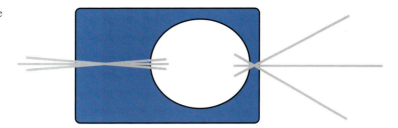

6. A traction test is highly recommended. This is carried out before draping, used to determine the force necessary to achieve adequate distraction of the hip. It is also used to signal the skin landmarks needed to find the entrance to the portals. Traction is released until surgery begins to diminish total length of traction.

## Intraoperative

### Related to Portal Creation and Instrument Introduction

Nerve and vascular injury can also occur secondary to direct laceration and can be avoided by in-depth knowledge of the anatomy and skin landmarks of the hip. The lateral femoral cutaneous nerve, however, is always at risk when the anterior portal is created, and a *nick and spread technique* should, therefore, be used. Even with a meticulous technique, however, neuropraxia has been reported following forceful instrument introduction or removal of large loose bodies [7].

Loss of a portal will usually require a new one to be made. Thus, employing slotted cannulas or flexible guides is useful so as not to lose arthroscopic access when changing portals. Flexible guidewire breakage is always a risk.

An extended capsulotomy starting at the capsular orifice for the portal will give greater mobility both to the arthroscope and to the other instruments used. Nonetheless, capsulotomy causes greater extravasation of irrigation fluid, and this will be aggravated by the use of arthroscopic pumps. Clinical concerns include hip dislocation secondary to extensive capsulotomies and overresection of the anterior acetabular rim in the case of pincer impingement.

The hip is a deep joint, with thick soft tissues around it. This makes portal placement more difficult and more important than in other joints (Fig. 13.1). It is more difficult because there are fewer skin references. It is more important because manageability of the instruments is more limited than in other joints. Many portals have been described, but only the anterolateral portal has been consistently maintained and is used routinely and systematically as the first portal. The other portals described are created depending on the condition to be treated and on the surgeon's preferences and familiarity and experience with each one.

The labrum can be pierced by the spinal needle while attempting to distract the joint. This type of injury can be avoided by removing the needle and reintroducing it into the joint after it has been distended with saline or air. Direct visualization of the needle is helpful to avoid labral damage.

Due to the risk of damage to the lateral femoral cutaneous nerve by the anterior portal, Philippon [10] recommends creating an accessory distal anterior or distal anterior-oblique portal. This portal is located 6–7 cm distally and anteriorly to the anterolateral portal and runs at an angle of about 60° to that portal. The accessory distal anterior portal also provides a good vantage point and a comfortable working angle for resection of the pathological prominence on the head–neck junction of the femur in patients with femoroacetabular impingement. The portals are not always at the same location in different patients. It is important to note that because of limited maneuverability within the hip joint, slight variations in their position are possible and additional portals may even be necessary to provide adequate exposure of the joint. Internal or external rotation of the hip can significantly alter the relationship between the greater trochanter and the femoral head.

### Recommendations

1. Always draw landmarks before draping, during the traction test.
2. Use of distention needle is mandatory. It helps to find the correct space and to avoid the labrum.
3. Anterior portal can be avoided using the accessory distal anterior or anterolateral distal portal instead.

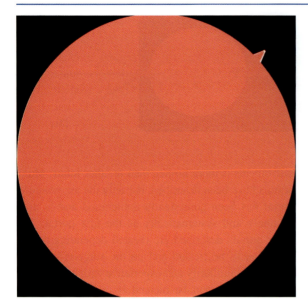

**Fig. 13.2** Red vision

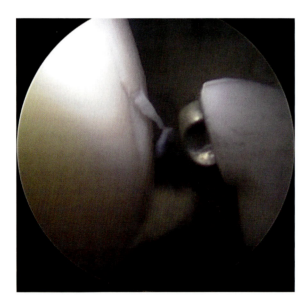

**Fig. 13.3** Femoral head cartilage scuffing

4. Achieve adequate capsulotomies to increase maneuverability and decrease iatrogeny to femoral and acetabular cartilage.

## Procedure Specific
### Red View
"Red view" is a stressful situation after proper placement of the first portal (Fig. 13.2). Structures can be damaged, the second portal cannot be well established,

and it is difficult to view things from only one portal. The clue for resolving the problem is easy: patience. A water pump can be handy, but using one is not always a guarantee that "red view" will not occur at the beginning of the procedure. Establishing two portals with air before starting irrigation serum can be a good trick. Any "red vision" can be easily solved if two portals are used.

### Chondral Damage
Although nerve injury is the most commonly reported complication following hip arthroscopy, most experienced surgeons contend that the single most common complication is actually damage to the articular and labral surfaces secondary to "scope trauma." Scuffing of the femoral head can occur to various extents with or without distraction (Fig. 13.3). Mild scope trauma to the femoral head, however, does not affect outcomes. Poor distraction and synovitis, frequent in degenerative osteoarthritis, may lead to chondral damage during portal placement. Patient positioning and adequate distraction are crucial to avoid this injury.

Patient selection is crucial during the learning curve. Tönnis type 2 and obese patients are at higher risk of chondral damage. Scope trauma can be minimized by training with a 70° scope in an easier articulation, like the knee joint, or in cadaver courses.

### Labral Damage
Examination of the central compartment determines the risk of labral perforation. To avoid labral damage, it is important to reenter the central compartment after initial insufflation of the joint. It is also important to note that when using the anterolateral portal, instruments should always be angled so that they penetrate the capsule below the labrum. The instruments can then be redirected superiorly to avoid scuffing the femoral head. It is also possible for instruments to break if vigorous levering is performed against the resistant envelope that surrounds the hip joint. Passing all arthroscopic instruments into the hip through strong metallic sheaths can help to minimize this complication.

Notwithstanding the above, portal placement can be carried out through labrum (Fig. 13.4). After creation of second portal, inspection of initial portal placement is mandatory. In the event of translabrum portal creation, the portal needs to be redirected and labrum damage should be assessed.

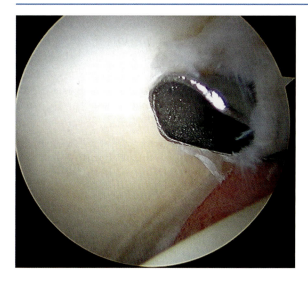

**Fig. 13.4** Translabral portal

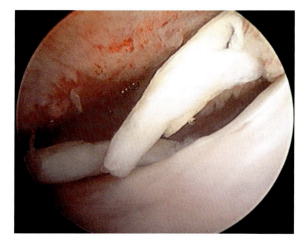

**Fig. 13.5** Articular loose bodies

### Rare But Potential Complications

Other rare but potential complications include heterotopic ossification (HO), avascular necrosis (AVN) of the femoral head, and fluid extravasation. HO is a relatively common complication of open surgery to the hip and pelvis. However, there is only one reported case of HO along the anterior portal tract after hip arthroscopy [11].

Although there have been no reports of AVN as a direct consequence of hip arthroscopy, there are at least two reports of the progression of AVN following arthroscopy [6, 7]. Whether this progression was secondary to the arthroscopic procedure or the natural history of the disease has not been determined.

Fluid extravasation into the pelvis or abdominal regions is an uncommon but potentially devastating complication that has been observed in the lateral decubitus position [12, 13]. To reduce the risk of fluid extravasation, careful attention should be paid to fluid management, especially when excessive OR time is necessary or the hip joint and capsule are compromised.

### Femoroacetabular Impingement

Failure to recognize and treat or incompletely reshape impingement deformities may be the most frequent cause for a second hip arthroscopy and redebridement of the deformity [14].

On the other hand, only one femoral neck fracture following arthroscopic cam remodeling has been reported in a large series of patients.

### Loose Bodies

The need for revision arthroscopy for incomplete removal of loose bodies because of poor intraoperative visualization is the main complication. The peripheral compartment can hold articular loose bodies (Fig. 13.5).

The camera must also be carefully maneuvered posteriorly to view the posterior aspect of the transverse ligament where it inserts into the posteromedial labrum. This is also a site where articular loose bodies can lodge.

### Related to General Arthroscopic Complications

Although infection is a risk with any surgical procedure, the overall incidence of infection after hip arthroscopy is only 0.05%.

In general, therefore, although surgeons should be keenly aware of the potential complications besetting hip arthroscopy, these are relatively uncommon, especially if early experience with hip arthroscopy is excluded.

Portal wound bleeding, portal hematoma, trochanteric bursitis, instrument breakage, and scope trauma are also possible.

## Guidelines to Becoming an Expert Hip Arthroscopist

Skill in arthroscopy is accepted by most surgeons as being directly related to experience. From a practical point of view we can differentiate three stages.

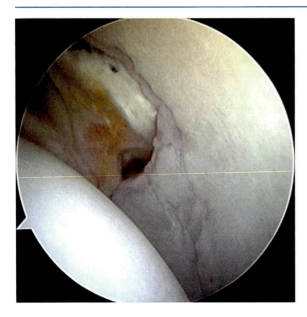

**Fig. 13.6** Triradiate scar

## Stage I

Beginning hip arthroscopy – limited experience with hip arthroscopy/limited exposure to arthroscopy of any joint.

### Recommendations

1. First cases: Performance of diagnostic arthroscopy procedures to evaluate the joint before open hip surgery. Attendance at a cadaveric course before the first diagnostic arthroscopy is highly recommended and should then be repeated after 20 cases have been performed.
2. Indications and contraindications for hip arthroscopy should be noted.
3. Surgeons must have an excellent understanding of patient anatomy and choose the safest approaches for portal insertion.
4. Surgeons must be aware of the normal variants in the hip: A physeal scar (area of old triradiate physis) should not be misinterpreted as an old fracture line. It is important to get used to the normal arthroscopic appearance of the paralabral sulcus, as certain disorders commonly give rise to adhesions at this site, obliterating the sulcus. The distinction between the sublabral sulcus and a labral lesion is not always clear; a labral lesion should be considered when there are compatible symptoms, or when there is an associated image of labral hemorrhage in acute

disorders or granulation tissue indicating attempted healing in chronic disorders [15] (Fig. 13.6).

5. Surgeons must carry out a systematic arthroscopic examination of the central and peripheral compartments of the hip to increase the accuracy and reproducibility of each hip arthroscopy. The use of a standardized, systematic approach ensures that all components of the hip are carefully inspected and makes it possible to document the procedure correctly so that it can be reviewed in the future.

Although the arthroscopic surgical technique is an adaptation of the open surgical procedure, there are a series of steps that are specific to hip arthroscopy and pose special challenges to the surgeon, opening the door to the appearance of complications directly related to these steps [16, 17, 18, 19, 20, 21, 22]. Proper tutelage in animal or cadaver labs can be provided with both a contextually relevant practice environment and the repetitions needed to develop the basic psychomotor skills associated with arthroscopy. In cooperation with anatomy departments, academic program-based arthroscopy-skills laboratories have access to an abundant supply of lightly embalmed anatomic specimens that better retain their life-like state.

## Stage II

Limited experience with hip arthroscopy/experienced arthroscopist in other joints.

### Recommendations

In addition to diagnostic arthroscopy and the recommendations in stage I listed previously, all of the following are reasonable procedures for this surgeon.

- Loose body removal
- Arthroscopic irrigation/debridement of contaminated joints
- Synovial biopsy
- Synovectomy for rheumatoid arthritis, chronic infectious arthritis, or other arthritides
- Labral debridement
- Posttraumatic intra-articular debris

Cadaveric practice, always beneficial becomes essential as surgical indications increase.

Training with simulators considerably improves surgeons' dexterity with arthroscopic instruments, reduces surgery times, increases surgical confidence, and enhances procedure safety, reducing the morbidity

of real interventions and making it possible to gain experience of a large variety of pathologies.

## Stage III

The experienced hip arthroscopist.

Procedures for this surgeon: Same as stage II plus the following:

Hip capsule laxity and instability, chondral lesions, osteochondritis dissecans, ligamentum teres injuries, snapping hip syndrome, iliopsoas bursitis, synovial chondromatosis, management of osteonecrosis of the femoral head, bony impingement, peritrochanteric space disorders, femoroacetabular impingement, adhesive capsulitis, microfracture of selected grade IV articular cartilage lesions (microfractures in the hip are not as easy as in other joints) and labral repair and refixation.

## Recommendations

1. Judicious patient selection: In rare cases, hip arthroscopy can be used to temporize the symptoms of mild-to-moderate hip osteoarthritis with associated mechanical symptoms, but there is moderate evidence from case series reports that the outcomes from hip arthroscopy are poor when the patient has osteoarthritis, and/or severe acetabular chondral damage (grade IV lesions using the Outerbridge classification system).
2. Severe osteoarthritis, large osteophytes surrounding the hip joint, arthrofibrosis, and a history of multiple open hip surgeries are contraindications.
3. Increased attention to the steep learning curve associated with arthroscopy should help minimize the frequency of patient cases with postoperative effusions, chondral lesions, and lengthened operative times.

In our first 100 hip arthroscopies performed for femoroacetabular impingement in the supine position, there was a remarkable decrease in complications from the first 30 cases compared to the remaining 70 operations. Five cases of chondral damage were noted in the first 30 cases, compared to 3 in the remaining 70 cases. The number of perineal injuries was noted to decrease from 5 cases in the first 30 operations to 3 in the subsequent 70 operations.

There was an overall decrease in operative time over the 100 cases, representing a gradual learning process throughout (from an average time of 195 min for the first 30 cases, to the average operative time of 140 min for the remaining 70 cases). We thus believe the learning curve to be 30 operations, but although the exact number of cases necessary is controversial, most surgeons will need a minimum of 100 cases of hip arthroscopy to reach this level III of expertise.

Becoming an Expert Hip Arthroscopist clearly involves a steep learning curve with pitfalls that can be divided into two categories: difficulties and complications.

## References

1. Clarke MT, Arora A, Villar RN (2003) Hip arthroscopy. Complications in 1054 cases. Clin Orthop Relat Res 406:84–88
2. Sampson TG (2001) Complications of hip arthroscopy. Clin Sports Med 20:831–836
3. Sussmann PS, Zumstein M, Hahn F, Dora C (2007) The risk of vascular injury to the femoral head when using the posterolateral arthroscopy portal: cadaveric investigation. Arthroscopy 23:1112–1115
4. Eriksson E, Arvidsson I, Arvidsson H (1986) Diagnostic and operative arthroscopy of the hip. Orthopedics 9:169–176
5. Byrd JWT (2005) Gross anatomy. In: Byrd JWT (ed) Operative hip arthroscopy, 2nd edn. Springer, New York, pp 69–83
6. Glick JM (1990) Complications of hip arthroscopy by the lateral approach. In: Sherman OH, Minkoff J (eds) Current management of complications in orthopaedics. Arthroscopic surgery. Williams and Wilkins, Baltimore, pp 193–201
7. Villar RN (1992) Hip arthroscopy. Butterworth-Heinemann, Oxford
8. Rodeo SA, Forster RA, Weiland AJ (1993) Neurological complications due to arthroscopy. J Bone Joint Surg Am 75A:917–926
9. Dienst M, Gödde S, Seil R, Hammer D, Kohn D (2001) Hip arthroscopy without traction. In vivo anatomy of the peripheral hip joint cavity. Arthroscopy 17:924–931
10. Philippon M (2006) Advances in hip Arthroscopy Meeting. Warwick, UK
11. Beck M, Leunig M, Parvizi J (2004) Anterior femoroacetabular impingement. Part II: midterm results of surgical treatment. Clin Orthop Relat Res 418:67–73
12. Bartlett CS, DiFelice GS, Buly RL, Quinn TJ, Green DS, Helfet DL (1998) Cardiac arrest as a result of intraabdominal extravasation of fluid during arthroscopic removal of a loose body from the hip joint of a patient with an acetabular fracture. J Orthop Trauma 12:294–299
13. Haupt U, Völkle D, Waldherr C, Beck M (2008) Intra- and retroperitoneal irrigation liquid after arthroscopy of the hip joint. Arthroscopy 24:966–968
14. Ilizaliturri VM Jr (2009) Complications of arthroscopic femoroacetabular impingement treatment: a review. Clin Orthop Relat Res 467:760–768, Epub Nov 19, 2008

15. Byrd JWT (1996) Labral lesions: an elusive source of hip pain case reports and literature review. Arthroscopy 12: 603–612

16. Byrd JWT (1994) Hip arthroscopy utilizing the supine position. Arthroscopy 10:275–280

17. Byrd JWT (1998) The supine position. In: Byrd JWT (ed) Operative hip arthroscopy. Thieme, New York, pp 123–138

18. Glick JM, Sampson TG, Gordon RB, Behr JT, Schmidt E (1987) Hip arthroscopy by the lateral approach. Arthroscopy 3:4–12

19. Sampson TG, Farjo L (1998) Hip arthroscopy by the lateral approach. In: Byrd JWT (ed) Operative hip arthroscopy. Thieme, New York, pp 105–122

20. Klapper RC, Dorfmann H, Boyer T (1998) Hip arthroscopy without traction. In: Byrd JWT (ed) Operative hip arthroscopy. Thieme, New York, pp 139–152

21. Miller WE (1985) Learning arthroscopy. South Med J 8:935–940

22. Sweeney HJ (1982) Teaching arthroscopic surgery at the resident level. Orthop Clin North Am 13:255–261

# My Experience of Hip Arthroscopy in the Lateral Position

# 14

Alexandros P. Tzaveas and Richard N. Villar

## Introduction

Femoroacetabular impingement (FAI) was described as early as 1936 by Smith-Petersen [1]. However, only recently it has been considered as a cause of early osteoarthritis of the hip [2, 3]. The mechanism is the abutment of the proximal femur to the anterior acetabular rim, leading to injury of the acetabular labrum and the adjacent acetabular articular cartilage. The aim of the excision of an impingement lesion is dual: the short-term management of pain and the long-term prevention of osteoarthritis.

FAI has originally been treated with open surgery, undertaking a hip dislocation and trochanteric osteotomy, with promising midterm results [4, 5]. The high incidence of FAI in young and active adults, as well as in high-class professional athletes, rendered a minimally invasive technique more attractive, in order to allow, perhaps, a shorter rehabilitation period and a quicker return to sport activities.

## Pre-operative Assessment

History and clinical examination are the main guides for patient selection. The impingement sign [6] is probably the strongest indicator for femoroacetabular

impingement. Extra-articular causes of pain should be excluded.

Routine radiographic examination includes antero-posterior and lateral views of hip joint, and the cross-over sign [7] and alpha angle [8] are evaluated. MRI is always useful not only to assess labrum but also to exclude avascular necrosis of the hip.

## Arthroscopic Treatment of FAI

All patients receive general anaesthetic for the procedure. In our practice, the lateral position for hip arthroscopy, as originally described by Glick et al. [9] is always used. Positioning of the patient is of great importance, not only for the avoidance of any complications but also for the better convenience of the surgeon during the procedure. Traction of the hip is accomplished through use of either the Smith and Nephew Hip Positioning Device (Smith & Nephew, Inc., Endoscopy Division, Andover, Massachusetts) or the McCarthy Hip Distractor (Innomed Inc., Savannah, Georgia, USA).

Special care is taken in the positioning to avoid any potential injuries (Fig. 14.1). The perineum and genitalia should be protected when lateralising the perineal bollard. Special padding is also applied in these regions, but wrinkles in the padding should be eliminated in order to avoid the development of pressure sores; impaction of the testicles or labia majora with the perineal bollard is a not infrequent danger. Contact with any metal parts of the distractor and the correct position of the diathermy plate on the contralateral limb should also be checked. Adequate space should be left between the bollard and the contralateral, underlying

A.P. Tzaveas • R.N. Villar (✉)
The Richard Villar Practice, The Wellington Hospital,
St. John's Wood, London, UK
e-mail: rnv1000@aol.com

Ó. Marín-Peña (ed.), *Femoroacetabular Impingement*,
DOI 10.1007/978-3-642-22769-1_14, © Springer-Verlag Berlin Heidelberg 2012

**Fig. 14.1** Lateral position with the Smith and Nephew Hip Positioning Device. (*1*) perineal bollard covered by padding. (*2*) firm contact of the foot in the boot. (*3*) Vectors showing the direction of lateralisation and traction (*red arrows*) and the resultant vector (*blue*). (*4*) adequate space has been left to prevent pressure on the contralateral limb

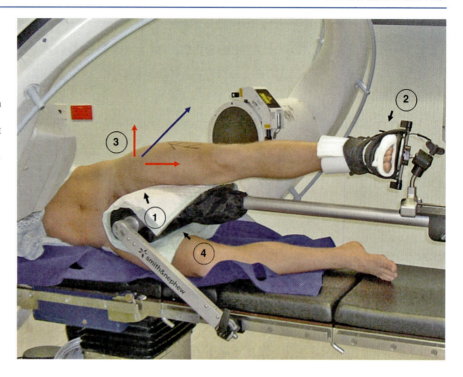

limb in order to avoid pressure ischaemia; the surgeon can check this by placing his hand between bollard and inner thigh. For the operated limb, the foot should be securely fixed by the special boot of the distractor so that it remains tightly bound even when distraction is applied.

The layout in the operating theatre is shown in Fig. 14.2. The surgeon should be able to simultaneously view easily the arthroscopy monitor and the image intensifier screen. The image intensifier is placed obliquely, allowing adequate space for the surgeon, who stands behind the patient. The layout of the instruments on the two trolleys is shown in Fig. 14.3. The deeply situated hip joint, surrounded by dense soft tissues, requires special instrumentation for the arthroscopic procedure. Instruments with extra length have been designed, curved instruments are inserted through slotted cannulae, burrs and shaver blades have been modified, and probes can be deflected to various angles to reach previously inaccessible areas of the joint. We routinely use a 70° arthroscope for both compartments. Occasionally, we use a 30° arthroscope.

The whole procedure is carried out under image intensifier guidance. A shower-type drape is used (Steri-Drape Ioban 2, Large Isolation Drape with Ioban 2 Incise Film and Pouch, 3 M Health Care, St. Paul,

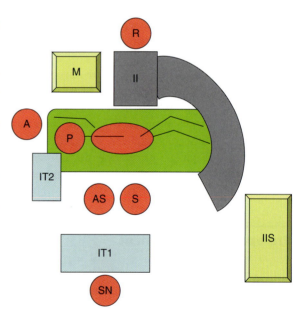

**Fig. 14.2** Layout of the operating theatre for arthroscopy of the right hip. *P* patient, *A* anaesthetist, *S* surgeon, *AS* assistant surgeon, *SN* scrub nurse, *IT1* instrument table 1, *IT2* instrument table 2, *M* monitor, *IIS* image intensifier screen, *II* image intensifier, *R* radiographer

MN, USA). A fluid pump is used throughout the operation (Fluid Management System Control Unit, Dyonics 25, Smith and Nephew, Inc., Andover, MA,

**Fig. 14.3** General layout of the instruments at instrument table 1 (**a**) and 2 (**b**), before surgery commences

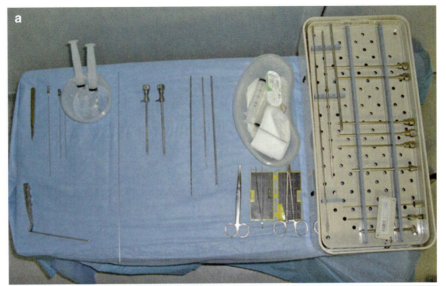

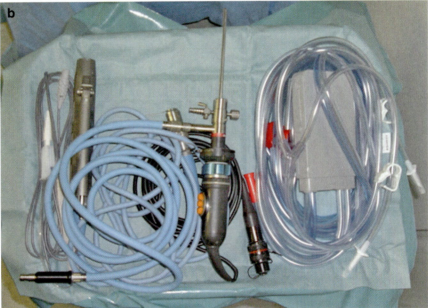

USA). We routinely add 1 mg of adrenaline to 3 L of irrigation fluid (saline) in order to reduce the chance of haemorrhage.

## Technique

Before passing instruments into the joint, the ability to distract the hip should be confirmed with the image intensifier. While the surgeon is unscrubbed, traction is applied with simultaneous palpation of the abductors at their greater trochanteric attachment, until the vacuum sign [10] appears (Fig. 14.4), which shows the negative intra-articular pressure. If the vacuum sign does not appear, the patient's position is checked as well as the foot placement in the special boot, to confirm that there is no loosening, and then traction is re-applied. After a vacuum sign appears, the traction is then released, to minimise its total duration, and preparation and draping are performed by the scrub nurse while the surgeon scrubs. When all instrumentation is ready, traction is then reapplied. In cases with a joint effusion, synovitis or degenerative change, the vacuum sign may not appear. Should this occur it is best to

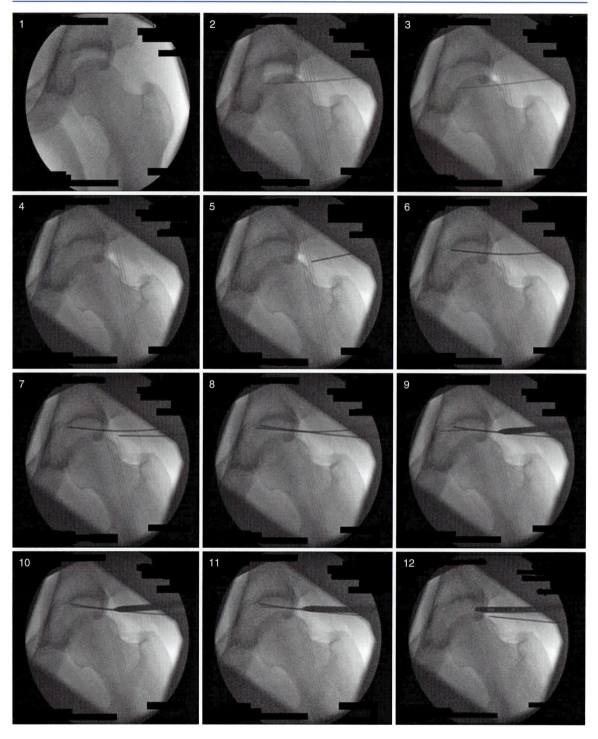

**Fig. 14.4** The full sequence of image intensifier images showing the insertion of needles and creation of portals. (*1*) The vacuum sign above the femoral head after traction has been applied, (*2*) insertion of the first needle (18-G), (*3*) saline instillation diminishes the white area, (*4*) 40 mL of saline has been injected, the joint has been distended and a small white area remains, showing the area inferolateral to the labrum, (*5*) a 17-G needle is inserted into the hip joint while keeping close to the femoral head, in order to miss the labrum, (*6*) the 17-G needle has been placed successfully, (*7*) insertion of a second 17-G needle, (*8*) the second 17-G needle has been placed successfully, (*9*) a blunt guide wire is passed down the first 17-G needle, the needle is removed, and a 4.5 mm cannulated trocar is passed over the guide wire, (*10*) the guide wire is pulled outwards slightly, in order to avoid its breakage against the acetabular floor on insertion of the trocar, (*11*) the trocar is pushed into the joint, (*12*) the trocar has been removed, and the arthroscope has been inserted through the cannula

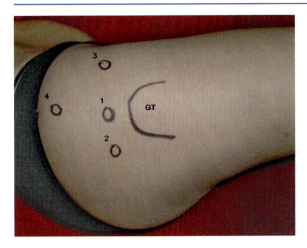

**Fig. 14.5** Representation of the portals. *GT* greater trochanter, *(1)* the supratrochanteric portal for the first needle and the saline injection, *(2)* posterior paratrochanteric portal for camera (*central compartment*), *(3)* anterolateral portal for instruments (*central and peripheral compartments*), *(4)* portal used for camera (*peripheral compartment*), forming an equilateral triangle with the other two

proceed directly to needle insertion, which may itself create a vacuum sign.

A long needle (18 G – 1.2 mm × 205 mm) is inserted into the hip through a supratrochanteric portal (Fig. 14.5), under image intensifier guidance, and the trocar is then removed. An audible 'hiss' is occasionally heard as air passes into the joint and the hip distracts, showing an air arthrogram on the screen. Then, 20–40 mL of normal saline is injected to cause distention. The elimination of the air arthrogram confirms the saline instillation, and a new image will show the articular space to be widened. The first needle is removed, and two shorter needles (17 G – 1.4 mm × 45 mm) are inserted, anteriorly and posteriorly to the entry point of the first needle, creating the two primary portals for the central compartment (Fig. 14.5). Caution is needed to avoid piercing the labrum at this stage: it is recommended to insert the needles more distally, aiming superiorly; another tip is to enter the joint through the 'white' area formed by the arthrogram, and not higher (Fig. 14.4). Piercing of the labrum creates a feeling of increased resistance during needle insertion, whereas piercing of the joint capsule is much smoother. The posterior paratrochanteric portal is used for arthroscope insertion and the anterolateral portal for the instruments. Clustering of these portals is a common pitfall for inexperienced arthroscopists, a distance of 4–5 cm between portals being adequate. Triangulation of these needles can be tricky. The positioning of the posterior paratrochanteric

needle is critical as its path will dictate the subsequent track of the arthroscope. For the anterolateral portal, some surgeons might choose to use an arthroscopic aiming device, although this is not an instrument used widely in the senior author's (RNV) practice. A long, blunt-ended, flexible Nitinol guidewire is next passed through the posterior needle, and the needle is then removed. A stab incision is then made around the base of the guidewire, and a cannulated 4.5 mm arthroscopy trocar and cannula are passed over the guidewire with gentle pushing and twisting movements. Withdrawing the guidewire by a few millimetres before inserting the trocar is helpful and may prevent possible breakage. Once in the joint the trocar and guidewire are removed and a 70° arthroscope is inserted. The position of the anterior needle can then be seen and adjusted accordingly. Once access has been gained anteriorly, a wide capsulotomy is made, connecting the two portals, and using a combination of sharp and radiofrequency dissection.

A systematic inspection of the central compartment is then performed, by viewing the labrum, acetabular articular cartilage, cotyloid fossa, ligamentum teres, anterior and posterior stellate creases, transverse ligament and central compartment portion of femoral head. We treat labral tears with partial labrectomy or repair, according to the configuration of the lesion. We perform direct labral repair, when indicated, with the employment of special sutures (FasT-Fix Suture System, Smith and Nephew, Inc., Andover, MA, USA). Labral reattachment, if performed, is undertaken using the Bioraptor anchor system (Bioraptor, Smith & Nephew Endoscopy, Andover, MA). Chondral defects are treated with a microfracture technique. In cases with a labral tear combined with chondral delamination, or chondral delamination alone, we use the microfracture technique combined with fibrin adhesive (Tisseel Kit, Baxter Healthcare Ltd, Norfolk, UK) in order to secure the articular cartilage to the underlying subchondral bone. Occasionally, we shrink a partially torn ligamentum teres with a radiofrequency probe.

In cases with a pincer-type impingement lesion, we aim to trim the ossified labrum or the acetabular rim beneath the labrum, by an acetabular recession (Fig. 14.6) while keeping the labrum still attached to the acetabular margin. This is performed while in the central compartment. We aim to visualise the area immediately anterior to the anterior acetabular labrum. Using a radiofrequency probe, all soft tissue adjacent to the anterior surface of the anterior acetabular labrum is removed developing the paralabral sulcus. At the

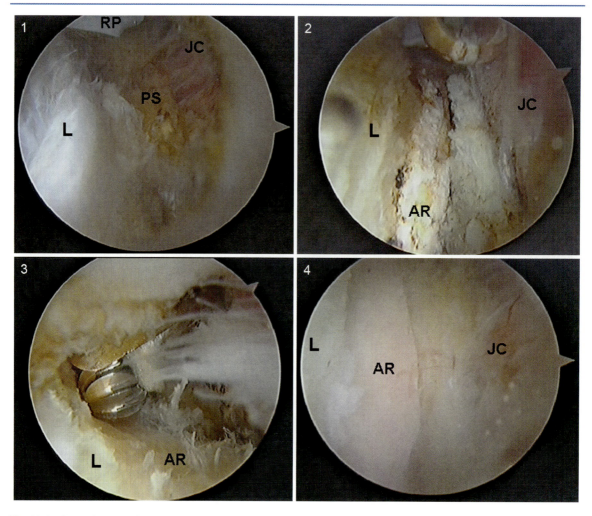

**Fig. 14.6** (*1*) Development of the perilabral sulcus with a radiofrequency probe, (*2*) the acetabular rim has been exposed, (*3*) the acetabular rim is trimmed with an arthroscopic burr, (*4*) the pincer lesion has been excised (*L* labrum, *RP* radiofrequency probe, *PS* perilabral sulcus, *JC* joint capsule, *AR* acetabular rim)

bottom of this area lies the bony acetabular rim. Special care is taken to avoid damaging the labrum itself. Upon identification of the bony acetabular rim, a 4.0 mm burr (DYONICS POWER, abrader burr, Smith and Nephew, Inc., Andover, MA, USA) is used for the recession. The use of an image intensifier is essential at this stage for the inspection of the recessed area (Fig. 14.7). If the labrum becomes detached during this process, it can be formally reattached using bone anchors [11].

Upon completion of the procedure in the central compartment, all instruments are removed, traction is released, and the hip is brought into 30° of flexion. A 17-G needle is used to gain access to the peripheral compartment using an entry point which is located superior to the two earlier portals, forming an equilateral triangle with them (Fig. 14.5). The needle is aimed

towards the femoral head–neck junction under image intensifier control; when the tip of the needle touches this area, the needle direction is changed, heading more anteriorly. The needle stylus is then removed, and backflow of saline confirms the position in the anterior peripheral compartment. It is occasionally possible to enter the posterior peripheral compartment by mistake. However, once in the anterior peripheral compartment, the arthroscope is then inserted through this portal using the guidewire-trocar combination as in the central compartment. For operating instruments, a second 17-G needle is inserted through the original anterolateral portal, the image intensifier being used for accurate triangulation. Essentially, the tip of the second needle should be approximated to the tip of the arthroscope on the image intensifier screen. Once this

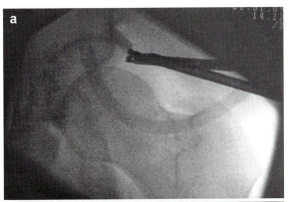

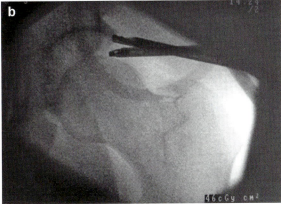

**Fig. 14.7** Pincer lesion. (**a**) The position of instruments is confirmed with an image intensifier, (**b**) trimming of the pincer lesion underway

is achieved, the second portal is complete, and any required operating instruments may be passed into the peripheral compartment. These portals, which may be interchanged as required, give good access to the femoral head–neck junction, the non-weight-bearing portion of the femoral head, the anterior capsule, the medial synovial fold and the zona orbicularis. After systematic observation of the whole peripheral compartment, an assistant flexes and rotates the joint in order to confirm the existence of FAI, the limb then being returned to 30° of hip flexion.

A further capsulotomy is critical at this stage, as well as dividing the zona orbicularis. This latter structure can limit the movement of instruments quite significantly until it has been divided. The next step is to delineate the true margins of the impingement lesion with a 90° radiofrequency probe (VULCAN SAPHYRE II, bipolar ablation probe – suction, Smith and Nephew, Inc., Andover, MA, USA), which denudes the bony prominence of all soft tissue. A 4.0 mm burr is then used for excision of the impingement lesion (DYONICS POWER, abrader burr, Smith and Nephew, Inc., Andover, MA, USA). A larger diameter burr may also be used but can sometimes create a significant quantity of debris which may obscure arthroscopic vision. The depth of resection is usually a minimum of about 5 mm, using the diameter of the burr as reference. The excision is continued (Fig. 14.8) until there is no evidence

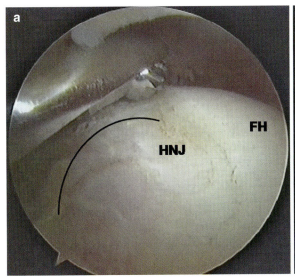

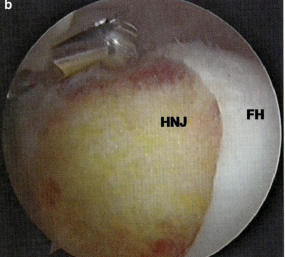

**Fig. 14.8** (**a**) Cam-type lesion (*FH* femoral head, *HNJ* head-neck junction). Black curved line showing the '*bump*'. (**b**) Post-resection of the lesion with the burr (*FH* femoral head, *HNJ* head–neck junction)

of impingement on hip movements. Distally, the resection is brought flush with the anterior cortex of the femur. The radiofrequency probe is then used for haemostasis of the resected bony surface.

Once the procedure is complete, the joint is thoroughly irrigated and local anaesthetic (bupivacaine plain 0.25%) or hyaluronic acid (60 mg) or both are instilled into the joint. The skin incisions are closed with interrupted nylon sutures, and dry dressings are applied. Pre-operatively, all patients are warned that there is a 5% possibility their symptoms may become worse after surgery, and a small chance that it will be impossible to gain access to the joint at all.

## Post-operative Rehabilitation

All patients are told that a long rehabilitation is likely to follow, ranging between 3 and 4 months. Touch weight-bearing is advised for the first 4 weeks, with the use of crutches. Hip flexion of more than 90° and extreme rotational movements are not allowed for this period. Physiotherapy input is essential, and patients attend 1–2 sessions weekly, according to their general progress. Isometric, core exercises and swimming are allowed during the first 6 post-operative weeks; range-of-movement exercises, stationary bicycle and cross-trainer are encouraged between 6 and 12 weeks after surgery. High-impact exercises are not recommended until the 3-month point.

## Results

A recent study conducted in our practice assessed the effect of femoral osteoplasty [12]. Two groups of patients were included: a study group of 24 patients (24 hips) with a cam-type FAI lesion who underwent excision of their lesion, and a control group of 47 patients (47 hips) who underwent an arthroscopic debridement but without excision of their impingement lesion. In both groups, the presence of FAI was confirmed on pre-operative plain radiographs. By the 1-year post-operative assessment, and using a modified Harris hip score, there was a statistically significant improvement in the osteoplasty group. It was concluded that additional symptomatic improvement may be obtained after hip arthroscopy for femoroacetabular impingement with the inclusion of femoral osteoplasty.

The peripheral compartment should not be ignored during surgery for FAI.

## Conclusions

For more than two decades, the lateral position has been extensively used in our practice for hip arthroscopic surgery and has proved very useful. Access to both the central and peripheral compartment can be easily achieved by an experienced arthroscopist, allowing inspection of all structures. A variety of procedures can be performed, the image intensifier can be easily used, and instruments do not fall to the floor when the surgeon removes his hands from them. That said, the authors realise that equally effective hip arthroscopic surgery may be performed with the patient in the supine position. There is a matter of surgical preference, nothing less and nothing more.

## References

1. Smith-Petersen MN (1936) Treatment of malum coxae senilis, old slipped upper femoral epiphysis, intrapelvic protrusion of the acetabulum, and coxa plana, by means of acetabuloplasty. J Bone Joint Surg Am 18:869–880
2. Ito K, Minka MA 2nd, Leunig M, Werlen S, Ganz R (2001) Femoroacetabular impingement and the cam-effect. A MRI-based quantitative anatomical study of the femoral head-neck offset. J Bone Joint Surg Br 83:171–176
3. Ganz R, Parvizi J, Beck M, Leunig M, Nötzli H, Siebenrock KA (2003) Femoroacetabular impingement: a cause for osteoarthritis of the hip. Clin Orthop Relat Res 417:112–120
4. Ganz R, Gill TJ, Gautier E, Ganz K, Krügel N, Berlemann U (2001) Surgical dislocation of the adult hip a technique with full access to the femoral head and acetabulum without the risk of avascular necrosis. J Bone Joint Surg Br 83:1119–1124
5. Beck M, Leunig M, Parvizi J, Boutier V, Wyss D, Ganz R (2004) Anterior femoroacetabular impingement: part II. Midterm results of surgical treatment. Clin Orthop Relat Res 418:67–73
6. Klaue K, Durnin CW, Ganz R (1991) The acetabular rim syndrome. A clinical presentation of dysplasia of the hip. J Bone Joint Surg Br 73:423–429
7. Reynolds D, Lucas J, Klaue K (1999) Retroversion of the acetabulum: a cause of hip pain. J Bone Joint Surg Br 81:281–288
8. Notzli HP, Wyss TF, Stoecklin CH, Schmid MR, Treiber K, Hodler J (2002) The contour of the femoral head-neck junction as a predictor for the risk of anterior impingement. J Bone Joint Surg Br 84:556–560
9. Glick JM, Sampson TG, Gordon RB, Behr JT, Schmidt E (1987) Hip arthroscopy by the lateral approach. Arthroscopy 3:4–12

10. Griffin DR, Villar RN (1999) Complications of arthroscopy of the hip. J Bone Joint Surg Br 81:604–606
11. Khanduja V, Villar RN (2006) Arthroscopic surgery of the hip: current concepts and recent advances. J Bone Joint Surg Br 88:1557–1566
12. Bardakos NV, Vacsoncelos JC, Villar RN (2008) Early outcome of hip arthroscopy for femoroacetabular impingement: the role of femoral osteoplasty in symptomatic improvement. J Bone Joint Surg Br 90(12):1570–1575

# Arthroscopic Treatment of FAI: Supine Position, My First Option

Marcelo Quieroz, Katrina DelaTorre, and Bryan T. Kelly

## Introduction

The concept of femoroacetabular impingement has been popularized by Ganz et al. as mechanical cause of hip pain and the development of osteoarthritis in the hip [1]. Contact resulting from the loss of anterior offset at the femoral head–neck junction has been termed "cam impingement," and contact due to increased coverage of the anterior aspect of the acetabulum has been termed "pincer impingement."

Cam impingement is due to a loss of the normal sphericity of the femoral head either from congenital, developmental, or posttraumatic changes in the shape of the proximal femur (Fig. 15.1).

The deformity usually occurs at the anterolateral aspect of the junction between the femoral head and neck, but can occur in any location around the circumference of the hip. Cam impingement results in a characteristic injury pattern to the transition zone cartilage of the acetabulum, where the labrum loses its structural attachment to the adjacent hyaline cartilage. In cases of pure CAM impingement, the labrum itself may be spared from injury.

Pincer impingement results from over coverage of the acetabulum resulting in a specific pattern of labral degeneration as the overhanging bone on the acetabulum crushes the labrum during movement resulting in one or more cleavage planes of variable depth within the substance of the labrum (Fig. 15.2).

Several subtypes of pincer morphology have been identified: anterosuperior overhang, coxa profunda, acetabular protrusio, and acetabular retroversion [2]. The pattern of damage seen in pincer impingement consists of intrasubstance delamination, cystic degeneration, and tearing of the labrum anterosuperiorly and has been termed a type II tear by Seldes et al. [3]. With repetitive injury, ossification of the labrum can occur resulting in further bony abutment against an even more prominent rim. Also, there can be an associated contrecoup lesion in the posterior inferior chondral surfaces of the hip joint [1]. The majority of cases involve a combination of both rim and cam impingement.

The labrum has been shown by Ferguson to protect the integrity of the hip joint by functioning as a fluid seal for the hip. By enabling fluid to stay within the joint, it reduces friction and contact stresses in the joint (Fig. 15.3).

The labrum also provides translational stability to the hip joint during motion [4–6]. Loss of this sealing function has been shown to increase cartilage consolidation due to decreases in the protective hydrostatic pressure provided by the indwelling synovial fluid. Repetitive contact between the femoral head and the acetabulum in impingement leads to the previously described injury pattern to the acetabular labrum, the adjacent transition zone cartilage, and ultimately leads to a progressive deterioration of the articular cartilage within the joint. Due to the mechanical effects of the bony impingement in conjunction with the damage to the labrum, patients with FAI have an increased risk for the development of hip arthritis requiring hip replacement.

Appropriate treatment of this mechanical process and refixation of any viable labral tissue is now recommended in symptomatic young adults. An initial trial

M. Quieroz • K.D. Torre • B.T. Kelly (✉)
Department of Orthopedic Surgery,
Hospital for Special Surgery,
New York, NY, USA
e-mail: kad9021@nyp.org

**Fig. 15.1** Three-dimensional reconstruction CT scan demonstrating an aspherical femoral head at the typical anterolateral location between the 1 o'clock (*superolateral*) and 4 o'clock (*inferomedial*) positions at the head–neck junction

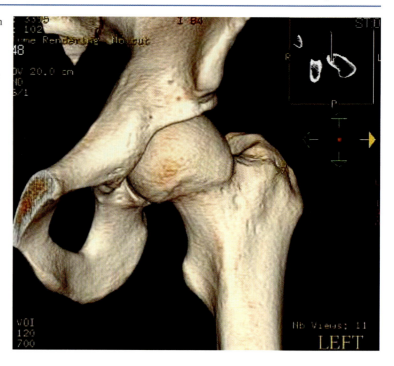

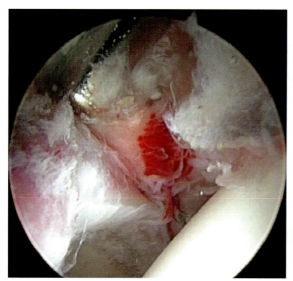

**Fig. 15.2** Arthroscopic image of a crushed labrum secondary to a pincer lesion. The primary injury in rim impingement results in intrasubstance damage to the labrum

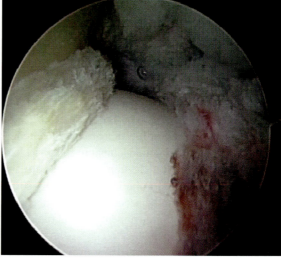

**Fig. 15.3** Demonstration of the suction seal effect of the labrum as the femoral head is brought back into the concavity of the acetabulum during preparation for evaluation in the peripheral compartment

of conservative management may be attempted prior to surgical intervention. Conservative management consists of activity restriction or modification and non-steroidal anti-inflammatory medications. Physical therapy strategies should focus on treating associated periarticular muscle dysfunction that may be present. Due to the young, athletic profile of patients suffering

from femoroacetabular impingement, and the increased association with progressive chondral damage, conservative treatment, in general, renders high rates of failure, especially in the setting of mechanical symptoms.

Surgical treatment can be performed through the traditional open approach using surgical dislocation [1], the mini-anterior approach, and through appropriate arthroscopic techniques [7, 8]. Arthroscopy requires significant technical expertise, and should be reserved for patients with cam lesions in the anterior aspect of the head–neck junction, and small pincer lesions with associated labral pathology [9]. If the patient has bony deformity that is not accessible by the surgeon, or if there are other associated bony abnormalities that are not correctable by arthroscopy, then alternative surgical approaches should be strongly considered [10]. Failure of arthroscopic techniques for FAI are most commonly associated with incomplete decompression of the associated bony anatomy [11].

## Surgical Technique

Hip arthroscopy can be performed in either the supine or the lateral position [12]. The positioning of the patient is based upon surgeon preference as there are pros and cons to each approach [13]. The most important factor is consistency and comfort level by the surgeon and the ancillary staff as the majority of complications associated with hip arthroscopy are associated with patient positioning and traction. Complications have been reported to be between 1% and 6% of cases with the most common reported complications involving neuropraxias affecting the lateral femoral cutaneous and pudendal nerves. The standard portals that are used are the anterolateral peritrochanteric, posterolateral peritrochanteric, and anterior or mid-anterior portals. Anatomical studies have demonstrated that the anterior portal has the greatest risk for nerve injury due to its close proximity to the lateral femoral cutaneous nerve. A variety of other portals have been described and are useful for more advanced technical procedures [14, 15]. Both 70° and 30° arthroscopes are helpful throughout specific procedures.

## Positioning and Assessment

The goal of surgery is adequate decompression of both the rim and cam impingement lesions, debridement of all nonviable labral tissue, refixation of all viable labral tissue, and treatment of associated chondral injury with either debridement and/or microfracture. Our preference is positioning in the supine position. The feet are well padded, and an extra-large perineal cushion is used to optimize distraction of the hip joint with the least amount of traction. Adequate traction typically

requires between 25 and 50 lb of force [16]. The force necessary for distraction can be reduced by releasing the vacuum within the joint with arthrocentesis and injecting saline into the joint. Traction is applied under direct fluoroscopic visualization. Adequate distraction is confirmed with fluoroscopic visualization of approximately 10 mm of joint space widening in the antero-posterior plane. The general position of the operative limb is 20° of flexion, neutral adduction, and maximal internal rotation. Gentle traction is also applied to the contralateral limb to provide counterforce. Minor variations in the specific position of the hip joint with regard to flexion and extension, abduction and adduction, and internal and external rotation, have been published.

The main advantage of the lateral position is that fat drops away from operative sight when the patient is placed on the side [17]. As in the supine position, a fracture table is required to apply the necessary joint distraction. The principles of joint distraction are identical in both positions. Compared with the supine position in which the anterior portal is often used, the lateral position provides comfortable access to the hip joint via just the anterolateral and posterolateral portals. Principles of portal placement and arthroscopic technique do not vary with position, and the choice of set-up is based primarily on surgeon preference and training. Traction attachments are now available so that standard operating tables can be used in the surgery center setting.

Surgery is initiated in the central compartment with the hip in traction. Entry into the central compartment is performed by inserting a 70° arthroscope through the anterolateral portal using fluoroscopic assistance. The posterolateral peritrochanteric and anterior portals can then be established under direct visualization to avoid iatrogenic injury to the labrum or the cartilage surfaces. The mid-anterior portal is helpful to access the central compartment in patients with acetabular retroversion, pincer impingement, and profunda.

## Treatment of the Labrum

The first step in arthroscopic treatment of impingement is to evaluate the pattern and location of labral pathology as this dictates the treatment of the associated bony pathology. An assessment of viable versus nonviable labral pathology will determine whether or not any portion of the labrum can be refixed. Degenerative or

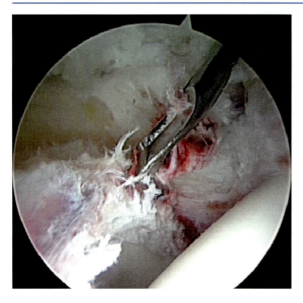

**Fig. 15.4** Nonviable labral tissue is debrided with the goal of maintaining as much healthy tissue as possible so that the suction seal effect can be reestablished

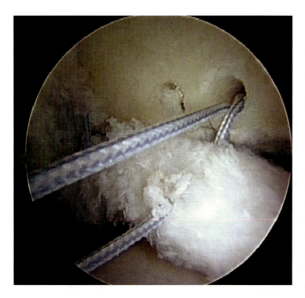

**Fig. 15.5** Passage of the suture from the base of the labrum to the tip of the labrum prevents eversion of the tissue and abrasion of the suture material against the articular surface

injured labral tissue is debrided of all nonviable tissue using extra-long arthroscopic shaver instrumentation (Fig. 15.4).

Labral tears localized laterally are most easily addressed with the 70° arthroscope in the anterior or mid-anterior portal while passing instruments through the anterolateral or posterolateral portal. Medial tears are addressed while viewing from the anterolateral portal and passing instruments through the anterior or mid-anterior portal. If the labral tissue is robust and is amenable to repair, the acetabular bed is first debrided to bleeding bone using an arthroscopic motorized burr [18]. Fluoroscopy is used to aid in proper suture anchor placement at the edge of the acetabulum. Once the anchor is placed and fixation strength is assessed, the suture is passed through the labral tissue using either an arthroscopic suture penetrator or other suture shuttling techniques. The suture should be passed from the base of the labrum at the bone interface to the tip of the labrum (Fig. 15.5).

The suture is tied on the capsular surface to avoid eversion of the labrum and articular cartilage abrasion from the suture material.

## Rim Decompression

Acetabular rim impingement is caused by either excessive acetabular retroversion or a "pincer" lesion that causes excessive contact of the acetabulum against the anterior femoral neck at extremes of motion of the hip joint. This type of lesion causes a characteristic crushing injury to the labrum against the femoral neck and is usually associated with a compressed, degenerative, or cystic labrum. The anterior portal can serve as the viewing portal to address pincer lesions located at the 12 o'clock position moving posteriorly on the face of the acetabulum. For lesions located more anteriorly and medially, the anterolateral portal serves as the best viewing portal. The pincer lesion is identified arthroscopically by probing the margins of the lesion with a flexible instrument (Fig. 15.6).

There are two ways in which the pincer lesion can be resected: First, the overlying labrum can be sharply incised and detached off the pincer lesion and protected while the pincer lesion is resected using an arthroscopic burr or shaver. Once the pincer lesion is excised, the labrum is reattached to the underlying acetabulum using labrum repair techniques as previously described. Second, the pincer lesion can be resected by cutting the capsule using a radiofrequency tissue ablator overlying the pincer

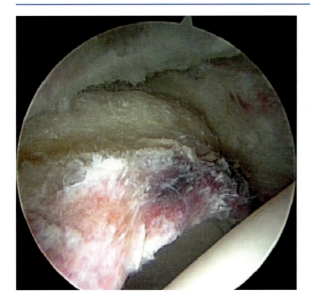

**Fig. 15.6** Arthroscopic visualization of the rim impingement lesion from the anterolateral portal. Fluoroscopic imaging is useful to confirm the location of the lesion and appropriate size and depth of resection

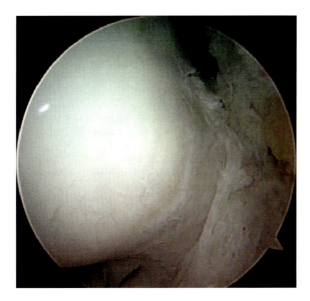

**Fig. 15.7** Arthroscopic visualization of the anterolateral cam lesion as seen from the peripheral compartment. Complete demarcation of the borders of the lesion is necessary to perform an adequate decompression

lesion without detachment of the labrum. Once the underlying bone is exposed, the pincer lesion is resected using either an arthroscopic burr or shaver. Both techniques should use fluoroscopic imaging to confirm the appropriate location and degree of bony resection. The goal is to restore the normal relationship between the anterior and posterior walls of the acetabulum.

## Cam Decompression

Treatment of the cam lesion is performed with the hip out of traction [19]. The location of the asphericity must be clearly delineated preoperatively using appropriate imaging tools. Arthroscopy can adequately access lesions present in the anterior aspect of the head–neck junction between the 12 (superolateral) and 6 o'clock (inferomedial) positions (Fig. 15.7).

Superolateral cam lesions are best decompressed with the hip in extension and internal rotation. Inferomedial lesions are best decompressed with the hip at 45° of flexion and external rotation. The surgical goal of decompression of the femoral head–neck junction (cam decompression) is restoration of the normal head–neck junction offset and clearance of the femoral head within the acetabulum with full flexion and rotation. Cadaver studies have proven that hip arthroscopy affords excellent visualization of the femoral head–neck junction, and osteoplasty can be performed with results comparable to those of the open procedure [20].

Once the size and location of the cam lesion are verified, the hip is appropriately positioned, and a 5.5 mm burr is introduced through a second portal. The boundaries of the cam impingement lesion are marked out, and then sequential removal of the cam lesion is performed to recreate a spherical femoral head. On completion of the bone resection, all bone debris are removed from the peripheral compartment, and dynamic arthroscopy and fluoroscopy are performed to confirm the absence of any residual impingement. A resection of less than 30% of the head–neck junction is recommended because this has shown to preserve the load-bearing capacity of the femoral neck (Fig. 15.8).

Good results have been reported in the literature for patients treated arthroscopically for labral tears and associated femoroacetabular impingement, with as high as 93% of patients able to return to sports and 78% able to remain active at 1.5 years after surgery [21].

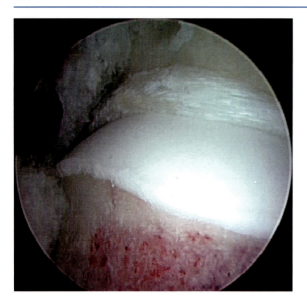

**Fig. 15.8** Completed bony resection of the cam lesion. The suction seal of the labrum is maintained. Dynamic arthroscopy and fluoroscopic imaging on multiple planes will confirm the adequacy of the resection

## References

1. Ganz R et al (2003) Femoroacetabular impingement, a cause for osteoarthritis of the hip. Clin Orthop Relat Res 417: 112–120
2. Beck M, Kalhor M, Leunig M, Ganz R (2005) Hip morphology influences the pattern of damage to the acetabular cartilage: femoroacetabular impingement as a cause of early osteoarthritis of the hip. J Bone Joint Surg Br 87: 1012–1018
3. Seldes RS et al (2001) Anatomy, histologic features, and vascularity of the adult acetabular labrum. Clin Orthop Relat Res 382:232–240
4. Ferguson SJ, Bryant R, Ganz R, Ito K (2000) The influence of the acetabular labrum on hip joint cartilage consolidation: a poroelastic finite element model. J Biomech 33:953–960
5. Ferguson SJ, Bryant JT, Ganz R, Ito K (2003) An in vitro investigation of the acetabular labral seal in hip joint mechanics. J Biomech 36:171–178
6. Ferguson SJ, Bryant JT, Ito K (2001) The material properties of the bovine acetabular labrum. J Orthop Res 19:887–896
7. Philippon MJ et al (2007) Arthroscopic management of femoroacetabular impingement: osteoplasty technique and literature review. Am J Sports Med 35:1571–1580
8. Guanche CA, Bare AA (2006) Arthroscopic treatment of femoroacetabular impingement. Arthroscopy 22(1):95–106
9. Kelly BT, Williams RJ 3rd, Philippon MJ (2003) Hip arthroscopy: current indications, treatment options, and management issues. Am J Sports Med 31(6):1020–1037
10. Wenger DE et al (2004) Acetabular labral tears rarely occur in the absence of bony abnormalities. Clin Orthop Relat Res 126:145–150
11. Heyworth BE, Shindle MK, Voos JE, Rudzki JR, Kelly BT (2007) Radiologic and intraoperative findings in revision hip arthroscopy. Arthroscopy 23(12):1295–1302
12. Byrd JW (2001) Hip arthroscopy. The supine position. Clin Sports Med 20(4):703–731; Byrd JW (1994) Hip arthroscopy utilizing the supine position. Arthroscopy 10(3):275–280
13. Mason JB, McCarthy JC, O'Donnell J, Barsoum W, Mayor MB, Busconi BD et al (2003) Hip arthroscopy: surgical approach, positioning, and distraction. Clin Orthop Relat Res 406:29–37
14. Robertson WJ, Kelly BT (2008) The safe zone for hip arthroscopy: a cadaveric assessment of central, peripheral, and lateral compartment portal placement. Arthroscopy 24(9):1019–1026
15. Byrd JW, Pappas JN, Pedley MJ (1995) Hip arthroscopy: an anatomic study of portal placement and relationship to the extra-articular structures. Arthroscopy 11(4):418–423
16. Dienst M, Seil R, Godde S, Brang M, Becker K, Georg T et al (2002) Effects of traction, distension, and joint position on distraction of the hip joint: an experimental study in cadavers. Arthroscopy 18(8):865–871
17. Glick JM, Sampson TG, Gordon RB, Behr JT, Schmidt E (1987) Hip arthroscopy by the lateral approach. Arthroscopy 3(1):4–12
18. Kelly BT, Weiland DE, Schenker ML, Philippon MJ (2005) Arthroscopic labral repair in the hip: surgical technique and review of the literature. Arthroscopy 21(12):1496–1504
19. Dienst M, Godde S, Seil R, Hammer D, Kohn D (2001) Hip arthroscopy without traction: in vivo anatomy of the peripheral hip joint cavity. Arthroscopy 17(9):924–931
20. Sussmann PS, Ranawat AS, Lipman J, Lorich DG, Padgett DE, Kelly BT (2007) Arthroscopic versus open osteoplasty of the head-neck junction: a cadaveric investigation. Arthroscopy 23(12):1257–1264
21. Bedi A, Chen N, Robertson W, Kelly BT (2008) The management of labral tears and femoroacetabular impingement of the hip in the young, active patient. Arthroscopy 24(10): 1135–1145

# Complications and Revision Surgery in Hip Arthroscopy

# 16

Bruno G.S. e Souza and Marc J. Philippon

## Complications

The development of hip arthroscopy began in the early 1930s, with Burman [1], although it was given little attention until the 1980s, when new approaches, specific techniques, and instruments were developed. This delay can be partially attributed to the difficulties that the anatomical characteristics of the hip joint presented to the surgeon [2]. Many complications seen at that time were related to the evolving technique, inadequate instrumentation, and lack of understanding of hip joint anatomy. Initial results showed complication rates of up to 13% in reported cases [3].

The surgeon beginning to perform hip arthroscopy is not likely to be confronted with all of the original complications experienced by pioneers of hip arthroscopy, as surgical protocols for a safe procedure have been created, and enhanced instruments have become readily available for both the lateral and supine positions [4, 5]. Most recent studies report complication rates varying from 0.5% to 6.4% [6]. Nonetheless, hip arthroscopy continues to be considered a defying procedure with a steep learning curve, only to be attempted under supervision of an experienced surgeon in the first few cases, and preferably after specific training [7, 8].

Debates as to whether this learning curve is due in part to complications are ongoing. While some surgeonst report a decrease in complications with experience in hip arthroscopy, others have not observed this trend, despite a large number of cases performed [9–12]. Some studies contend that the types of complications vary within the learning curve, such that as different arthroscopic procedures in the hip are added to the surgeon's portfolio, new complications may be expected [12].

Complications can be classified into articular (referring to all musculoskeletal complications that can occur in the articular topography, not excluding complications in the extra-articular space, but with close relation to the joint), neurological (comprising all types of damage to peripheral nerves), and vascular-ischemic (including any possible damage or compression of arteries, veins, or lymph vessels) [12]. The potential mechanism of each complication provides the subdivisions for this classification (Table 16.1).

## Articular

Articular complications used to be considered minor, causing low levels of morbidity. However, as more complex procedures were developed, more severe complications were reported [12, 13, 14]. Awareness of these new events is of high importance, even for the most experienced surgeon, in order to prevent a repetition of technical flaws.

### Instrument Breakage

Instrument breakage within the joint was much more frequent in the early stages of hip arthroscopy. Breakage

B.G.S. e Souza • M.J. Philippon (✉)
Steadman Hawkins Research Foundation,
Vail, CO, USA
e-mail: drphilippon@steadman-hawkins.com;
brunogss01@yahoo.com.br

Ó. Marín-Peña (ed.), *Femoroacetabular Impingement*,
DOI 10.1007/978-3-642-22769-1_16, © Springer-Verlag Berlin Heidelberg 2012

**Table 16.1** Classification of complications following hip arthroscopy

| Complication type | Examples |
|---|---|
| *Articular* | |
| Instrument breakages | Guide wire breakage |
| | Forceps breakage |
| Intra-articular structures damage | Articular cartilage scuff |
| | Iatrogenic labral lesion |
| Extra-articular structures damage | Iatrogenic muscle lesion |
| | Iatrogenic tendon lesion[a] |
| | Myositis ossificans |
| | HO of the iliopsoas tendon |
| | Pericapsular HO |
| | Trochanteric bursitis |
| Adhesions | Adhesion |
| Fractures | Femoral neck stress fractures |
| Joint instability | Hip dislocation (macroinstability) |
| | Hip instability[a] (microinstability) |
| Infections | Superficial wound infection |
| | Pyarthrosis |
| *Neurological* | |
| Related to portal placement | Meralgia paresthetica |
| | Neurapraxia of LCFN |
| | Femoral nerve injury[a] |
| Related to articular distraction | Sciatic nerve palsy |
| | Femoral nerve palsy |
| | Sympathetic reflex |
| Related to compression | Pudendal nerve palsy |
| | Loss of erection |
| Related to manipulation | Direct injury of the femoral nerve[a] |
| | Direct injury of the sciatic nerve[a] |
| | Direct injury of the gluteus superior nerve[a] |
| *Vascular and ischemic* | |
| Related to venous stasis | Deep venous thrombosis |
| | Vulvae edema |
| Related to ischemia | Skin necrosis of the perineum |
| | Osteonecrosis of the femoral head |
| Related to fluid extravasation | Cardiac arrest |
| | Edema |
| Related to bleeding | Wound bleeding |
| | Perineal lacerations |
| | Hematomas |
| | Grand vessel injuries[a] |

*HO* heterotopic ossification, *LCFN* lateral cutaneous femoral nerve

[a]Have not yet been reported to date

was often attributable to inadequate instruments and technique. In general, fragments are easily removed at the time of arthroscopy, without further morbidity [14]. However, one case of unattainable removal of a forceps fragment was reported. The metallic body was seen in the cotyloid fossa in the postoperative roentgenogram and remained there at follow-up, causing no symptoms or articular problems thereafter [15].

In order to avoid this complication, use of instruments specifically designed for hip arthroscopy is preferred. A gentle technique, without levering movements or excessive strength, is also advisable. Pulling back the guide wire, as the cannulated instrument is inserted, prevents bending and breakage in the joint (Fig. 16.1). Guide wires made of nitinol are almost unbreakable and help prevent such occurrences [12, 16].

## Intra-articular Structural Damage

The most common intra-articular structure damaged during hip arthroscopy is the articular cartilage. Articular scuffing may carry no clinical relevance; however, visualization of the joint may be impaired [17]. Few authors have reported incidence of such occurrence; however, one study has reported femoral head abrasions in 3% of cases [7]. Clark et al. estimated that the upper limit of risk of intra-articular damage was 18%, as access to the joint in these cases was considered difficult [11]. Frequency of these events may be underreported and unknown; however, there is general consensus that such lesions should be avoided [11]. A careful surgical technique, sufficient articular distraction, use of blunt instruments, and assistance of an image intensifier may contribute to avoiding these complications [16].

Another structure susceptible to injury is the labrum. Serious iatrogenic lesions can occur at many stages of the procedure [7]. The labrum may be damaged during insertion of the instruments if vigilant technique is not applied. Resistance should not be felt as the needle penetrates the capsule during insertion into the first portal, which is done without direct visualization. If resistance is felt, this indicates that the labrum has been pierced and the needle should be repositioned. An image intensifier can aid in avoiding this complication, decreasing the number of attempts to obtain safe access into the joint [16]. Creating the following portals under direct visualization should avoid labral damage at this stage of the arthroscopic procedure (Fig. 16.2). The same advice is applicable when performing the capsulotomy and labral takedown, during which the

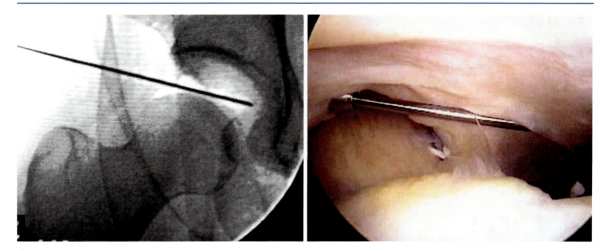

**Fig. 16.1** The guide wire should be retrieved as the cannula is inserted; otherwise it will progress further into the joint, bending and eventually breaking. Both the cannula obturator and the wire should then be retrieved together when the cannula is inside the joint. That also decreases the chances of breaking

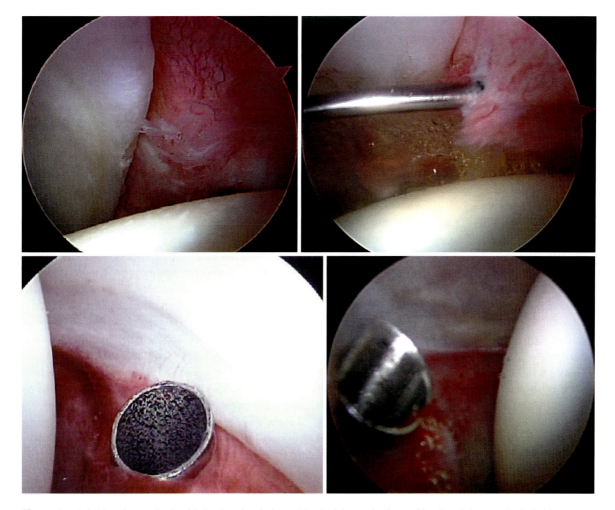

**Fig. 16.2** Right hip: The needle should aim the triangle formed by the labrum, the femoral head, and the capsule. Switching portals allows observing the anterolateral portal position in order to reassure no damage to the labrum has occurred

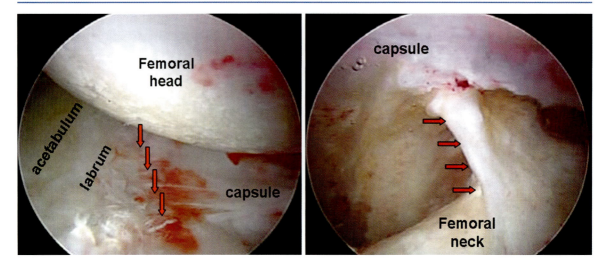

**Fig. 16.3** Adhesions (*red arrows*) may occur between the labrum and the capsule or between the capsule and the femoral neck, causing symptoms

labrum can be inadvertently disrupted if visualization is not adequate and manipulation is not gentle [16].

### Extra-articular Structural Damage

All types of surgery, including minimally invasive surgery, are expected to cause some measure of tissue damage. In hip arthroscopy, excessive manipulation has been reported to cause trochanteric bursitis [11]. In some refractory cases, treatment with local steroid injections may be necessary.

Cases of heterotopic ossification have been reported as a response to soft tissue damage [18]. In most cases, this condition is related to open approaches to the joint [19]. However, it has also been reported in hip arthroscopy, especially in extensive extra-articular procedures. Sampson reported an incidence of 0.6% symptomatic heterotopic ossification, which demanded additional surgery for removal [20]. Concomitant treatment of extra-articular pathologies and a predominately extra-articular approach to the capsule seem to be risk factors. In susceptible patients and those in which extra-articular procedures, such as bursectomies and tendon releases, are performed, prophylaxis should be seriously considered [21]. One study reported a case of myositis ossificans after treatment of synovial chondromatosis. Surgical removal was necessary 23 months after the index procedure [22].

### Adhesions

Postoperative intra-articular adhesions have been blamed for the failure of open treatment of femoroac-

etabular impingement [23, 24] (Fig. 16.3). Although rare, this condition has also been reported in hip arthroscopy [20, 25, 26]. Although no study has determined risk factors for the development of this condition, an analogy to similar conditions, such as treatment of articular fractures, may be applied. Postoperative immobilization and suboptimal rehabilitation protocols may be responsible for most of these types of adhesions. In order to avoid adhesions, we recommend an aggressive physical therapy protocol to obtain early range of motion [25].

### Fractures

No fractures related to hip arthroscopy had been reported until the beginning of treatment of femoroacetabular impingement [14]. Some studies have determined that the amount of resection of the head-neck junction that could be considered safe is 30% of the offset [27]. Another study showed that the accuracy of arthroscopic osteoplasty is similar to that obtained through an open approach [28]. Even so, four cases of femoral neck fracture have been reported after an arthroscopic approach to FAI by two different groups [12, 20]. These reports attributed the failures to poor patient compliance with weight-bearing restrictions following osteoplasty, presence of osteoporotic bone, or excessive bone removal. The treatment of that condition may vary from conservative treatment in compression-type stress fractures to reduction and fixation in displaced fractures. Therefore, surgeons should be aware of this potentially hazardous complication and perform to keep their osteoplasty within safe limits. An

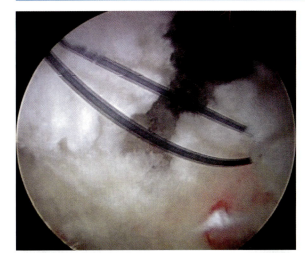

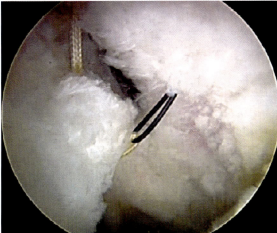

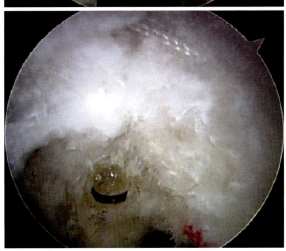

**Fig. 16.4** Capsular closure is performed to prevent potential instability and to accelerate healing

image intensifier can help achieve this objective. Patient education can also be a good strategy to avoid fractures [20, 29].

## Joint Instability

The importance of the hip capsule and its ligaments has long been investigated and is yet ill understood. Capsulotomies are necessary to obtain optimal joint visualization for most modern treatments of femoroacetabular impingement. Previous literature has described different regimens for treatment of femoroacetabular impingement, with debates on the cause of hip microinstability [14]. In fact, some studies have addressed the role of the capsule, and specifically the iliofemoral ligament, as stabilizing elements of the hip [30]. It was not until recently that the macroinstability of the joint was discussed. A hip dislocation, which occurred 2 months after treatment of a labral tear and cam impingement in a patient with an underlying capsular laxity, was attributed to the capsulotomy performed at the index procedure [31]. A revision arthroscopy was carried out when the patient showed no improvement at follow-up. A capsular plication resolved apprehension symptoms and, to a certain extent, the pain. Caution is recommended when performing capsulotomies in patients with risk factors for hip instability. Attentive capsular closure and postoperative restraints may be necessary in order to avoid failure of the capsule repair and anterior dislocation (Fig. 16.4).

Excessive acetabular rim trimming can also lead to dislocation of the joint [12]. The acetabular rim seems to be extremely sensitive to bone removal. Excessive resection may lead to dysplastic conformation, worsening joint biomechanics, or ultimately result in a hazardous complication such as hip dislocation with persistent instability. There is a correlation between the amount of resection and the value of the center-edge angle, so a formula should be used to predict the amount of trimming desired. The formula CE angle$=1.8+(0.64 \times$ rim reduction in millimeters) was obtained in a prospective study and provides an excellent parameter for the resection. Put more simply, 1 mm rim trimming will decrease the CE angle by approximately $2.4°$, while 5 mm rim trimming will decrease the CE angle by approximately $5°$. The resection should never reduce the center-edge angle to less than $25°$ [32].

## Infections

Infections in hip arthroscopy are extremely rare with a reported incidence of less than 1 per 1,000 cases. One case of pyarthrosis due to *Staphylococcus aureus* was documented in a patient arthroscopically treated for synovial chondromatosis [11]. Treatment included open drainage and debridement, in addition to antibiotic therapy.

Although rare, infection is a potentially devastating complication, and no efforts should be spared to avoid its occurrence. It has been reported that more complex procedures lead to higher infection rates, even in arthroscopic procedures [33]. Therefore, an aseptic technique is recommended, especially in more extensive procedures.

## Neurological

Since the beginning of hip arthroscopy, neurological complications have been recognized and feared by surgeons. In the last couple of decades, many attempts have been made to prevent neurological complications, although none seem to have completely resolved this issue.

### Related to Portal Placement

Various arthroscopic portals have been previously described around the hip joint. Nonetheless, the medial, anterior, and posterolateral approaches are considered to be the most critical [2, 34, 35]. Usage of the medial portal has been reported in the pediatric population, but has not been established as a standard approach in adults. The anterior approach poses direct risk to the femoral nerve and lateral cutaneous femoral nerve. In fact, nerve section, laceration, and palsy have been reported in connection with that approach [14]. In order to avoid lesions to the lateral cutaneous femoral nerve, more lateral and distal portals have been recommended [17]. However, surgeons should be aware of the multiple branches and anatomical variations of that structure, which may explain the occurrence of meralgia paresthetica (pain and skin numbness), even with these modified approaches. A superficial incision and subsequent blunt dissection may decrease the risk of nerve section, but not palsy, due to proximity to the portal [36]. Currently, there is no documentation of portal related injury to the femoral nerve. Although it has not yet been reported in the literature, the posterior trochanteric (posterolateral) portal is also considered risky, due to potential sciatic nerve injury [35, 36].

### Related to Articular Distraction

Adequate distraction during hip arthroscopy is necessary so that the joint space permits insertion of the instrumentation within the joint [37]. Temporary palsies of the sciatic and femoral nerves have been reported as a consequence of excessive articular distraction [9, 11, 16]. Excessive hip flexion, of more than 10° in the lateral position, has been related to temporary impairment of the sciatic and peroneal nerves, with excessive distraction [3]. A maximum of 60 lb (27.2 kg) and 60 min have been suggested as the safe limit for distraction [4]. We currently perform an alternative approach to the central and peripheral compartments, which allow us to both dynamically evaluate our bone resections and labral repair and decrease the length of continued distraction.

One anecdotal case of reflex sympathetic dystrophy persisted for at least 2 years in a series of 20 hip arthroscopies [38]. Investigation of predisposing factors and avoidance of excessive joint distraction might be able to prevent further cases.

### Related to Compression

Perineal nerve impairment often occurs in hip arthroscopy. Incidence varies from 0% to 13% of cases in both supine and lateral approaches [3]. This complication is regarded as temporary, although in some cases complete recovery may take up to 12 weeks [12, 39]. Erectile dysfunction may also occur in male patients. Although this condition is uncommon, recovery may take months [12, 40]. In traumatic patients, with the same complication due to compression by the perineal post, palsy of the pudendal nerve was considered to be more related to magnitude of traction than length of the procedure [40]. Eccentric positioning of the perineal post, adequate padding with a specific foam roll, general anesthesia for complete patient relaxation, limiting time of procedure, and rational use of traction have all been described as pearls to prevent such complications [6, 7, 12, 14] (Fig. 16.5).

### Related to Manipulation

No complications related to direct manipulation of nerve structures have been reported in the literature. As endoscopic approach to extra-articular conditions evolves, new complications are to be expected. Vicinity of the sciatic nerve for the treatment of piriform syndrome and vicinity of femoral nerve in iliopsoas release for internal snapping syndrome should be kept in mind by the surgeon performing these surgeries endoscopically [41].

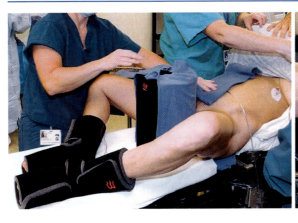 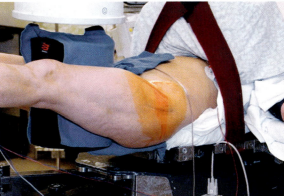

**Fig. 16.5** The eccentric position of the perineal post, adequate padding of at least 9 cm, and rational use of traction should be able to prevent most complications related to articular distraction

## Vascular and Ischemic

Vascular and ischemic complications in hip arthroscopy are often overlooked. Although major bleeding complications have not yet been reported in the literature, other potentially severe complications may occur.

### Related to Venous Stasis

Deep venous thrombosis is not considered a common complication in hip arthroscopy [42]. Currently, we are aware of only two cases. In one of these, the DVT was diagnosed 1 month after surgery in a patient with factor V Leiden deficiency [7]. No coagulation disturbances were reported in the other patient who developed symptoms in the immediate postoperative period [12]. No pulmonary embolism has been described to date [42]. There are no fundamentals to recommend chemical prophylaxis to all patients [14]. Individual recommendations should guide the clinical option for mechanical, chemical, or no prophylaxis [29, 42]. We currently recommend the use of a strong nonsteroidal anti-inflammatory drug for 2 weeks postoperatively to limit the risk of heterotopic ossification and DVT. Mechanical compression devices and drug therapy are used for 4 weeks. Drug therapy options include high-dose aspirin, warfarin, and low-molecular-weight heparin in higher-risk patients [25].

Another rare complication is the genital edema found after the inappropriate positioning of the patient against the perineal post [12]. This condition seems to be induced by local venous stasis due to compression and is generally resolved at 1 week postoperatively. Careful positioning should prevent such occurrences.

### Related to Ischemia

Skin necrosis in the perineal region has been reported after extended traction [12, 16, 43]. Contrary to neurological symptoms that are more sensitive to the amount of traction than the duration of the procedure, there seems to be a clear and obvious relation between ischemia and time of traction against the perineal post (Fig. 16.5).

Another potentially severe ischemic complication is femoral head osteonecrosis. We are aware of only one case reported in the literature in a patient treated for labral tear [9]. The exact relation between hip arthroscopy and this phenomenon has yet to be investigated. Impairment of blood supply to the femoral head could originate from injury of the medial circumflex artery branches. This injury could occur during instrument insertion or an intra-articular procedure. An anatomical study demonstrated that, as long as the anatomy is preserved, the posterolateral approach is relatively safe since instruments pass at an average of 10 mm (minimum 3 mm) from that structure [44]. The lateral retinacular vessels are major contributors to the perfusion of the femoral head [45]. The lateral synovial fold, which contains these vessels, is visible during arthroscopy [34, 46]. All efforts should be made to avoid damaging these vessels during an intra-articular procedure, due to the potential risk of causing osteonecrosis of the head [29] (Fig. 16.6).

### Related to Fluid Extravasation

Fluid extravasation to the surrounding tissues is not a rare condition in hip arthroscopy. Excessive fluid pressures, extra-articular procedures, and extended procedure time

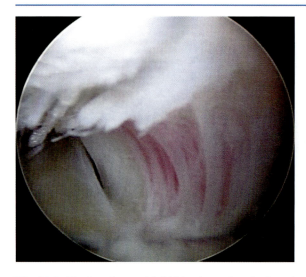

**Fig. 16.6** The lateral synovial fold is observed at the lateral aspect of the femoral neck and should be avoided under for the potential risk of avascular necrosis of the femoral head

are risk factors for local edema. The absorption of liquid often occurs in hours and happens uneventfully [14].

More rare extravasations to the abdominal compartment are accompanied by higher morbidity. One study reported on a patient with an acetabular fracture who was operated on 12 days after the trauma. Five weeks later, this patient underwent an arthroscopic procedure in the lateral position, and went into cardiac arrest 2 h after the surgery had begun. The condition was attributed to liquid extravasation into the abdominal compartment, which induced compartment syndrome and cardiovascular symptoms. The abdomen was drained of 8 L of fluid, which was followed by a spontaneous and abrupt return of circulation [47]. A constant decrease in body temperature during surgery should raise the suspicion of that complication [48]. Acetabular fractures are risk factors for potentially devastating complications related to fluid extravasation. To avoid this complication, it is advisable to postpone arthroscopy in patients at risk as well as to decrease operating time [14].

### Related to Bleeding

There are no reports in the current literature of major bleeding episodes related to hip arthroscopy, although an incorrect surgical technique and anatomical aberrancies could lead to injury of important vessels.

Moderate bleeding through established portals has been reported in some cases [11].

Local hematomas may develop in the perineal area as a consequence of trauma against the perineal post [2, 10]. Careful positioning and padding of the perineal post often help to avoid this problem.

## Revision Surgery

Revision surgery in hip arthroscopy can be defined as failed primary arthroscopic or open surgery requiring re-intervention. The reason for grouping those situations together is that the causes for intervention and the technical difficulties encountered are similar. The primary reasons for patient dissatisfaction and the main cause for revision surgery include persistent pain or recurrence of symptoms [25]. Revision surgery for hip arthroscopy is usually performed in referral centers worldwide. Ganz showed that femoroacetabular impingement can be a cause of labral tears in nondysplastic hips [49]. This observation revolutionized the way nonarthritic hips are treated. Many cases previously unresolved by conservative treatment or even by some surgical approaches gained a new perspective. Revision surgery of symptomatic patients, who were originally treated surgically without addressing bony abnormalities, has demonstrated good results thus far [25, 26].

Patients who also seem to benefit from revision surgery are those with bony deformities that were previously undertreated and have remained with persistent impingement. This has been reported as the major cause of revision hip arthroscopy in two recent studies [25, 26]. Despite initial studies demonstrating good results for the isolated treatment of labral lesions, more recent studies have shown a direct correlation between labral lesions and femoroacetabular impingement [50]. Revision surgery was performed mainly in patients with undertreated bone deformities, reinjuries, persistent pain, or return of symptoms. This reinforces the idea that these deformities are often the cause of symptoms, and emphasizes the need for revision surgery.

A common cause of symptoms after hip arthroscopy [25, 26] or more frequently, open treatment of hip conditions [23, 24] are adhesions (Fig. 16.3). Adhesions have been found in many arthroscopic revision cases and seem to be the only cause of symptoms for some patients. The location of these adhesions may vary, but they are often found between the manipulated labrum and the capsule [25]. Adhesions were also reported to occur between the femoral neck and the capsule on the site of the previous incision [23]. After hip dislocation for treatment of FAI, adhesions were described as an important source of groin pain [23]. Revision arthroscopy provided improvement of pain and better functional scores at short-term follow-up after both open or arthroscopic index procedures [24–26].

The intraoperative findings in arthroscopic revision surgery include labral tears, chondral defects, capsular laxity, ligamentum teres tears, loose bodies, recurrent disease, in addition to bone abnormalities, and the adhesions previously described [25].

At revision surgery, labral lesions can be debrided, repaired, or reconstructed. Previously debrided labra have been correlated with poorer results after revision surgery. Re-repair of the labrum due to failed repair is extremely rare [25, 26]. Failed labrum repair could be due to inadequate suture placement. New injuries in patients who suffered from a traumatic lesion or a previously unaddressed deformity are the most common causes for labral lesions seen at revision surgery. Iliopsoas impingement was also reported as a cause for labral lesions, though mechanism of injury was not clear [26]. An attempt to reattach the labrum must be made whenever possible, as long as the repaired structure is expected to heal and be functional. Debridement, however, may be the only option in degenerative, thin, and manipulated labra. All torn tissue must be debrided, but as much healthy labrum as possible must be left in place. In certain patients, especially athletes, labral reconstruction can be performed when limited labral tissue is seen at time of revision [51] (Fig. 16.7). Regardless of the type of labral treatment selected, not addressing the cause of the lesion will result in poorer outcomes [25, 26].

Repair of chondral lesions from sutures has shown variable results. The degenerative joint can be reapproached, and symptoms may be relieved for an extended period of time [25]. Joint space of less than 2 mm was correlated to poorer outcomes. Due to these results, there is no indication for further arthroscopic treatment [52]. Other factors for poor prognosis are concomitant full-thickness chondral defects in the femoral head and acetabulum known as kissing lesions [53] (Fig. 16.8). However, good results can be expected from the treatment of isolated chondral lesions, especially in the acetabulum. The microfracture technique (Fig. 16.9) has shown good long-term results in the knee [54] and has obtained promising early outcomes in the hip [53]. Focal lesions in young patients, even in the presence of degenerative changes, are good indications for this procedure.

Hip instability may be caused by traumatic lesions, overuse or systemic hyperlaxity [30]. However, iatrogenic micro- and macroinstability may occur after capsulotomy and capsulectomy in hip arthroscopy [14, 31]. This is especially true in patients with risk factors for instability, in which the iliofemoral ligament was sectioned and adequate capsular closure was not obtained in the index procedure. This was reported in a single case of hip dislocation [31]. In a series of 37 revisions, the senior author performed 13 procedures to treat hip instability: three thermal capsulorrhaphies and ten capsular plications [25].

An untreated degenerated or torn ligamentum teres may cause pain leading to revision arthroscopy [25, 26]. These lesions were noted in up to 59.4% of the revision cases in one series [25]. Debridement is the standard treatment this type of lesion. Some attempts of reconstruction have been made; however, the cases are anecdotal and indications for that procedure have not yet been defined [25].

Loose body removal was recognized in 10 of 37 revision arthroscopies. Loose bodies are commonly found in association with other lesions [25]. Conditions like pigmented villonodular synovitis and synovial chondromatosis may be treated in staged procedures or they may recur, needing additional surgeries [26].

Overall success rates in hip arthroscopy revisions stand at 86.5%. Among the successful cases, an average 77-point improvement in the Harris Hip Score has been documented in the first year. Patients who reported a new traumatic injury and had normal abduction of the hip before the revision surgery obtained the best scores [25]. Previous resection of the labrum in the first surgery, lower HHS before

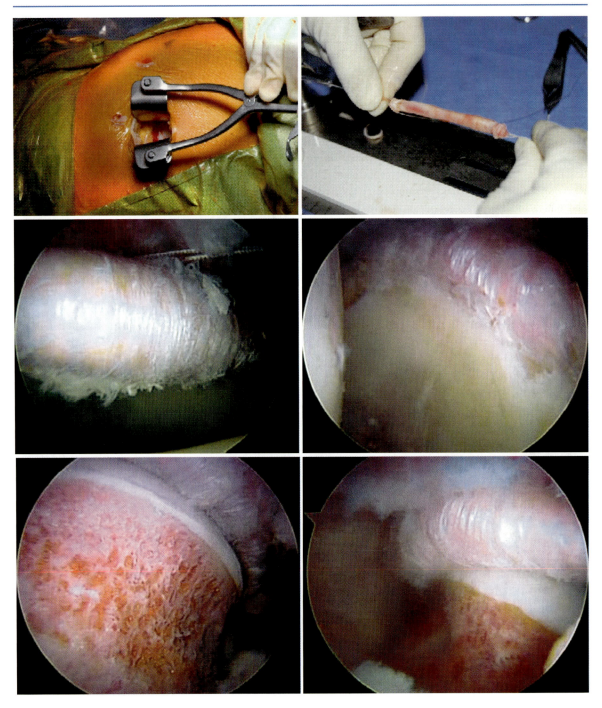

**Fig. 16.7** Iliotibial band autologous graft used in labral reconstruction in a left hip. Graft harvest, preparation, fixation and aspect after traction release (*good seal*)

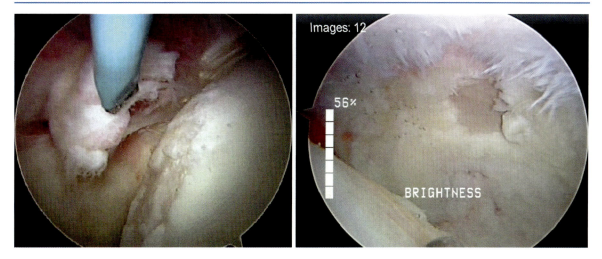

**Fig. 16.8** Simultaneous chondral defects in the femoral heal and in the acetabulum, known as kissing lesion, are factors for poor prognosis in revision arthroscopy

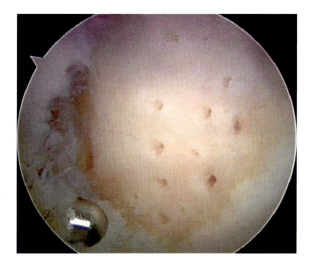

**Fig. 16.9** Chondral defects noticed at revision can be treated with microfractures

revision, radiographic signs of advanced osteoarthritis, and longer time between index procedure and revision were factors related to poorer results following revision [24, 25].

# References

1. Burman MS (1931) Arthroscopy or the direct visualization of joints. J Bone Joint Surg 4:669–695
2. Funke EL, Munzinger U (1996) Complications in hip arthroscopy. Arthroscopy 12(2):156–159
3. Rodeo SA, Forster RA, Weiland AJ (1993) Neurological complications due to arthroscopy. J Bone J Surg Am 75A(6):917–926
4. Glick JM, Sampson TG, Gordon RB, Behr JT, Schmidt E (1987) Hip arthroscopy by the lateral approach. Arthroscopy 3(1):4–12
5. Byrd JW (1994) Hip arthroscopy utilizing the supine position. Arthroscopy 10(3):275–280
6. Smart LR, Oetgen M, Noonan B, Medvecky M (2007) Beginning hip arthroscopy: indications, positioning, portals, basic technique, and complications. Arthroscopy 23(12):1348–1353
7. McCarthy JC, Lee JA (2005) Hip arthroscopy: indications, outcomes, and complications. J Bone Joint Surg 87(5):1138–1145
8. Shetty VD, Villar RN (2007) Hip arthroscopy: current concepts and review of the literature. Br J Sports Med 41(2):64–68
9. Sampson TG (2005) Complications of hip arthroscopy. Tech Orthop 20:63–66
10. Griffin DR, Villar RN (1999) Complications of arthroscopy of the hip. J Bone Joint Surg Br 81(4):604–606
11. Clarke MT, Arora A, Villar RN (2003) Hip arthroscopy: complications in 1054 cases. Clin Orthop Relat Res 406:84–88
12. Souza BGS, Polesello G, Honda E, Ono NK, Guimaraes RP, Ricioli Jr W, Dani WS (2009) Complications in hip arthroscopy. Proceedings of the 2009 Meeting of the American Academy of Orthopaedic Surgeons, Las Vegas, NV
13. Sampson TG (2001) Complications of hip arthroscopy. Clin Sports Med 20(4):831–835
14. Ilizaturri VM Jr (2009) Complications of arthroscopic femoroacetabular impingement treatment: a review. Clin Orthop Relat Res 467(3):760–768
15. Glick JM (1991) Hip arthroscopy. In: McGinty JB (ed) Operative arthroscopy. Raven, New York, pp 663–676
16. Byrd JTW (ed) (1998) Operative hip arthroscopy. Thieme, New York

17. Dorfman H, Boyer T (1999) Arthroscopy of the hip: 12 years of experience. Arthroscopy 15(1):67–72

18. Walton M, Rothwell AG (1983) Reactions of thigh tissues of sheep to blunt trauma. Clin Orthop Relat Res 176:273–281

19. Graves ML, Mast JW (2009) Femoroacetabular impingement: do outcomes reliably improve with surgical dislocations. Clin Orthop Relat Res 467(3):717–723

20. Sampson TG (2008) Arthroscopic treatment of femoroacetabular impingement. Am J Orthop 37(12):608–612

21. Polkowski GG, Jones KS (2009) Endoscopic management of the snapping iliopsoas tendon. Proceedings of the 2009 Meeting of the American Academy of Orthopaedic Surgeons, Las Vegas, NV

22. Byrd JTW, Jones SJ (2000) Prospective analysis of hip arthroscopy with 2-year follow-up. Arthroscopy 16(6):578–587

23. Beck M (2009) Groin pain after open FAI surgery: the role of intraarticular adhesions. Clin Orthop Relat Res 467:769–774

24. Krueger A, Leunig M, Siebenrock KA, Beck M (2007) Hip arthroscopy after previous surgical hip dislocation for femoroacetabular impingement. Arthroscopy 23(12):1285–1289

25. Philippon MJ, Schenker ML, Briggs KK, Kuppersmith DA, Maxwell RB, Stubbs AJ (2007) Revision hip arthroscopy. Am J Sports Med 35:1918–1921

26. Heyworth BE, Shindle MK, Voos JE, Rudzki JR, Kelly BT (2007) Radiologic and intraoperative findings in revision hip arthroscopy. Arthroscopy 23(12):1295–1302

27. Mardones RM, Gonzalez C, Chen Q, Zobitz M, Kaufman KR, Trusdale RT (2005) Surgical treatment of femoroacetabular impingement: evaluation of the size of the resection. J Bone Joint Surg Am 87:273–279

28. Mardones R, Lara J, Donndorff A, Barnes S, Stuart MJ, Glick J, Trousdale R (2009) Surgical correction of "cam-type" femoroacetabular impingement: a cadaveric comparison of open versus arthroscopic debridement. Arthroscopy 25(2):175–182

29. Philippon MJ, Stubbs AJ, Schenker ML, Maxwell RB, Ganz R, Leunig M (2007) Arthroscopic management of femoroacetabular impingement: osteoplasty technique and literature review. Am J Sports Med 35(9):1571–1580

30. Philippon MJ, Schenker ML (2005) Athletic hip injuries and capsular laxity. Oper Tech Orthop 15:261–266

31. Ranawat AS, McClincy M, Sekiya JK (2009) Anterior dislocation of the hip after arthroscopy in a patient with capsular laxity of the hip: a case report. J Bone Joint Surg Am 91A(1):192–197

32. Philippon MJ, Wolff AB, Briggs KK, Zehms CT, Kuppersmith DA (2009) Rim reduction for the treatment of pincer-type FAI correlates with pre & postoperative CE angle. Proceedings of the 2009 Meeting of the American Academy of Orthopaedic Surgeons, Las Vegas, NV

33. Villar RN (1994) Arthroscopy. BMJ 308(6920):51–53

34. Dvorak M, Duncan CP, Day B (1990) Arthroscopic anatomy of the hip. Arthroscopy 6(4):264–273

35. Elsaidi GA, Ruch DS, Schaefer WD, Kuzma K, Smith BP (2004) Complications associated with traction on the hip during arthroscopy. J Bone Joint Surg Br 86(6):793–796

36. Byrd JW, Pappas JN, Pedley MJ (1995) Hip arthroscopy: an anatomic study of portal placement and relationship to the extra-articular structures. Arthroscopy 11(4):418–423

37. Byrd JWT, Chern KY (1997) Traction versus distension for distraction of the joint during hip arthroscopy. Arthroscopy 13:346–349

38. Kim SJ, Choi NH, Kim HJ (1998) Operative hip arthroscopy. Clin Orthop Relat Res 353:156–165

39. Merrel G, Medvecky M, Daigneault J, Jokl P (2007) Hip arthroscopy without a perineal post: a safer technique for hip distraction. Arthroscopy 23(1):107e1–107e3

40. Brumback RJ, Ellison TS, Molligan H, Molligan DJ, Mahaffey S, Schmidhauser C (1992) Pudendal nerve palsy complicating intramedullary nailing of the femur. J Bone Joint Surg Am 74(10):1450–1455

41. Dezawa A, Kusano S, Miki H (2003) Arthroscopic release of the piriformis muscle under local anesthesia for piriformis syndrome. Arthroscopy 19(5):554–557

42. Bushnell BD, Anz AW, Bert JM (2008) Venous thromboembolism in lower extremity arthroscopy. Arthroscopy 24(5):604–611

43. Eriksson E, Arvidsson I, Arvidsson H (1986) Diagnostic and operative arthroscopy of the hip. Orthopedics 9(2):169–176

44. Sussmann PS, Zumstein M, Hahn F, Dora C (2007) The risk of vascular injury to the femoral head when using the posterolateral arthroscopy portal: cadaveric investigation. Arthroscopy 23(10):1112–1115

45. Gautier E, Ganz K, Krugel N, Gill T, Ganz R (2000) Anatomy of the medial femoral circumflex artery and its surgical implications. J Bone Joint Surg Br 82B(5):679–683

46. Dienst M, Godde S, Seil R, Hammer D, Kohn D (2001) Hip arthroscopy without traction: in vivo anatomy of the peripheral joint cavity. Arthroscopy 17:924–931

47. Bartlett CS, DiFelice GS, Buly RL, Quinn TJ, Green DS, Helfet DL (1998) Cardiac arrest as a result of intraabdominal extravasation of fluid during arthroscopic removal of a loose body from the hip joint of a patient with an acetabular fracture. J Orthop Trauma 12(4):294–299

48. Haupt U, Volkle D, Waldherr C, Beck M (2008) Intra- and retroperitoneal irrigation liquid after arthroscopy of the hip joint. Arthroscopy 24(8):966–968

49. Ganz R, Parvizi J, Beck M, Leunig M, Notzli H, Siebenrock KA (2003) Femoroacetabular impingement: a cause for osteoarthritis of the hip. Clin Orthop Relat Res 417:112–120

50. Wenger DE, Kendell KR, Miner MR, Trousdale RT (2004) Acetabular labral tears rarely occur in the absence of bony abnormalities. Clin Orthop Relat Res 426:145–150

51. Philippon MJ, Kuppersmith D, Wahoff M, Briggs KK (2009) Outcomes of arthroscopic acetabular labral reconstruction in the hip in professional athletes. Proceedings of the 2009 Meeting of the American Academy of Orthopaedic Surgeons, Las Vegas

52. Philippon MJ, Schenker ML, Briggs KK, Maxwell RB (2008) Can microfracture produce repair tissue in acetabular chondral defects? Arthroscopy 24(1):46–50

53. Lienert JJ, Rodkey WG, Steadman JR, Philippon MJ, Sekiya JK (2005) Microfracture techniques in hip arthroscopy. Oper Tech Orthop 15:267–272

54. Steadman JR, Briggs KK, Rodrigo JJ, Kocher MS, Gill TJ, Rodkey WG (2003) Outcomes of microfracture for traumatic chondral defects of the knee: average 11-year follow-up. Arthroscopy 19:477–484

# Combined Techniques in FAI: Hip Arthroscopy Followed by Mini-Anterior Approach

# 17

Nader A. Nassif and John C. Clohisy

## Introduction

A proper relationship between the proximal femur and acetabulum is essential for normal hip biomechanics. Subtle anatomic variations on either side of the joint may result in a pathomechanical environment leading to increased pressure on the acetabular labrum and acetabular articular cartilage. This concept of femoroacetabular impingement (FAI) has been refined by Ganz et al. and is postulated to result in osteoarthritis secondary to repetitive microtrauma to the femoral head–neck junction and/or the acetabular rim complex [1].

FAI lesions can present on the femur and acetabulum. Femoral-sided, or cam-type, lesions are due to reduced head–neck offset, Perthes deformity, or slipped capital femoral epiphysis deformity. Acetabular-sided or pincer-type impingement results from acetabular overcoverage as present in coxa profunda, protrusio, and acetabular retroversion. Surgical management has been proposed for FAI in order to address the structural mismatch and associated intra-articular abnormalities (i.e., labral tears and chondromalacia). Surgical hip dislocation initially recommended by Ganz et al.

has been the gold standard since it provides a safe and effective technique in exposing the femoral head and acetabulum with preservation of blood supply to the femoral head [2].

Recent advances in arthroscopy have allowed surgeons to examine the hip joint and address certain impingement features through minimally invasive techniques [3–5]. Hip arthroscopy allows the surgeon to assess the labrum, acetabular, and femoral cartilage as well as the femoral head–neck junction. With hip arthroscopy, labral tears and defects in the acetabular articular cartilage can be addressed directly [6–8]. Deformity correction of femoral-sided abnormalities exclusively through the arthroscope has also been described [4, 9–12]. This all-arthroscopic technique can be technically challenging. One potential limitation of the all-arthroscopic technique is inadequate resection of the femoral head–neck junction since visualization of the femoral head–neck junction may be compromised. With increasing experience, however, complete arthroscopic osteochondroplasty has been shown to be equivalent to open procedures [13, 14]. Combined with a limited open anterior approach, hip arthroscopy provides the ability to precisely assess and address intra-articular lesions, while the limited open exposure provides direct access to and visualization of the head–neck junction. This combined arthroscopic and limited open technique may reduce risks associated with surgical hip dislocation including bleeding, avascular necrosis, heterotopic ossification, or trochanteric nonunion. We present this surgical technique as one alternative for the surgical management of hip impingement disease. In this chapter, we summarize the indica-

N.A. Nassif • J.C. Clohisy (✉)
Department of Orthopaedic Surgery,
Washington University School of Medicine,
St. Louis, MO, USA
e-mail: jclohisy@wustl.edu

Ó. Marín-Peña (ed.), *Femoroacetabular Impingement*,
DOI 10.1007/978-3-642-22769-1_17, © Springer-Verlag Berlin Heidelberg 2012

**Table 17.1** Advantages and disadvantages of limited open osteochondroplasty

*Advantages*
- Ability to directly visualize and correct cam deformities
- Less technically demanding than arthroscopic osteochondroplasty
- Able to directly palpate and dynamically test for adequacy of decompression
- Avoid trochanteric osteotomy
- Avoid hip dislocation
- Assess joint prior to open procedure

*Disadvantages*
- Limited ability to work on acetabular rim
- Risk of injury to the lateral femoral cutaneous nerve
- Inadequate exposure for complex deformities

tions, surgical technique, and preliminary results of this combined arthroscopic and limited open approach (Table 17.1).

## History and Physical Exam

Patients with impingement disorders usually present with intermittent, activity-related groin pain [15]. They are typically active young to middle-aged adults. Patients often report pain during cutting and pivoting moves while participating in sports, as well as groin pain with prolonged sitting or squatting. Labral symptoms including locking and catching within the hip joint are sometimes reported [16].

On physical exam, patients often avoid sitting with an erect posture to prevent impingement in flexion. A slight limp may be observed, and abductor weakness is common. Careful hip range of motion examination is performed to detect limited flexion and internal rotation. It is essential to stabilize the pelvis and to note forced pelvic motion as the endpoint of hip flexion. Most patients with symptomatic FAI have less than 100° of hip flexion and less than 15° of internal rotation at 90° of flexion. A positive impingement sign can often be elicited at 90° of flexion, slight adduction, and internal rotation. This maneuver produces abutment of the anterolateral femoral head–neck junction on the acetabular rim complex. The presence of posterior hip impingement can be tested with hip extension, external rotation, and adduction. An examination of the lumbar spine is also performed to eliminate a neurological etiology of hip symptoms. Buttock and lower lumbar discomfort commonly coexist with hip impingement disease [15].

## Imaging Studies

Plain films including an AP pelvis, false profile, cross-table lateral, frog-leg lateral, 45° Dunn view, and 90° Dunn view can be considered in evaluating FAI patients [17]. In our practice, we currently obtain an AP pelvis, frog lateral, false profile, and 45° Dunn view for FAI hips. Since the typical cam lesion is usually located on the anterolateral aspect of the femoral neck, we find the frog-leg view and 45° Dunn views to be useful in evaluating the femoral-sided deformity. High-resolution computed tomography with 3-D reconstruction is becoming increasingly popular to assess the extent of the acetabular and femoral deformity preoperatively. MR arthrograms are recommended for evaluation of labral and articular cartilage lesions. Magnetic resonance studies are very important in assessing the integrity of the articular cartilage in borderline cases when joint preservation is being considered relative to nonsurgical or arthroplasty options.

## Indications

Limited open osteochondroplasty is indicated in patients with cam or combined cam/pincer impingement disorders. If present, acetabular-sided impingement lesions are treated during the arthroscopic portion of the procedure, and femoral-sided lesions are connected via the limited open approach. Ideal candidates for surgery have symptomatic FAI, are less than 50 years of age, and have little to no evidence of secondary arthritis. Obese patients or those with significant comorbidities may benefit from this limited procedure to reduce the morbidity associated with a surgical hip dislocation.

## Surgical Technique

The overall goals of surgery are to provide pain relief, enhance function and activity, and improve patient quality of life. The technical aims of surgery are to correct the structural impingement abnormalities and to address associated soft tissue problems (i.e., labral or chondral pathology). Hip arthroscopy is performed first in order to evaluate and treat intra-articular disease and the acetabular rim. A limited open anterior approach is then performed following the arthroscopy to address the femoral impingement deformity [18, 19].

**Fig. 17.1** Positioning of the patient. The operative leg is placed in traction, neutral abduction, slight flexion, and neutral rotation. Nonoperative leg is placed stir-up without traction

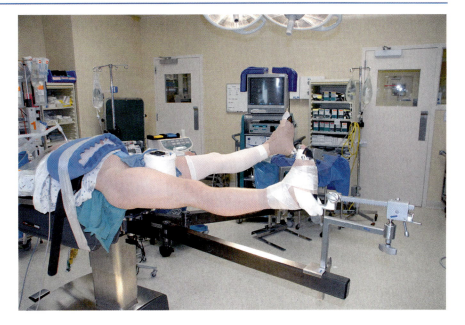

**Fig. 17.2** Draping and positioning of the patient. A shower curtain drape is used to cover the extremity. The Image intensifier is positioned between the legs

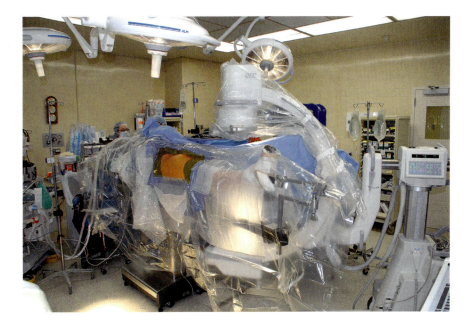

## Patient Positioning

The patient is induced under general anesthesia with relaxation and placed supine on a traction table. After the patient is asleep, an exam under anesthesia is performed. Special attention is paid to flexion and internal rotation with flexion motion. A well-padded perineal post is placed between the legs. The operative leg is placed in neutral abduction, 0–10° of internal rotation, and slight flexion (10–15°). The nonoperative leg is placed 30–40° of abduction and neutral rotation (Figs. 17.1 and 17.2). Traction of the joint is applied under fluoroscopic guidance to achieve 8–10 mm of joint distraction.

## Hip Arthroscopy

After positioning, the surgical field is prepped and draped. Landmarks are palpated and marked. The anterior

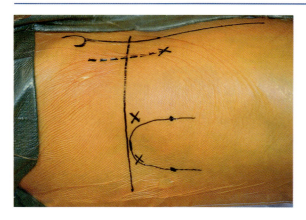

**Fig. 17.3** The anterior superior iliac spine, greater trochanter are outlined. The portals are indicated by the (x). The anterior approach is indicated by the *dashed*

superior iliac spine is outlined, and a line extending distally is drawn. A perpendicular line is drawn at the level of the superior border of the greater trochanter (Fig. 17.3). The superior, anterior, and posterior borders of the greater trochanter are identified and marked. Portals are established using standard 4.0, 4.5, or 5.0 mm hip arthroscopic cannulas. The anterolateral portal is established first under fluoroscopic visualization. The posterolateral portal is placed under direct visualization after the arthroscopic camera is inserted. Finally, the anterior portal is then made slightly lateral to the direct anterior line in order to protect the lateral femoral cutaneous nerve and facilitate intra-articular techniques. As our method has evolved, the position of the anterior portal has changed. Presently, this portal is made approximately 2 cm lateral to the anterior line and 2–3 cm distal to the anterolateral portal. The location of the anterior portal is made such that it can be incorporated into the mini open anterior approach. After the portals are established, the capsulotomies are extended with a beaver blade. This facilitates mobility of the arthroscope and access to various aspects of the joint. During the arthroscopic procedure, care is taken to avoid prolonged traction and excessive fluid extravasation.

Diagnostic arthroscopy is initiated after establishing the portals. The acetabular cartilage, labrum, femoral cartilage, acetabular fossa, and joint recesses are visualized and probed for abnormalities. Specific attention is given to the labrochondral junction of the anterior and superolateral acetabular rim. Labral tears, disruption of the labrochondral junction, articular cartilage debonding, and detachments are common findings in

FAI. Acetabular labral disease findings are variable, and arthroscopic management is dictated by the characteristics of the labrum and the associated impingement deformity (cam, pincer, or combined cam/pincer) [6, 8, 20]. For hips with isolated cam impingement, acetabular rim trimming is not required. Labral fraying and small labral irregularities are treated with partial resection or recontouring. More extensive labral detachments are repaired arthroscopically if the labral tissue appears healthy. If the labral tissue has major degenerative changes, labral recontouring is usually performed. In hips with a pincer deformity, the labrum is detached, the rim trimming performed with an arthroscopic burr, and the labrum refixed with suture anchors. Again, if the labral tissue is unhealthy, we prefer partial resection/recontouring.

Articular cartilage lesions also vary in depth, size, and location. In early impingement, the majority of articular cartilage disease is encountered at the acetabular rim. As the joint disease progresses, it extends centrally in the acetabulum and also involves the femoral head. Debonded articular cartilage without detachment or a flap is left untreated. Partial thickness cartilage fraying is debrided with an arthroscopic shaver. Full-thickness articular cartilage lesions and flaps are treated with debridement of unstable tissue and microfracture if the articular degeneration is not too extensive.

## Limited Open Osteochondroplasty

The arthroscopic portion of the procedure assesses the joint and precisely treats the acetabular labrum, acetabular rim, and articular cartilage disease of both the femur and acetabulum. Attention is then turned to the limited open anterior approach for management of the femoral impingement deformity. An 8–10-cm incision is made approximately 2 cm lateral to the anterosuperior iliac spine over the tensor fascia latae (TFL); this incision incorporates the anterior portal. Subcutaneous dissection is taken to the fascia of the TFL, which is incised and the muscle belly retracted laterally. The sartorius and superficial fascia layer are retracted medially (Fig. 17.4). The medial soft tissue sleeve contains the lateral femoral cutaneous nerve which should be protected. We do not dissect to identify or isolate the lateral femoral cutaneous nerve. The interval between the tensor and sartorius is developed. The reflected head of the

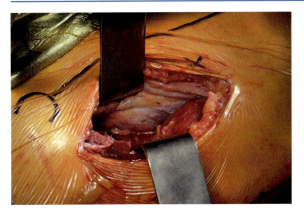

**Fig. 17.4** The tensor fascia is opened, retracted laterally and the interval between tensor and sartorius is developed

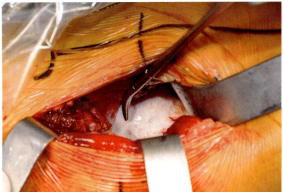

**Fig. 17.6** After the arthrotomy is performed, the femoral head and head–neck junction are visible. An impingement trough is often seen on the femoral head (indicated by the *point of the clamp*)

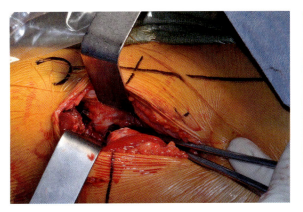

**Fig. 17.5** The reflected head of the rectus is identified (*arrow*), isolated, and transected. The direct head of the rectus can be left intact

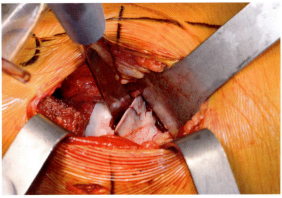

**Fig. 17.7** A quarter-inch curved osteotome is used to perform the osteochondroplasty of the femoral head–neck junction in a gentle slopping manner

rectus is transected with an adequate cuff to allow for repair during closure (Fig. 17.5). The interval between the direct head of the rectus and the underlying hip capsule is established. A cobra retractor is passed under the rectus to expose the capsule. The capsule is then directly visualized and the arthroscopy portals identified. The arthrotomy is completed in a "capital I-shaped" fashion creating large medial and lateral flaps for closure. The femoral head–neck junction is exposed and inspected (Fig. 17.6).

The femoral head articular cartilage is examined to look for areas of chondromalacia and/or an impingement trough, as these findings can guide the location of the osteochondroplasty. The extent of the impingement lesion of the head–neck junction is determined with careful examination. The anteromedial region is best

visualized with the extremity in slight flexion, abduction, and maximal external rotation. The more lateral aspect is visualized in extension and internal rotation. An osteotome is then used to produce a gentle sloping osteochondroplasty in the region of insufficient offset (Fig. 17.7). A burr is utilized to refine the osteochondroplasty site (Fig. 17.8) with special attention to establishing a smooth transition at the articular cartilage femoral neck junction. Although the ideal resection amount can vary, cadaveric study by Mardones et al. demonstrated that resection less than 30% of the femoral neck is safe and does not increase the potential risk for femoral neck fracture [21]. Most cases require far less resection than 30%. After completion of the osteochondroplasty, fluoroscopic images are obtained. AP radiographs are taken in neutral, internal, and external rotations. Fluoroscopic

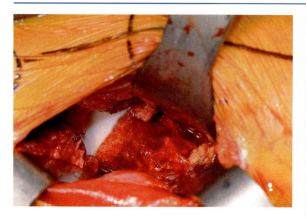

**Fig. 17.8** The osteochondroplasty is refined with a burr

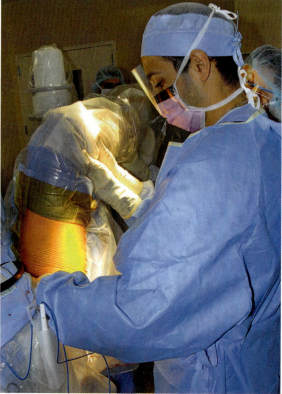

**Fig. 17.10** The hip is put through a range of motion under direct palpation to assess any residual impingement. Specifically, the hip is assessed in flexion and combined flexion and internal rotation

frog-leg lateral and Dunn views are also obtained to assess the adequacy of the resection at the anterolateral head–neck junction (Fig. 17.9). This region is also manually palpated with combined flexion and internal rotation to assess for residual impingement (Fig. 17.10).

The wound is copiously irrigated. The capsulotomy is closed using #1 Vicryl suture. A 1/8-in. Hemovac drain is placed into the wound exterior to the capsule. The reflected head of the rectus is repaired using a 2–0 Ethibond suture. The tensor fascia is closed using #1 Vicryl with care not to encroach on the lateral femoral cutaneous nerve. Subcutaneous closure with 2–0 Vicryl and either subcuticular Monocryl suture or staples. The remaining portal sites are closed with subcutaneous and 3–0 Monocryl or staples.

## Postoperative Care

The patient is given standard perioperative antibiotics. Compression stockings and aspirin twice daily for 6 weeks are used for DVT prophylaxis. Patients are toe-

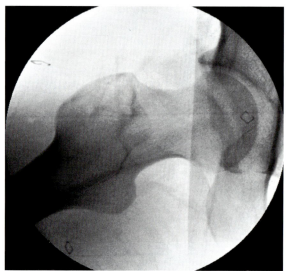

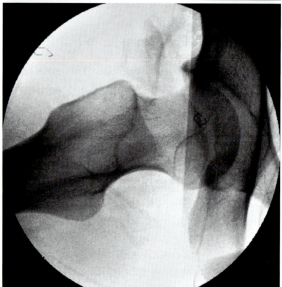

**Fig. 17.9** Fluoroscopic Dunn view and frog-leg view following osteochondroplasty demonstrating the improved head–neck offset and the gentle sloping shape of the resection

touch weight bearing if they had a labral repair. Patients who exclusively had an osteochondroplasty are made 50% weight bearing. The patient is placed in a CPM for hip flexion 0–60° for 6 h per day for 4 weeks. Physical therapy focuses on gentle hip range of motion with the patient starting on postoperative day #1. Hip flexion is limited to 90° for 4 weeks. The patient is placed on Naproxen 500 mg PO twice a day for 4 weeks for heterotopic bone prophylaxis. At 4 weeks, the patient is allowed to increase weight bearing as tolerated, and the strengthening program is accelerated. Patients are released to full activity at 3–4 months after surgery.

## Complications

Although hip arthroscopy is a generally safe procedure, there are known complications [22]. Neuropraxia of the pudendal nerve, femoral nerve, or sciatic nerve can result from excessive traction. Irritation of the lateral femoral cutaneous nerve can occur during placement of the anterior portal or with the anterior dissection. Avascular necrosis is an uncommon complication as arthroscopy should not encroach on the femoral head blood supply. However, care should be taken to preserve the posterolateral retinacular vessels when extending the osteochondroplasty posteriorly. Femoral neck fracture associated with osteochondroplasty is a potential risk, and care should be taken not to resect more than 30% of the femoral neck [21]. Heterotopic ossification and DVT can occur, and prophylaxis should be considered.

## Results/Outcomes

Recent studies suggest that the combined arthroscopic and limited anterior approach is efficacious in treating FAI. Laude et al. examined 100 hips in 97 patients who underwent hip arthroscopy with a limited anterolateral open osteochondroplasty with a mean follow-up of 58 months [23]. Patients improved their NAHS score significantly from 54 to 83 points. In his series, 13 patients required revision arthroscopy for persistent hip pain with 8 patients requiring labral refixation and 6 requiring revision of the osteochondroplasty site. There were several complications noted in this study. One patient sustained a femoral neck fracture which was treated nonoperatively. Eleven percent of the hips were converted to a total hip at a mean follow-up time of 29 months.

Hartman et al. looked at 33 patients with FAI who underwent a limited open osteochondroplasty at a mean follow-up of 15 months [24]. The average Harris hip score improved from 64 to 85 postoperatively with only one patient requiring a conversion to a total hip. Radiographically, the alpha angle improved from 77° to 39° postoperatively. Two patients had transient femoral nerve palsy; two patients had transient pudendal nerve irritation; and 15 patients (45%) had irritation of the lateral femoral cutaneous nerve. There were no cases of avascular necrosis of the femoral neck.

Clohisy et al. similarly demonstrated improvement in a cohort of 41 hips [25]. In this series, the measured alpha angle improved from 63° to 38° with a concurrent improvement of modified Harris hip score by 24 points. No neurapraxias, femoral neck fractures, or avascular necrosis were noted in this study.

## Conclusion

Hip arthroscopy combined with a limited open anterior approach provides a useful tool in the management of femoroacetabular impingement. Early studies demonstrate good results and acceptable complication rates. This technique combines precise arthroscopic management of intra-articular and acetabular disease with femoral deformity correction under direct visualization via the limited open approach. The procedure may serve as a surgeon's primary technique or can be utilized in selected cases when an all-arthroscopic procedure or surgical dislocation is less appealing. In our practice, mild to moderate impingement deformities with a cam component are managed with an all-arthroscopic technique. Cases with more extensive or severe deformities are treated with combined arthroscopy and limited open osteochondroplasty. Severe, combined cam/pincer impingement deformities (e.g., Perthes deformity) all undergo surgical hip dislocation to provide comprehensive reconstruction on both sides of the joint. All of these procedures need further investigation to determine long-term efficacy.

## References

1. Ganz R et al (2003) Femoroacetabular impingement: a cause for osteoarthritis of the hip. Clin Orthop Relat Res 417: 112–120
2. Ganz R et al (2001) Surgical dislocation of the adult hip a technique with full access to the femoral head and acetabulum without the risk of avascular necrosis. J Bone Joint Surg Br 83(8):1119–1124

3. Byrd JW (2006) Hip arthroscopy by the supine approach. Instr Course Lect 55:325–336

4. Philippon MJ et al (2007) Arthroscopic management of femoroacetabular impingement: osteoplasty technique and literature review. Am J Sports Med 35(9):1571–1580

5. Bardakos NV, Vasconcelos JC, Villar RN (2008) Early outcome of hip arthroscopy for femoroacetabular impingement: the role of femoral osteoplasty in symptomatic improvement. J Bone Joint Surg Br 90(12):1570–1575

6. Bedi A et al (2008) The management of labral tears and femoroacetabular impingement of the hip in the young, active patient. Arthroscopy 24(10):1135–1145

7. Philippon MJ et al (2009) Outcomes following hip arthroscopy for femoroacetabular impingement with associated chondrolabral dysfunction: minimum two-year follow-up. J Bone Joint Surg Br 91(1):16–23

8. Philippon MJ, Schenker ML (2006) A new method for acetabular rim trimming and labral repair. Clin Sports Med 25(2):293–297, ix

9. Larson CM, Giveans MR (2008) Arthroscopic management of femoroacetabular impingement: early outcomes measures. Arthroscopy 24(5):540–546

10. Ilizaliturri VM Jr et al (2008) Arthroscopic treatment of cam-type femoroacetabular impingement: preliminary report at 2 years minimum follow-up. J Arthroplasty 23(2):226–234

11. Philippon MJ et al (2008) Early outcomes after hip arthroscopy for femoroacetabular impingement in the athletic adolescent patient: a preliminary report. J Pediatr Orthop 28(7):705–710

12. Byrd JW, Jones KS (2009) Arthroscopic femoroplasty in the management of cam-type femoroacetabular impingement. Clin Orthop Relat Res 467(3):739–746

13. Sussmann PS et al (2007) Arthroscopic versus open osteoplasty of the head-neck junction: a cadaveric investigation. Arthroscopy 23(12):1257–1264

14. Mardones R et al (2009) Surgical correction of "cam-type" femoroacetabular impingement: a cadaveric comparison of open versus arthroscopic debridement. Arthroscopy 25(2):175–182

15. Clohisy JC et al (2009) Clinical presentation of patients with symptomatic anterior hip impingement. Clin Orthop Relat Res 467(3):638–644

16. Burnett RS et al (2006) Clinical presentation of patients with tears of the acetabular labrum. J Bone Joint Surg Am 88(7):1448–1457

17. Clohisy JC et al (2008) A systematic approach to the plain radiographic evaluation of the young adult hip. J Bone Joint Surg Am 90(Suppl 4):47–66

18. Clohisy JC, McClure JT (2005) Treatment of anterior femoroacetabular impingement with combined hip arthroscopy and limited anterior decompression. Iowa Orthop J 25:164–171

19. Pierannunzii L, d'Imporzano M (2007) Treatment of femoroacetabular impingement: a modified resection osteoplasty technique through an anterior approach. Orthopedics 30(2):96–102

20. Espinosa N et al (2007) Treatment of femoro-acetabular impingement: preliminary results of labral refixation. Surgical technique. J Bone Joint Surg Am 89(Suppl 2 Pt. 1):36–53

21. Mardones RM et al (2005) Surgical treatment of femoroacetabular impingement: evaluation of the effect of the size of the resection. J Bone Joint Surg Am 87(2):273–279

22. Ilizaliturri VM Jr (2009) Complications of arthroscopic femoroacetabular impingement treatment: a review. Clin Orthop Relat Res 467(3):760–768

23. Laude F, Sariali E, Nogier A (2009) Femoroacetabular impingement treatment using arthroscopy and anterior approach. Clin Orthop Relat Res 467(3):747–752

24. Hartmann A, Gunther KP (2009) Arthroscopically assisted anterior decompression for femoroacetabular impingement: technique and early clinical results. Arch Orthop Trauma Surg 129:1001–1009, Epub 2009 Jan 6

25. Clohisy JC et al (2010) Combined hip arthroscopy and limited open osteochondroplasty for the treatment of anterior femoroacetabular impingement. J Bone Joint Surg Am 92:1697–1706

# Femoroacetabular Impingement Management Through a Mini-Open Anterior Approach and Arthroscopic Assistance: Technics and Mid-Term Results

# 18

Frédéric Laude and Elhadi Sariali

## Introduction

Femoroacetabular impingement (FAI) was first described in the late 1990s by Rheinhold Ganz [2, 3, 12, 19] in Bern, Switzerland, as abnormal contact between the anterior acetabular rim and the femoral neck. It has been described as a common cause of hip pain in young adults and has been proposed as a cause of osteoarthritis. In 2001, Ganz also described a safe technique [11] to dislocate the hip joint to modify the shape of the femoral head at the head–neck junction and to correct the abnormalities on the acetabular side (lesions of the labrum, overcoverage of the anterior acetabular rim and cartilage damage) [8].

This technique came to enjoy wide acceptance, and many surgeons like Beck et al. [3], Murphy et al. [22] or Beaulé et al. [1] embraced it to treat FAI. Even if the preliminary results are encouraging, the surgical exposure carries some morbidity in terms of length of incision and post-operative recovery. Furthermore, the need to remove the hardware is common, with Beaulé and associates reporting the need to remove the internal fixation in 9 out of 34 patients because of persistent bursitis.

Even though the surgical dislocation technique as described by Ganz has demonstrated itself to be safe and capable of maintaining femoral head vascularity, when

Ganz started to report on the surgical dislocation approach in the late 1990s, no data was available, and the risk of femoral head necrosis was unknown. This is why, in 1999, we developed a technique using the Hueter mini-invasive anterior approach with arthroscopic assistance. The purpose of the present study is to report on the mid-term results of this technique in the treatment of FAI.

## Materials and Methods

Between April 1999 and December 2004, 100 hips in 97 patients with persistent hip pain secondary to femoroacetabular impingement were treated in our department. The cohort was composed of 50 men and 47 women with an average age of 33.4 years (range, 16–56). Ninety-one patients were reviewed with an average follow-up of 57 months (ranging from 13 to 104). Although six patients were lost to follow-up, all had an average follow-up of 43 months (range 70–13).

All patients presented with persistent hip pain of more than 6 months' evolution, and five had been painful for more than 10 years. All patients had a positive impingement test [12, 14] (pain was elicited in flexion, adduction and internal rotation). All patients had at least an MRI arthrography or a CT-scan arthrography of the hip performed in order to analyse potential labral tears. The final decision to proceed with surgery was based on clinical examination (even if the radiologic examination was not conclusive). From 2001, patients who showed joint space narrowing on a Lequesne false-profile view [16, 17] were no longer considered for surgical correction because of poor clinical outcomes in this kind of patients in our early experience. Sixty-seven patients had a Tonnis grade 0, 30 patients had grade 1,

F. Laude (✉)
Department of Othopedic Surgery,
CMC Paris V, Paris, France
e-mail: flaude@mac.com

E. Sariali
Department of Orthopedic Surgery,
Hopital la Pitié Salptrière,
Paris, France

Ó. Marín-Peña (ed.), *Femoroacetabular Impingement*,
DOI 10.1007/978-3-642-22769-1_18, © Springer-Verlag Berlin Heidelberg 2012

**Fig. 18.1** The patient is positioned in supine position with the traction device. The traction is only applied on the operated lower limb during the acetabular time. All of the approach is done with a light flexion. No fluoroscopy is needed. The incision is antero-lateral and sized approximately 2–4 cm. The skin incision is parallel to the classic incision described by Hueter but moved downwards by approximately 1.5 cm to prevent injury of the lateral nerve of the thigh. The incision is centred on the summit of the great trochanter. Another more lateral and lower portal is used for the scope

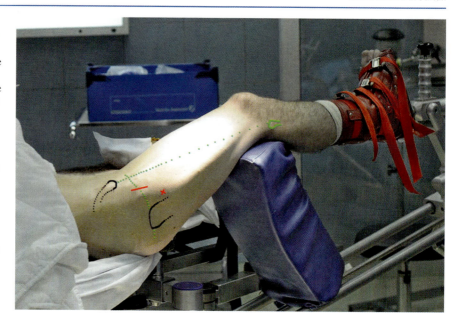

and three patients had grade 2. Five patients had had prior hip surgery: one had had a previous femoral neck fracture; one had a mild femoral head deformity following trauma at age 14; one had had previous labral resection; one had already been operated for FAI but had persistent hip pain; one had been subjected to in situ pinning of slipped capital femoral epiphysis.

All patients were given a clinical evaluation preoperatively and at the last follow-up. Quality of life was assessed with the Christensen score (NAHS) using a self-administered questionnaire filled in by the patients. Videos and photographs were taken in each case, and the acetabular lesions were characterised according to the criteria of Beck et al. The depth of the acetabular cartilage lesions was measured; the lesions were classified using the Beck score. Clinical result was considered very good if the NAHS score was above 90, good if it ranged between 80 and 90, average between 70 and 80 and poor under 70.

## Surgical Technique

All 100 hips underwent surgery with the same procedure. We used a scope to see the acetabulum in all but two of the patients. Patients were positioned supine on a regular table to which an extension was attached, allowing traction along the axis of the operated lower limb. The other leg was free so if too much traction was applied, the pelvis would tilt, preventing traction

damage. The size of the perineal post is a minimum of 12 cm. We have never used fluoroscopy. The knee was slightly flexed to relax the anterior structure of the hip (capsule, rectus femoris and psoas).

The skin incision was parallel to the classic incision described by Hueter but moved downwards by approximately 1.5 cm to prevent injury of the lateral nerve of the thigh. The incision was centred on the summit of the great trochanter (Fig. 18.1). There is no problem in making the incision longer, which could even provide better visualisation of the anterior part of the joint. A 7-cm incision provides a very large view. As the surgeon becomes more confident with this procedure, he can diminish the size of the skin incision.

The superficial fascia of the thigh is opened along the tensor fascia latae. The access continues inside the muscle girdle of the fascia lata towards the lateral side of the rectus (Fig. 18.2). The deep fibres of the rectus run straight down to an aponeurosis. At the upper part of this aponeurosis, just below the reflected part of the proximal tendon, there is a gap where one sees the capsule surrounded by fat. The innominate fascia is open (Fig. 18.2). No muscle is attached to this part of the fibrous capsule. There is a fat pad that can be removed (Fig. 18.2). We do not detach the gluteus minimus nor the iliocapsularis from the capsule. The dissection is easily done with a finger. This is an avascular space and usually does not bleed. This approach also has the advantage that it passes between two innervation territories: the muscles innervated by the femoral nerve (rectus psoas) and the

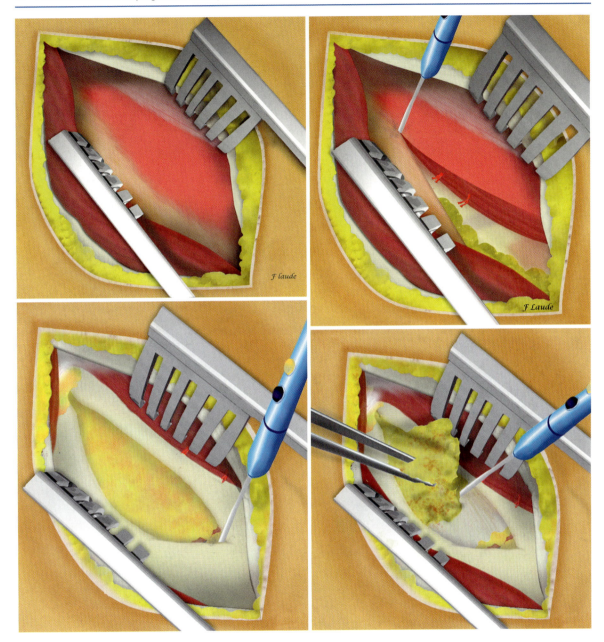

**Fig. 18.2** Description of the approach

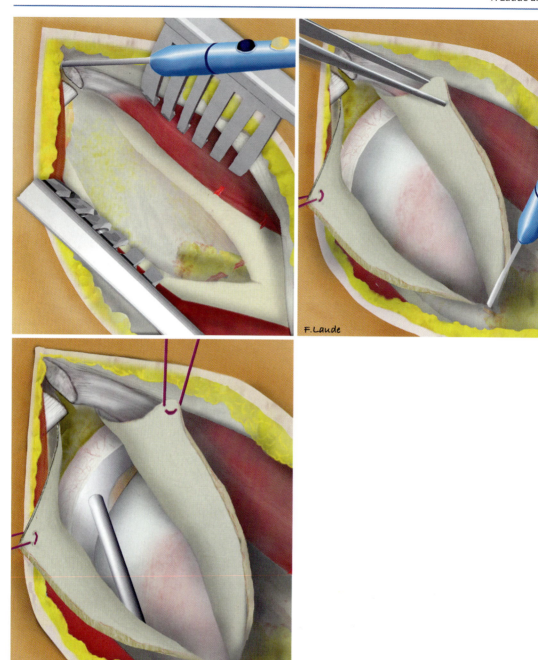

**Fig. 18.2** (continued)

muscles innervated by the gluteal nerve (gluteus minimus, gluteus medius and tensor fascia latae).

The articular capsule is opened along the upper border of the acetabulum from 10 and 2 o'clock, just over the labrum. In most cases, it is advisable to cut the pars reflecta of the rectus femoris to have a better view on the upper part of the acetabulum (Fig. 18.2). Then, a short vertical incision is performed along the medial band of the ilio-femoral ligament (Fig. 18.2). This vertical incision stops when the lateral circumflex artery becomes visible. If the surgeon wants to have a very good view of the lower part of the femoral neck, the lateral circumflex artery may be sectioned and ligated. This will allow better debridement of the capsula to see the lower part of the femoral neck. Section of this artery does not interfere with blood supply to the femoral head. The joint is usually kept open with a Gillis retractor during the procedure. The scope (a 30° scope at the beginning of our experience and a 70° scope thereafter) is inserted into the joint through another more lateral and distal portal (Fig. 18.2). At this time of the procedure, traction is applied to the lower limb in order to open and distract the joint. The distraction is usually less than 1 cm, with the scope permitting exploration of the acetabular cartilage and examination of the deeper region of the labrum. All the lesions were described, and a short video and some pictures were taken for all the patients. Cartilage lesions were assessed according to the criteria laid down by of Beck et al.

From 1999 to 2001, if the labrum was damaged, debridement was carried out, and then an acetabuloplasty was performed. Labral debridement consisted in a minimal excision of the damaged labrum. Since 2002, if we found debonded cartilage with loss of fixation to the sub-chondral bone (Beck type 3), the labrum was detached in order to perform an acetabuloplasty. If the labrum was intact, we tried, if possible, to refix it to the acetabular rim using two or three 2.9-mm suture anchors (Mitek R).

When present, delaminated cartilage and big flaps were not debrided. If an acetabuloplasty was performed, only unstable cartilage was removed. If a flap was present, a small curette and a chondral pick were used in order to perform micro-fractures, and then the flap was replaced. In one case of a 19-year-old male, the flap was so large that we had to stabilise it with non-absorbable monofilament (Prolene 5/0, Ethicon), and the labrum was refixed afterwards (Fig. 18.3).

The femoral side is probably the most critical time of the procedure. In our experience, it is fairly easy to determine the location of the bump on the femoral head. In fact, the conflictual cartilage was redder and more inflammatory than the normal cartilage, so it was quite easy to know where to perform the osteotomy of the femoral head–neck junction. We used a burr and a small chisel to perform the osteochondroplasty. In our early experience, we used a regular arthroscopic burr, but this instrument does not work very well when in contact with air, and it is sometimes easier to finish the trim-

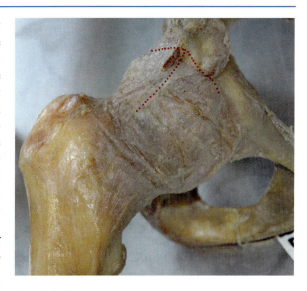

**Fig. 18.3** T-shaped opening of the capsulae. It may be sometimes necessary to cut the pars reflecta of the rectus femoris to have a better access to the acetabulum

ming of the femoral head with water. This is easily done by removing the retractor; in these cases, the water flows gently out through the anterior section without any consequence. In this case, trimming of the femoral head is performed only with arthroscopic visualisation.

Trimming of the femoral head usually extends from the medial synovial fold to the insertion of the retinacular vessel. This vessel can be seen clearly in most cases and must be preserved.

Duration of traction ranged between 5 and 45 min and was used only during the acetabular time (average time was about 32 min when the labrum was refixed and about 11 min otherwise). For the femoral preparation, it is usually easy to work with no traction and slight flexion of the thigh. Sometimes, light traction may be applied to allow better visualisation of the more lateral part of the femoral head.

If there are posterior lesions on the femoral head, it is advisable to establish another posterior portal for the scope or the instrument used to access the lesions. In our practice, we only had to resort to such a portal on two occasions.

Post-operatively, patients used crutches for 5 days on average. Full weight-bearing was allowed when they felt confident. Patients were encouraged to start biking as soon as they could. Impact sport practice was not allowed before 4–6 months. The procedure was always the same, even if we had to perform labral reattachment.

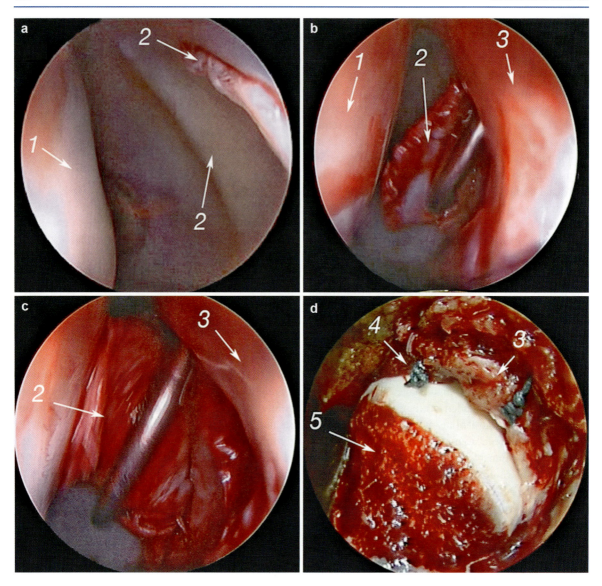

**Fig. 18.4** Scope view inside the acetabulum of a 19-year-old male (martial art performer) with a normal femoral head (1) and a huge flap (a–c). This big flap (2) is not removed. The labrum (3) is first fixed with two suture anchors (4), and the flap is fixed to the labrum with some non-absorbable monofilament (Prolene 5/0, Ethicon). The osteochondroplasty (5) of the femoral head–neck junction can then be performed with a chisel or a bur (d). This young patient had a very good result (NAHS improvement, 35 = >95) at 55 months

## Results

### Global Results

At the last follow-up analysis, mean NAHS score increased significantly by 29.6 points (84.3 ± 16 versus 54.5 ± 12, $p<0.000001$). The clinical result was very good in 40 cases, good in 38 cases, fair in 8 cases and poor in 14 patients. Eleven hips that developed osteoarthritis were eventually subjected to a total hip replacement. The final functional result was obtained after a mean period of 6.2 ± 3 months, with values ranging from 1 to 18 months. 67% of patients reached their final score before 6 months, but 14% needed more than 1 year to do so. Refixation of the labrum was not significantly correlated with a higher NAHS score (87 ± 11 versus 82 ± 19, $p<0.13$) at the last follow-up. In the group of patients under 40 and with a Tonnis grade of 0 (53), 90% obtained a very good or good result at a mean follow-up of 55 months (Fig. 18.4).

**Table 18.1** Details on patient with very good result: comparison between labrum fixation and others

| Patient with a final NAHS over 90 | Labrum refixation | No fixation |
|---|---|---|
| Number of cases | 17 | 23 |
| Age at surgery (years) | 29 | 34.1 |
| Follow-up (months) | 47.8 | 66.5 |
| Depth of the lesions | 6.41 | 4.7 |
| Revision | 2 | 0 |
| Tonnis grade = 1 at the time of surgery | 3/17 | 4/23 |
| Number of months before final score | 6.19 | 5.41 |

**Table 18.2** Details on patients with a good result: comparison between labrum fixation and others

| Patient with a final NAHS 80–90 | Labrum refixation | No fixation |
|---|---|---|
| Number of cases | 17 | 21 |
| Age at surgery (years) | 29.7 | 35 |
| Follow-up (months) | 48 | 62.6 |
| Depth of the lesions | 5.23 | 6.8 |
| Revision | 5 | 3 |
| Tonnis grade = 1 at the time of surgery | 1/17 | 8/21 |
| Number of months before final score | 6.19 | 6.29 |

## Sub-Group with Very Good Results

At the last follow-up analysis (58 months), 40 patients had a very good result, with a final score of more than 90 points (average pre-op 56.2± versus 97±) Table 18.1). The mean age for this special group was 32. The mean acetabular lesion depth was 5.5 mm. These patients were able to resume their regular sport activities with nearly no limitations. In this group, 21 hips were considered perfect with no pain even with strenuous sport activity. 13 of those 21 patients were professional athletes. They all returned to high-level sports with no limitations. 17 patients had a labral refixation. The NAHS score showed no significant difference between the sub-group with labral refixation ($p=0,1$) and the sub-group with no labral refixation.

Two patients had an average initial result at 1-year follow-up, so they were subjected to a complementary arthroscopic debridement. The first one was a 25-year-old professional ballet dancer who was reoperated at 17 months post-operatively for an arthroscopic resection of the bump on the femoral head. At the last follow-up analysis, she had a NAHS score of 95 and was still dancing professionally. The second patient was a 16-year-old woman who initially had a labral refixation. She underwent revision arthroscopic labral debridement at 1 year post-operatively. At the last follow-up, the score was 92. The pain also disappeared.

## Sub-group with Good Results

At the last follow-up (56.1±), 38 hips had a good result (Table 18.2). Mean age was 33. The average acetabular lesion depth was 6.1 mm. Those patients had normal daily life activities and performed gentle sport activities, such as biking or tracking.

Eight patients in this group had another hip arthroscopy because of recurrent pain. The average time between the two procedures was 33.2 months (range 87–1,5). One of those cases was our first case in 1999. The patient had already been operated in 1998 for an acetabular cyst in another institution. He was 19 at that time and was totally disabled (score less than 40). In 1999, we grafted the cyst and performed osteochondroplasty of the head–neck junction. The result was very good for 6 years, but some pain came back in 2006. He had an undetected retroversion of the acetabulum in 1999. The recurrent procedure was simply an acetabuloplasty with arthroscopic labral debridement. He had a good result at 15 months' follow-up. There was no significant difference between the patients with labral fixation and the sub-group with no labral refixation ($p=0.1$).

## Sub-group with Average Results

At the last follow-up visit (42), eight patients had a score between 70 and 80, with a significant improvement of 23.3 points (51 ± 6.4 versus 73 ± 3.4). Mean age was 33. At the last follow-up, these patients had limitations only during their sport activities. They could only do low-level physical activities. They had a normal daily life but were occasionally in pain. Only 11 patients had Tonnis grade 0, 6 had grade 1, and 1 had grade 2. The average depth of the acetabular lesion was 8.1 mm. In this group, two patients underwent labral refixation.

**Table 18.3** Details on patients who underwent an additional reconstructive surgery

| Case | Gender, age at surgery | Pertinent finding | Beck type | Depth of the lesions | Tonnis grade | Delay (months) | Type of surgery |
|---|---|---|---|---|---|---|---|
| 1 | F, 48 | The other hip was pain free at the time of the procedure and had a THA previously | 5 | 10 | 1 | 75 | THR |
| 2 | M, 39 | Moderated slipped capital epiphysis. Other hip had a THR in 1989 for the same problem | 3 | 10 | 1 | 52 | THR |
| 3 | M, 38 | Judoka. Actually, the 2 hips had THR | 5 | 10 | 2 | 25 | THR |
| 4 | M, 40 | Triathlete, marathon runner. Still very active | 4 | 5 | 1 | 16 | THR |
| 5 | M, 34 | Karateka. Never stop karate even after resurfacing | 5 | 10 | 1 | 58 | Hip resurfacing |
| 6 | F, 29 | International ballet dancer. Mild dysplasia. Refuse the periacetabular osteotomy | 5 | 15 | 0 | 36 | Hip resurfacing |
| 7 | F, 24 | Severe slipped capital epiphysis | 5 | 15 | 2 | 10 | THR |
| 8 | M, 42 | Mixed FAI (pincer and cam) | 5 | 10 | 1 | 5 | THR |
| 9 | F, 45 | Previous arthroscopy for osteochondromatosis | 3 | 15 | 0 | 15 | THR |
| 10 | F, 56 | Fracture of the femoral neck at 3 weeks treated conservatively with moderate varus malunion. Had a very good hip for 18 months | 3 | 10 | 0 | 26 | THR |
| 11 | M, 48 | The other hip already had a THR | 4 | 10 | 1 | 70 | THR |

## Sub-group with Poor Results and No THR

At the last follow-up (62), three patients had a poor outcome, with a mean improvement of 11 points. This poor result was surprising in two patients who had nearly no cartilage lesion pre-operatively. Both of them underwent labral refixation. One of them had revision arthroscopy, during which a torn and detached labrum was found. After resection, the patient seemed to experience a huge improvement, but the procedure was performed too recently to remove her from the poor-results list. The problem was probably due to a technical failure with inadequate labral fixation or insufficient osteochondroplasty of the femoral neck. The third patient (a 38-year-old female) had a femoral neck fracture in childhood. Initially, she had a very good result; however, pain reappeared at 3 years post-operatively.

She had another arthroscopic procedure which demonstrated a worsening of her cartilage damage. At the last follow-up, she was still in pain with a low score (50).

## Sub-group with Poor Results and THR

Eleven patients (11 hips) underwent an additional reconstructive hip surgery (Table 18.3). Nine patients had a total hip arthroplasty, and two had a resurfacing hip arthroplasty. Mean age of those patients was 40.3 (max, 56; min, 25). They all had showed severe acetabular cartilage lesions during the examination of their hip, with an average Beck score of 4. The mean acetabular lesion depth was about 10.9 mm.

However, some patients had quite good hip function for a while, and most of them do not regret the surgery.

## Surgical Complications

At 3 weeks post-operatively, one patient aged 56 sustained a femoral neck fracture. X-rays showed an undisplaced fracture of the femoral neck. We treated it conservatively, and she healed after 3 months but with slight varus malunion. She had a good result for 15 months but was eventually subjected to total hip replacement at 26 months. At the time of THR, the joint space was judged to be nearly normal.

Two patients had a deep infection treated successfully with surgical debridement and adapted antibiotic therapy for a period of 3 months.

One patient underwent a revision at 33 months post-operatively for a heterotopic ossification (Brooker 2), and ten patients had a revision for a complementary arthroscopic debridement 30 months ± 24 after the initial surgery. In seven cases, the initially reattached labrum was eventually debrided during the revision procedure.

## Predictive Parameters for Poor Results Treated with THR

THR risk was significantly correlated with a higher mean age (40 versus 32 $p < 0.01$), deeper acetabular lesions (33% of THR if depth was more than 10 mm, $p < 0.000001$) and Beck grade 5 (60% of THR, $p < 0.000001$). Refixation of the labrum was correlated with a lower rate of total hip replacement at the last follow-up (2.5% versus 18%, $p < 0.015$), but those who had a refixation of their labrum usually had healthier cartilage than those where the labrum was debrided.

In addition, poor clinical results were significantly correlated with a Tonis grade 1 or 2 ($p < 0.001$). There was no significant difference of age between the 4 groups; however, the poor-results group had a tendency towards a higher mean age (38 versus 32, $p = 0.09$). On the other hand, poor results were correlated with deeper acetabular lesions ($p < 0.001$).

## Discussion

We used the Christensen Non-arthritic Hip Score [6] (NAHS) in this study. The classic scores (Harris Hip Score and Merle d'Aubigné score) do not provide a clear idea of the patient's quality of life. A possible solution could be to combine different scores, like the WOMAC, the Harris and the UCLA activity score [1, 28]; the Christensen score (NAHS) could be considered to be a "simplified WOMAC" with many questions about sport activities. The questionnaire is easy to fill out and very sensitive. To simplify the review for our study, the questionnaire was installed on a secure Web site, allowing patients to fill it out online. Authors think that this is of great interest in order to follow those young patients who frequently move to different places.

Although the hip dislocation technique developed in Berne by Ganz et al. [11] is efficient and safe, the authors shied away from it at the beginning of their learning curve as no available data were reported in the literature at that time (1999). In addition, due to our vast experience with the Hueter approach in performing [27] THR, we felt that the latter could afford adequate visualisation of the impingement lesion and allow performance of a femoral head–neck junction osteochondroplasty with minimal soft tissue dissection. After the first two cases, it appeared that we had poor exposure on the acetabular side, so we started to use a 30° scope to explore the acetabular cavity. Arthroscopy allows full visualisation of the acetabular cavity without dislocation using minimal traction. Furthermore, arthroscopy allows the capture of video images that can be useful for analysis. A minimal opening of the joint is possible using an anterior mini-Hueter approach in order to assess and treat the lesions inside the acetabular cavity. Traction is applied only at that step, which is probably why we did not have any of the complications associated with traction in hip arthroscopy in our study [5].

We still use the surgical dislocation approach when confronted with large deformities in order to perform an osteotomy of the femoral neck or the femoral metaphysis.

Many authors [1, 3, 7, 11] recommend delamination of the cartilage to a stable edge. In this study, cartilage flaps on the acetabular side were not removed. In fact, micro-fractures of the sub-chondral bone were done under the flap which was repositioned in its normal position. In case of instability, the flap was fixed to the sub-chondral bone with a non-resorbable monofilament. Only the cartilage on the site of the acetabuloplasty was removed.

In contrast to the findings by Espinosa et al. [9, 10], our study showed no significant differences in terms of the clinical results between the group with labral refixation and the group with no labral refixation, even though there was a tendency towards a higher NAHS score in the cases of labral fixation. It is important to note that we never resected the whole labrum and our debridement applied only to the torn portion. This is different from Espinosa et al.'s paper where they compared resection to labral refixation. Thus, it is still unclear if labral refixation is necessary when the acetabular rim does not need trimming and requires further study. However, we keep on performing labral refixation only if the labrum is not damaged. In fact, we think that refixation of a damaged labrum could be responsible of pain, and so revision for debridement could be needed. Furthermore, all the patients had full immediate weight-bearing post-operatively, and this may prevent labral healing. This is why many authors [26] propose no weight-bearing for a period of 4–6 weeks.

Recently, some patients treated for FAI with a removal of their labrum had an arthroscopic exploration. We were very surprised to discover around the acetabulum soft tissue acting like a normal labrum. We postulate that good results may be achieved even in case of labrum removal.

The length of the recovery period varied widely in our study. Early intensive rehabilitation may allow quick achievement of the final functional result. In fact, Phillipon et al. [26] used continuous passive motion for more than 8 h a day during the first 4 weeks. This is probably a very good idea even if it does not seem easy to set up. According to our experience, cycling seems to lead to better functional results; unfortunately, we do not have enough data to support this. We prefer to use our own technique rather than the Bernese dislocation technique in order to avoid the complications related to trochanterotomy [1]. Furthermore, we think that our minimal invasive technique allows a shorter hospital stay because patients seem to be in less pain.

One femoral neck fracture was found in this cohort. The 56-year-old patient was the oldest in the series. In this case, the femoral head–neck junction osteochondroplasty was not very large and below the 30% safety threshold that Mardones et al. [20] recommend. We treated it conservatively, and the patient healed in 3 months, albeit with slight varus malunion. She obtained a good result during the first 15 months, but pain came back, making a total hip replacement necessary at 26 months. At the time of THR, the joint space width was nearly normal.

The good results in this cohort reinforce many of the previous studies on femoroacetabular impingement and its treatment [1, 3, 4, 7, 12, 13, 15, 18, 21–25, 29].

Very good results can be achieved with our technique, which is much less invasive than the Bernese surgical approach. The mini-open approach allowed us to get used to hip arthroscopy techniques, and so we have progressively switched to a fully arthroscopic technique. The all-arthroscopic technique is attractive because FAI can be better visualised under arthroscopy in full hip flexion. Furthermore, osteochondroplasty seems to be more easy to perform under arthroscopy, probably because of the liquid environment.

## References

1. Beaule PE, Le Duff MJ, Zaragoza E (2007) Quality of life following femoral head-neck osteochondroplasty for femoroacetabular impingement. J Bone Joint Surg Am 89(4):773–779
2. Beck M, Kalhor M, Leunig M, Ganz R (2005) Hip morphology influences the pattern of damage to the acetabular cartilage: femoroacetabular impingement as a cause of early osteoarthritis of the hip. J Bone Joint Surg Br 87(7):1012–1018
3. Beck M, Leunig M, Parvizi J, Boutier V, Wyss D, Ganz R (2004) Anterior femoroacetabular impingement: part II. Midterm results of surgical treatment. Clin Orthop Relat Res 418:67–73
4. Bizzini M, Notzli HP, Maffiuletti NA (2007) Femoroacetabular impingement in professional ice hockey players: a case series of 5 athletes after open surgical decompression of the hip. Am J Sports Med 35(11):1955–1959
5. Byrd JW, Pappas JN, Pedley MJ (1995) Hip arthroscopy: an anatomic study of portal placement and relationship to the extra-articular structures. Arthroscopy 11(4):418–423
6. Christensen CP, Althausen PL, Mittleman MA, Lee JA, McCarthy JC (2003) The nonarthritic hip score: reliable and validated. Clin Orthop Relat Res 406:75–83
7. Clohisy JC, McClure JT (2005) Treatment of anterior femoroacetabular impingement with combined hip arthroscopy and limited anterior decompression. Iowa Orthop J 25:164–171
8. Crawford JR, Villar RN (2005) Current concepts in the management of femoroacetabular impingement. J Bone Joint Surg Br 87(11):1459–1462
9. Espinosa N, Beck M, Rothenfluh DA, Ganz R, Leunig M (2007) Treatment of femoro-acetabular impingement: preliminary results of labral refixation. Surgical technique. J Bone Joint Surg Am 89(Suppl 2 Pt.1):36–53
10. Espinosa N, Rothenfluh DA, Beck M, Ganz R, Leunig M (2006) Treatment of femoro-acetabular impingement: preliminary results of labral refixation. J Bone Joint Surg Am 88(5):925–935
11. Ganz R, Gill TJ, Gautier E, Ganz K, Krugel N, Berlemann U (2001) Surgical dislocation of the adult hip a technique with full access to the femoral head and acetabulum without the risk of avascular necrosis. J Bone Joint Surg Br 83(8):1119–1124
12. Ganz R, Parvizi J, Beck M, Leunig M, Notzli H, Siebenrock KA (2003) Femoroacetabular impingement: a cause for osteoarthritis of the hip. Clin Orthop Relat Res 417:112–120

13. Guanche CA, Bare AA (2006) Arthroscopic treatment of femoroacetabular impingement. Arthroscopy 22(1):95–106

14. Klaue K, Durnin CW, Ganz R (1991) The acetabular rim syndrome. A clinical presentation of dysplasia of the hip. J Bone Joint Surg Br 73(3):423–429

15. Laude F, Boyer T, Nogier A (2007) Anterior femoroacetabular impingement. Joint Bone Spine 74(2):127–132

16. Lequesne M, de S (1961) [False profile of the pelvis. A new radiographic incidence for the study of the hip. Its use in dysplasias and different coxopathies.]. Rev Rhum Mal Osteoartic 28:643–652

17. Lequesne M, Samson M, Gerard P, Mery C (1990) Pain-function indices for the follow-up of osteoarthritis of the hip and the knee. Rev Rhum Mal Osteoartic 57(9 (Pt 2)):32S–36S

18. Leunig M, Beck M, Dora C, Ganz R (2006) Femoroacetabular impingement: trigger for the development of coxarthrosis. Orthopade 35(1):77–84

19. Leunig M, Ganz R (2005) Femoroacetabular impingement. A common cause of hip complaints leading to arthrosis. Unfallchirurg 108(1):9–10, 12–17

20. Mardones RM, Gonzalez C, Chen Q, Zobitz M, Kaufman KR, Trousdale RT (2005) Surgical treatment of femoroacetabular impingement: evaluation of the effect of the size of the resection. J Bone Joint Surg Am 87(2):273–279

21. May O, Matar WY, Beaule PE (2007) Treatment of failed arthroscopic acetabular labral debridement by femoral chondro-osteoplasty: a case series of five patients. J Bone Joint Surg Br 89(5):595–598

22. Murphy S, Tannast M, Kim YJ, Buly R, Millis MB (2004) Debridement of the adult hip for femoroacetabular impinge-ment: indications and preliminary clinical results. Clin Orthop Relat Res 429:178–181

23. Nogier A (2003) Le conflit fémoro-acétabulaire antérieur. Thèse de médecine. [Thèse de médecine.] Paris, Université Paris 7

24. Parvizi J, Leunig M, Ganz R (2007) Femoroacetabular impingement. J Am Acad Orthop Surg 15(9):561–570

25. Philippon M, Schenker M, Briggs K, Kuppersmith D (2007) Femoroacetabular impingement in 45 professional athletes: associated pathologies and return to sport following arthroscopic decompression. Knee Surg Sports Traumatol Arthrosc 15(7):908–914

26. Philippon MJ, Stubbs AJ, Schenker ML, Maxwell RB, Ganz R, Leunig M (2007) Arthroscopic management of femoro-acetabular impingement: osteoplasty technique and litera-ture review. Am J Sports Med 35(9):1571–1580

27. Sariali E, Leonard P, Mamoudy P (2008) Dislocation after total hip arthroplasty using Hueter Anterior approach. J Arthroplasty 23(2):266–272

28. Stucki G, Sangha O, Stucki S, Michel BA, Tyndall A, Dick W, Theiler R (1998) Comparison of the WOMAC (Western Ontario and McMaster Universities) osteoarthritis index and a self-report format of the self-administered Lequesne-Algofunctional index in patients with knee and hip osteoar-thritis. Osteoarthritis Cartilage 6(2):79–86

29. Zebala LP, Schoenecker PL, Clohisy JC (2007) Anterior femoroacetabular impingement: a diverse disease with evolving treatment options. Iowa Orthop J 27:71–81

# Part IV

# FAI and Hip Dysplasia

# Differentiating FAI from Dysplasia

**19**

Wadih Y. Matar and Javad Parvizi

## Introduction

Young adult patients presenting with hip pain can pose a challenging diagnostic dilemma for the inexperienced physician. A thorough history and physical examination followed by the appropriate imaging can often lead to the right diagnosis. In this chapter, distinguishing between two of the most common hip pathologies affecting the young adult, namely, hip dysplasia and femoroacetabular impingement (FAI), will be discussed. Diagnosing these two types of mechanical hip disorders can be at times challenging since they can coexist in the same patient [1–3] (Fig. 19.1).

The etiology of hip dysplasia has been studied extensively and been shown to implicate intrauterine, environmental, and genetic factors [4, 5]. FAI, on the other hand, is a much newer diagnosis that was first described by Ganz et al. [3, 6]. It is, however, similar to hip dysplasia in that they both have abnormal morphology of the hip joint leading to repetitive shear stress at the level of the acetabular rim [1]. In fact, FAI and hip dysplasia represent the two most common causes of acetabular rim syndrome. The increase in mechanical stress can eventually lead to degenerative osteoarthritis of the hip: an association that was first postulated by Harris in the 1980s and further studied by Ganz et al.

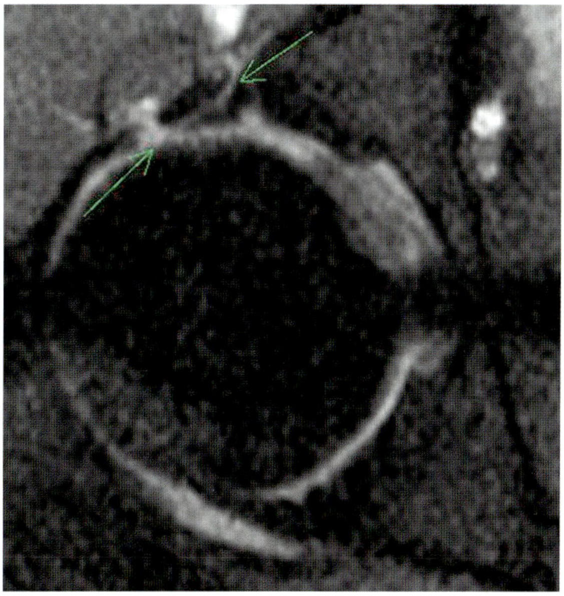

**Fig. 19.1** A 35-year-old patient with mild dysplasia of the hip who also has femoroacetabular impingement (a bump on the femoral neck) leading to labral tear and detachment (see *arrows*)

during the last decade [6–8]. It remains that being able to diagnose these two conditions early on prior to disease process can potentially give the orthopedic surgeon a method to alter and maybe halt the progression toward end-stage degeneration of the hip joint.

## History

Patient's interview should be focused on determining the etiology of the hip symptoms. This usually starts off by careful history taking with regard to the pain

W.Y. Matar • J. Parvizi (✉)
Department of Orthopaedic Surgery,
The Rothman Institute of Orthopaedics,
Thomas Jefferson University Hospital,
Philadelphia, PA, USA
e-mail: parvj@aol.com

Ó. Marín-Peña (ed.), *Femoroacetabular Impingement*,
DOI 10.1007/978-3-642-22769-1_19, © Springer-Verlag Berlin Heidelberg 2012

characteristics, location, onset, duration, and nature of the pain, as well as provoking and alleviating factors (treatment). The patient should also be questioned regarding all previous hip pathologies and their corresponding treatments. Family as well as occupational history, hobbies, and sports should be questioned as they can be important for the diagnosis. Finally, patient age, comorbidities, and overall physical conditioning should also be obtained.

Previous hip complaints in early childhood or a positive family history, first born, female, frank breech, and left sidedness are significant risk factors for developmental dysplasia of the hip [4, 5]. FAI can be usually found in young patients (<50 years) with abnormal hip anatomy (described below) who complain about pain in the seated position or with deep flexion and internal rotation of the hip [2, 9]. In this position, the abnormal proximal femur abuts against the acetabular rim leading to excessive shear stress. The pain is usually localized to the groin area, but can at times be present in the gluteal or the trochanteric areas secondary to abnormal gait biomechanics [9]. FAI can also be found in patients with excessive range of motion (ROM) of the hip (ballet, gymnastics, yoga). Furthermore, any history or catching or locking may be indicative of intra-articular hip pathology such as a labral tear or a chondral flap that are common with FAI [10, 11]. It is, however, important to develop a wide differential diagnosis when faced with a patient with hip pain, including radicular pain from disc disease, sacroiliac joint disease, traumatic and stress fractures, and greater trochanter bursitis to name a few.

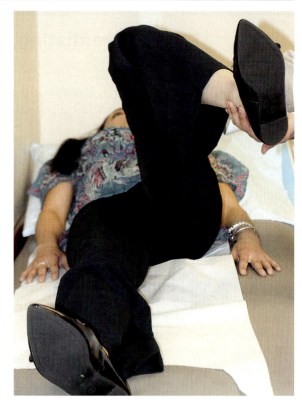

**Fig. 19.2** Anterior impingement sign: the hip is flexed to 90° while internally rotating and adducting the leg in a patient lying supine. A positive sign elicits groin pain in the FAI patient as the femoral head with decreased anterior head/neck offset abuts against the damaged cartilage of the acetabular rim

## Physical Examination

The postulated differential diagnosis obtained from the history can be narrowed down by a careful physical examination. The latter starts off by an assessment of the patient's overall physical conditioning and gait pattern. Some patients ambulate with an increased foot progression angle (>10°) secondary to an externally rotated leg from a slipped capital femoral epiphysis (SCFE) during adolescence [9]. FAI patients can present with an antalgic gait which should be distinguished from the Trendelenburg gait pattern seen with hip dysplasia secondary to weak abductors. An abductor lurch, on the other hand, can be suggestive of advanced hip arthritis. The patient's lower extremities are then assessed for any leg length discrepancy (LLD) or fixed deformities.

A severe case of hip dysplasia can present with a significant LLD. The pelvis is also examined for any pelvic tilt and lumbosacral flexibility.

Range of motion of both hips is also assessed actively and passively. It is important to keep a hand over the anterior superior iliac spine to detect the true limit of hip motion and the beginning of pelvic motion due to abutment. In general, patients with developmental hip dysplasia have good flexion and internal rotation in flexion, whereas FAI patients are restricted in both [1, 2]. Additionally, anterior FAI should be examined for by performing the impingement sign maneuver in the supine position (Fig. 19.2) [12, 13]. The affected hip is flexed to 90° while maximally internally rotating and adducting the leg. A positive sign reproduces groin pain in the FAI patient as the femoral head with a deficient anterior head/neck offset abuts against the damaged cartilage or acetabular rim. On the other hand, posterior impingement can be examined for by externally rotating a hyperextended hip. This posterior impingement test is usually positive in

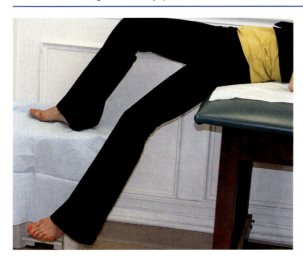

**Fig. 19.3** Posterior impingement test: the hip is externally rotated and hyperextended while the contralateral hip is maintained in a maximally flexed position. The test is done with both of the patient's limbs dangling over the end of the examination table. A positive test usually elicits buttock pain caused by the femoral head abutting against the posterior acetabular rim

the presence of posterior acetabular cartilage injury secondary to the impingement [9]. The test is done with the patient in the supine position and both legs dangling over the end of the examination table: the affected hip is extended and externally rotated, while the contralateral hip is maintained in a maximally flexed position by the patient (Fig. 19.3). A positive test usually reproduces buttock pain from the femoral head abutting against the posterior acetabular rim. Beck et al. showed that this test can also be positive in the presence of acetabular retroversion with FAI and a contrecoup lesion, which results from posterior subluxation of the femoral head secondary to anterior impingement with the acetabular rim [12]. Patient with acetabular retroversion also presents with decreased internal rotation [1]. In these patients, when the hip is brought into flexion, an obligatory external rotation of the limb occurs as the proximal femur contacts the prominent anterior rim of the acetabulum [9]. The physical examination is then completed with a thorough neurological and vascular examination of the lower extremity.

## Radiological Assessment

Every radiological assessment should include a plain anteroposterior (AP) radiograph of the pelvis along with an AP and cross-table or frog-leg lateral view of both hips. In most cases, these views are adequate in assessing hip morphology. However, in certain situations, specialized lateral radiographs such as Dunn's view [14] or the false-profile view of Lequesne [15] are necessary to assess anterior acetabular coverage. In other situation such as preoperative planning, a hip abduction view or a computerized tomography (CT-SCAN) will be useful in the dysplastic patient to better delineate the bony anatomy and the degree of dysplasia. In FAI patients, magnetic resonance imaging (MRI) arthrography of the hip is used commonly to measure femoral head asphericity and in diagnosing intra-articular labral or chondral pathologies [16–19]. Finally, when facing an uncertain diagnosis, a fluoroscopically guided diagnostic hip injection followed by a physical examination after the injection may help in the diagnosis.

With regard to the radiographs, it is important to ascertain that these are of good quality showing a clear outline of the acetabulum and done in a standardized fashion assuring proper patient positioning. A standard AP view of the pelvis should include the iliac crests and extend distally to include the proximal third of both femora. Furthermore, the distance between the tip of the coccyx and the top of the symphysis pubis should be between 1 and 2 cm to assure proper pelvic tilt [20]. Pelvic rotation is assured by obturator foramina symmetry and by making sure the tip of the coccyx is bisecting the symphysis pubis. Any discrepancy within these parameters should prompt the surgeon to repeat the AP radiograph prior to proceeding. The pelvic AP view is assessed for gross bony abnormality with careful attention to the structural anatomy of the hip joint: femoral head sphericity, contour of the head/neck junction, weight-bearing sourcil, anterior and posterior walls, medial teardrop, and the lateral edge of the acetabulum should be evaluated. The hip joint is further examined for the presence of any degenerative changes.

## Dysplastic Hips

The dysplastic hip represents several common deformities on both the acetabular and femoral side. Typical pelvic deformities include a shallow anteverted socket, lateralized hip center of rotation, and anterior and superolateral bony deficiency. The femur, on the other hand, can have a short, valgus neck with excessive anteversion, posteriorly displaced greater trochanter and a narrow intramedullary canal.

It is imperative that the orthopedic surgeon evaluates the radiographs for these changes. On the acetabular

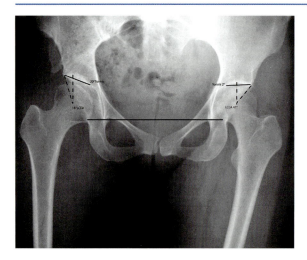

**Fig. 19.4** The LCE angle of Wiberg is contained between a line drawn from the center of the femoral head to the lateral aspect of the acetabular roof and a vertical line drawn through the center of the femoral head (*dashed line*). An angle less than 20° is diagnostic of dysplasia. The Tönnis angle is calculated by drawing a horizontal line across the medial edge of the weight-bearing portion of the acetabulum (*sourcil*) and a second line from this point out to the lateral edge of the acetabulum (*solid line*); its normal value is less than 10°

side, the following parameters should be measured: lateral center-edge angle of Wiberg (LCEA), anterior center-edge angle of Lequesne (ACEA), Tönnis angle, excursion distance (migration index), and finally, the

percentage of subluxation/dislocation to classify the extent of the disease. On the femoral side, the neck-shaft angle (normal 120–140°) and the percentage of femoral head coverage (dysplastic <75%) should be evaluated.

LCEA is measured between a line drawn from the center of the femoral head to the lateral aspect of the acetabular roof and a vertical line drawn through the center of the femoral head (Fig. 19.4) [21]. An angle greater than 25° is normal, whereas an angle less than 20° is diagnostic of dysplasia and angle between 20° and 25° is considered borderline. ACEA is measured on a false-profile view as described by Lequesne [15]. To obtain this image, the pelvis is positioned at 65° from the cassette with the affected hip proximal to the film (Fig. 19.5a). A good study should have the equivalent of one femoral head diameter distance between the two femoral heads (Fig. 19.5b). ACAE is measured in a similar fashion as described for the LCEA and is considered abnormal if less 25°. In addition to assessing for anterior coverage, the false-profile view also provides information on joint space integrity at the antero-superior and posteroinferior aspects of the hip joint, as well as on the presence of osteophytosis. The Tönnis angle is formed between the weight-bearing zone of the acetabular roof (sourcil) and a horizontal line (Fig. 19.4). It is considered dysplastic if greater than 10°. The excursion distance (migration index) is the amount of

**Fig. 19.5** (**a**) False-profile view of Lequesne [15]: the pelvis is positioned at 65° from the cassette with the affected hip more proximal to the film. (**b**) The ACE angle defined by a line drawn from the center of the femoral head to the lateral aspect of the acetabular roof and a vertical line drawn through the center of the femoral head (*dashed line*). An angle less than 25° is diagnostic of dysplasia

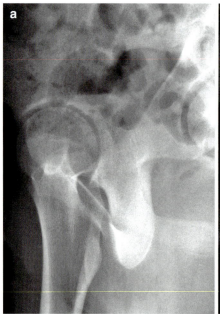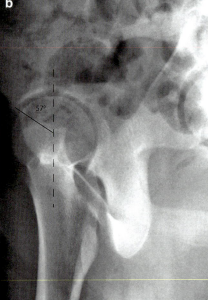

**Table 19.1** Dysplastic hip classifications as described by Crowe et al. [22] and Hartofilakidis et al. [23]

| Crowe | Crowe | Hartofilakidis |
|---|---|---|
| I | <50% of femoral head or <10% of pelvic height | Dysplasia (true acetabulum with sup deficit) |
| II | 50–75% of femoral head or 10–15% pelvic height | |
| III | 75–100% of femoral head or −20% pelvic height | Low dislocation (overlap of false and true acetab – ant and lat deficiency) |
| IV | 100% of femoral head or >20% pelvic height | High dislocation |

In the Crowe classification, the percentage of proximal femoral head displacement is estimated by measuring the distance from the inter-teardrop line to the inferomedial head–neck junction and dividing it by the height of the femoral head. If the femoral head is deformed, pelvic height can be used instead

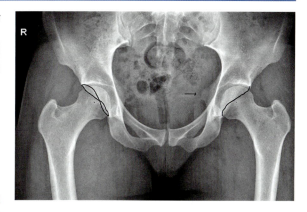

**Fig. 19.6** Pelvic AP view of a patient with bilateral acetabular retroversion. A crossover sign can be seen in the right hip: the junction of the anterior and posterior acetabular walls is distal to the lateral margin of the acetabular roof. The posterior wall sign, represented by the acetabular wall that lies medial to the center of the femoral head, is shown on the left hip. Also note the protrusion of the ischial spine into the pelvic cavity, which constitutes the third sign of a retroverted acetabulum

femoral head uncoverage divided by the width of femoral head. Normally, it should be less than 20%.

Two classification systems based on the proximal migration of the femoral head have been described (Table 19.1) [22, 23]. We tend to favor that of Hartofilakidis as it represents a better treatment algorithm. In this classification, the hip can be dysplastic (equivalent to Crowe I and II), low dislocation (equivalent to Crowe III), or a high dislocation (equivalent to Crowe IV).

## FAI

Femoroacetabular impingement has been divided into two types: Cam and Pincer [6]. Even though they have been described as separate entities, the majority of patients may have a combination of both [2, 9, 12]. Cam-type FAI is caused by the abutment of an abnormally shaped head/neck junction lacking in anterior offset against the acetabular rim. The typical patient with Cam-type impingement is a heavy laborer who is active and may have a previous history of SCFE, post-traumatic deformity, or coxa vara. Pincer type, on the other hand, is caused by acetabular retroversion or the presence of coxa profunda leading to excessive contact between the acetabular rim and the femoral head/neck junction ultimately leading to a decreased ROM. The majority of these patients are younger females engaged in activities that require excessive hip ROM such as ballet and gymnastics [6, 7, 12].

Several radiological signs have been identified to distinguish between the two entities. Radiological assessment should start with an AP view of the pelvis to identify acetabular version. In an anteverted socket, the anterior and posterior walls join at the proximal lateral margin of the acetabulum, whereas in the retroverted acetabulum, the junction is more distal. This sign has been termed the "crossover sign" by Reynolds et al. as an indicator for acetabular retroversion (Fig. 19.6) [24]. The "posterior wall sign" is a second radiological evidence of acetabular retroversion [3, 24]. It is present when the posterior wall of the acetabulum lies medially to the center of the femoral head. A third sign of retroversion has recently been identified by Kalberer et al. who have shown that the projection of the ischial spine into the pelvic cavity is more common in the setting of acetabular retroversion [25]. Comparing this to the crossover sign, they found a 91% sensitivity, 98% specificity, and positive predictive values.

Once acetabular version has been identified, the depth of the socket should be determined. Coxa profunda is identified when the medial wall or floor of the acetabular fossa lies in line with the ilioischial line (Kohler's line). However, if it lies medial to this line, then acetabular protrusio is present. This can be idiopathic (e.g., Otto's pelvis) or secondary to labral failure and degeneration in pincer impingement leading to a lower degree of overcoverage [9]. A classification system for acetabular protrusion has been described by Sotelo-Garza and Charnley [26]. Of note is that ACEA is usually increased in the setting of protrusio.

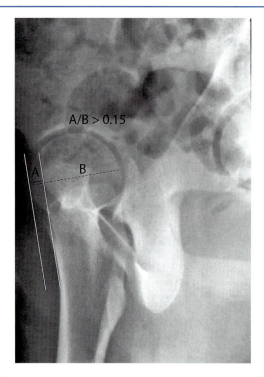

**Fig. 19.7** Eijer's ratio is calculated by dividing the anterior off-set distance "*A*" by the diameter of the femoral head "*B*" on a cross-table lateral view of the hip. An offset ratio <0.15 is diagnostic of FAI

Proximal femoral anatomy should then be assessed for deformities consistent with Cam impingement. These include pistol grip deformity [27] – convex superolateral head/neck junction secondary to a "bump" extension on the base of the neck – SCFE [28], and malunited femoral neck fractures [29]. Leunig et al. also identified fibrocystic changes ("herniation pits") at the anterosuperior aspect of the head/neck junction in one third of patient with FAI [30]. However, to truly assess the anterior head/neck offset and the asphericity of the femoral head, a lateral view is warranted (cross-table lateral or Dunn's view). Dunn's view is obtained by taking an AP of the hip with the leg at 45° of flexion (can also be done at 90°), neutral rotation, and 20° of abduction [14]. In this view, the lack of anterior head/neck offset and the presence of a "bump" rendering the normally concave surface more convex can be easily seen. Meyer et al. compared six different radiographic views to determine the best method to identify femoral head/neck asphericity [14]. They concluded that the latter is highly dependent on the radiological view at hand: the

Dunn's view at 45° or 90° of flexion and the cross-table view in internal rotation were best at showing femoral head/neck asphericity, while an AP or externally rotated cross-table views were likely to miss the asphericity.

Two methods are commonly used to quantify femoral head asphericity. The first is the offset ratio as described by Eijer et al. [31]. It is calculated on a cross-table lateral or Dunn's view by dividing the anterior offset distance by the diameter of the femoral head (Fig. 19.7) [31]. A ratio <0.15 is diagnostic of FAI.

The lack of anterior offset can also measured with the α-angle of Nötzli et al. [16]. This angle is measured on an axial MRI view taken parallel to the axis of the femoral neck and head. The α-angle is measured between a line drawn from the center of the femoral head bisecting the neck and a line from the center of the femoral head to a point where the anterior head/neck concavity transects a circle representing the radius of the head. In the original series, the FAI group of patients had an α-angle of 74° compared to 42° in the control group. It is now commonly accepted that an α-angle >50.5° is diagnostic of FAI (Fig. 19.8).

MRI scans are also used to obtain three-dimensional reconstructions of the head/neck junction to better visualize the "bump" and assist in surgical planning [32]. However, with added hip arthrography, the strength of the MRI scan rests in its ability to provide information on intra-articular pathologies, such as labral tears or cysts, articular damage and delamination, and intraosseous cyst formation; all of which are important factors in the treatment algorithm.

## Conclusion

The understanding of hip pathology in the young patient has progressed immensely over the last two decades especially due to the work of Prof. Ganz both on dysplasia, through periacetabular osteotomies, and on FAI as outlined above. However, the basic principles of obtaining a proper history and performing a physical examination have withstood the test of time and both remain crucial steps in obtaining a proper diagnosis. Improvements in imaging of the hip have allowed us to gain better insight into various pathologies of the hip joint. Further, improvements are needed to better visualize the articular cartilage and better define normal hip morphology.

**Fig. 19.8** The α-angle of Nötzli is measured by drawing a line between the center of the femoral head and the point at which the anterior head/neck concavity transects a circle representing the radius of the head. The angle between this line and the longitudinal axis of the femoral neck represents the α-angle of Nötzli. An α-angle >50.5° is diagnostic of FAI

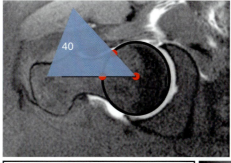

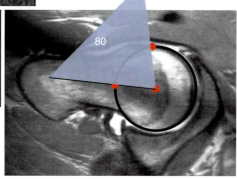

1. Draw a circle at head
2. Draw line through neck
3. Note where femoral head 'leaves circle'
4. Alpha angle: from here to femoral neck line

## References

1. Klaue K, Durnin CW, Ganz R (1991) The acetabular rim syndrome. A clinical presentation of dysplasia of the hip. J Bone Joint Surg Br 733:423–429
2. Clohisy JC, Beaule PE, O'Malley A, Safran MR, Schoenecker P (2008) AOA symposium. Hip disease in the young adult: current concepts of etiology and surgical treatment. J Bone Joint Surg Am 9010:2267–2281
3. Siebenrock KA, Schoeniger R, Ganz R (2003) Anterior femoro-acetabular impingement due to acetabular retroversion. Treatment with periacetabular osteotomy. J Bone Joint Surg Am 85-A2:278–286
4. Guille JT, Pizzutillo PD, MacEwen GD (2000) Development dysplasia of the hip from birth to six months. J Am Acad Orthop Surg 84:232–242
5. Dezateux C, Rosendahl K (2007) Developmental dysplasia of the hip. Lancet 3699572:1541–1552
6. Ganz R, Parvizi J, Beck M, Leunig M, Notzli H, Siebenrock KA (2003) Femoroacetabular impingement: a cause for osteoarthritis of the hip. Clin Orthop Relat Res 417:112–120
7. Lavigne M, Parvizi J, Beck M, Siebenrock KA, Ganz R, Leunig M (2004) Anterior femoroacetabular impingement: part I. Techniques of joint preserving surgery. Clin Orthop Relat Res 418:61–66
8. Harris WH (1986) Etiology of osteoarthritis of the hip. Clin Orthop Relat Res 213:20–33
9. Sierra RJ, Trousdale RT, Ganz R, Leunig M (2008) Hip disease in the young, active patient: evaluation and nonarthroplasty surgical options. J Am Acad Orthop Surg 1612:689–703
10. Peelle MW, la Rocca GJ, Maloney WJ, Curry MC, Clohisy JC (2005) Acetabular and femoral radiographic abnormalities associated with labral tears. Clin Orthop Relat Res 441:327–333
11. Wenger DE, Kendell KR, Miner MR, Trousdale RT (2004) Acetabular labral tears rarely occur in the absence of bony abnormalities. Clin Orthop Relat Res 426:145–150
12. Beck M, Kalhor M, Leunig M, Ganz R (2005) Hip morphology influences the pattern of damage to the acetabular cartilage: femoroacetabular impingement as a cause of early osteoarthritis of the hip. J Bone Joint Surg Br 877:1012–1018
13. Beaule PE, Le Duff MJ, Zaragoza E (2007) Quality of life following femoral head-neck osteochondroplasty for femoroacetabular impingement. J Bone Joint Surg Am 894:773–779
14. Meyer DC, Beck M, Ellis T, Ganz R, Leunig M (2006) Comparison of six radiographic projections to assess femoral head/neck asphericity. Clin Orthop Relat Res 445:181–185
15. Lequesne M, de Seze S (1961) False profile of the pelvis. A new radiographic incidence for the study of the hip. Its use in dysplasias and different coxopathies. Rev Rhum Mal Osteoartic 28:643–652
16. Notzli HP, Wyss TF, Stoecklin CH, Schmid MR, Treiber K, Hodler J (2002) The contour of the femoral head-neck junction as a predictor for the risk of anterior impingement. J Bone Joint Surg Br 844:556–560
17. Leunig M, Werlen S, Ungersbock A, Ito K, Ganz R (1997) Evaluation of the acetabular labrum by MR arthrography. J Bone Joint Surg Br 792:230–234
18. Leunig M, Podeszwa D, Beck M, Werlen S, Ganz R (2004) Magnetic resonance arthrography of labral disorders in hips with dysplasia and impingement. Clin Orthop Relat Res 418:74–80
19. Kassarjian A, Yoon LS, Belzile E, Connolly SA, Millis MB, Palmer WE (2005) Triad of MR arthrographic findings in patients with cam-type femoroacetabular impingement. Radiology 2362:588–592
20. Siebenrock KA, Kalbermatten DF, Ganz R (2003) Effect of pelvic tilt on acetabular retroversion: a study of pelves from cadavers. Clin Orthop Relat Res 407:241–248

21. Wiberg G (1939) Studies on dysplastic acetabula and congenital subluxation of the hip joint. Acta Chir Scand 58(Suppl 83):7

22. Crowe JF, Mani VJ, Ranawat CS (1979) Total hip replacement in congenital dislocation and dysplasia of the hip. J Bone Joint Surg Am 611:15–23

23. Hartofilakidis G, Stamos K, Karachalios T, Ioannidis TT, Zacharakis N (1996) Congenital hip disease in adults. Classification of acetabular deficiencies and operative treatment with acetabuloplasty combined with total hip arthroplasty. J Bone Joint Surg Am 785:683–692

24. Reynolds D, Lucas J, Klaue K (1999) Retroversion of the acetabulum. A cause of hip pain. J Bone Joint Surg Br 812:281–288

25. Kalberer F, Sierra RJ, Madan SS, Ganz R, Leunig M (2008) Ischial spine projection into the pelvis: a new sign for acetabular retroversion. Clin Orthop Relat Res 4663:677–683

26. Sotelo-Garza A, Charnley J (1978) The results of Charnley arthroplasty of hip performed for protrusio acetabuli. Clin Orthop Relat Res 132:12–18

27. Murray RO (1965) The aetiology of primary osteoarthritis of the hip. Br J Radiol 38455:810–824

28. Leunig M, Casillas MM, Hamlet M, Hersche O, Notzli H, Slongo T, Ganz R (2000) Slipped capital femoral epiphysis: early mechanical damage to the acetabular cartilage by a prominent femoral metaphysis. Acta Orthop Scand 714:370–375

29. Eijer H, Myers SR, Ganz R (2001) Anterior femoroacetabular impingement after femoral neck fractures. J Orthop Trauma 157:475–481

30. Leunig M, Beck M, Kalhor M, Kim YJ, Werlen S, Ganz R (2005) Fibrocystic changes at anterosuperior femoral neck: prevalence in hips with femoroacetabular impingement. Radiology 2361:237–246

31. Eijer H, Leunig M, Mahomed N, Ganz R (2001) Cross-table lateral radiographs for screening of anterior femoral head-neck offset in patients with femoro-acetabular impingement. Hip Int 11:37–41

32. Locher S, Werlen S, Leunig M, Ganz R (2002) MR-arthrography with radial sequences for visualization of early hip pathology not visible on plain radiographs. Z Orthop Ihre Grenzgeb 1401:52–57

# Advances in PAO Surgery: The Minimally Invasive Approach

Anders Troelsen and Kjeld Søballe

## Background

Until the early 1980s, several reorienting triple or spherical acetabular osteotomies for treatment of hip dysplasia had been introduced [1–3]. None of these techniques gained popularity as the obvious joint-preserving treatment in young adults with hip dysplasia. In 1983, a group led by Professor Reinhold Ganz from Bern, Switzerland, started the development of a new periacetabular osteotomy for the treatment of hip dysplasia [4]. This technique has become the joint-preserving treatment of choice in young adults with symptomatic hip dysplasia [5–15]. It is often referred to as the "Bernese" or "Ganz" periacetabular osteotomy.

## Periacetabular Osteotomy

In periacetabular osteotomy, the acetabulum is reoriented to enhance the coverage of the femoral head, and the aim is to achieve congruity, to stabilize the hip joint, to medialize the hip joint center, and to reduce contact pressures [4, 11, 16, 17] (Fig. 20.1). This will relieve pain, improve function, and is likely to prevent further overload of the labrum, cartilage, and soft tissues, thereby delaying or preventing the development of osteoarthritis [5, 6, 8, 10, 12, 13]. As outlined by Ganz et al. [4], periacetabular osteotomy has several

A. Troelsen • K. Søballe (✉)
Orthopaedic Research Unit, Aarhus University Hospital,
Aarhus, Denmark
e-mail: a_troelsen@hotmail.com; kjeld@soballe.com

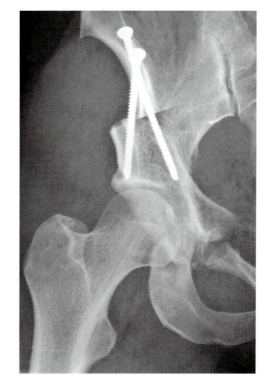

**Fig. 20.1** Part of an anterior-posterior pelvic radiograph showing the right hip following periacetabular osteotomy

technical advantages compared to existing techniques: The posterior column remains intact, leaving the pelvis stable, allowing partial weight-bearing immediately postoperative and minimal internal fixation; extensive three-dimensional mobilization of the acetabular fragment is possible; the blood supply of the acetabulum is unaffected, and the dimensions of the true pelvis are maintained. In general, periacetabular osteotomy is performed in patients after closure of the triradiate cartilage, but the exact indications for periacetabular osteotomy may differ between institutions. For daily clinical practice, the following indications have been developed: (1) symptomatic acetabular dysplasia defined by persistent pain, (2) a center edge angle of <25°, (3) a congruent hip joint, (4) maintained range of motion with hip flexion of >110°, and (5) preoperative osteoarthritis corresponding to Tönnis grades 0–1.

## Surgical Approaches and Technique

Since the development of periacetabular osteotomy, several surgical approaches have been used. Most surgeons prefer the ilioinguinal or modified Smith-Petersen (iliofemoral) approaches [6, 12, 18–20]. The surgical techniques are shortly outlined in Appendix. These "classic" approaches inflict an extensive trauma to the tissues, and some involve detachment of muscles, such as the rectus femoris and sartorius. The type of surgical approach may affect the occurrence of complications, duration of surgery, intraoperative blood loss, transfusion requirements, the ability of obtaining an optimal acetabular reorientation, and length of hospital stay [6, 20, 21]. The learning curve associated with periacetabular osteotomy is well documented, and technical and neurovascular complications have been reported by experienced surgeons [4, 8, 17, 20–22].

## Acetabular Reorientation

Achieving an optimal acetabular reorientation is the cornerstone of periacetabular osteotomy. Under- or overcorrection of the acetabulum can cause symptoms such as the feeling of instability and impingement respectively [9, 22, 23] and negatively influence the joint-preserving goals of the procedure [6, 13, 14]. The aim of the reorientation is to achieve an acetabular index angle between 0° and 10°, a center edge angle between 30° and 40°, and appropriate acetabular anteversion.

## Outcomes of Surgery

Studies reporting the outcome of periacetabular osteotomy often represent heterogenic patient populations in terms of diagnosis, severity of dysplasia, preoperative osteoarthritis, simultaneous surgical procedures, and duration of follow-up [5–8, 10–14, 18, 24–29]. The modified Smith-Petersen, ilioinguinal, and direct anterior approaches have been used [5–8, 10, 12–15, 18, 21, 24, 27]. Parameters such as duration of surgery, intraoperative blood loss, and transfusion requirements reflect the invasive characteristics of periacetabular osteotomy (Table 20.1). Mean duration of surgeries are reported to be approximately 3–4½ h [6, 12, 14, 18, 21], and mean intraoperative blood losses are reported to be approximately 700–2,300 mL [6, 8, 11, 12, 14, 18, 28]. One study reports a requirement of mean 4 units of blood following all procedures [14]. Length of hospital stay is rarely reported; however, approximately 5–10 days of admission seems normal [12, 18, 28]. Moderate and severe neurovascular complications are most frequently reported to occur at a rate of approximately 0–5% using different surgical approaches [4–8, 10, 12, 18, 25, 30]. The learning curve related to the occurrence of complications [4, 8, 17, 20, 21] affects the outcome in some studies. Based on this, periacetabular osteotomy can, in classical terms, be considered and extensive surgical procedure with a risk of disabling complications.

In most studies, the aim of the reorientation has been achieved when considering mean postoperative center edge and acetabular index angles [5, 10–13, 25, 27]. The short-term hip joint survival rates in most studies are >90%. Few studies report the medium- and long-term hip joint survival [11, 13, 14]. Recently, a hip joint survival rate of 60.5% has been reported at a mean follow-up of 20.4 years [13]. Clinical scores improve following periacetabular osteotomy, and there is evidence that significant improvements last up to 10 years [14]. A controversy in contemporary periacetabular osteotomy is whether arthrotomy and necessary labral intervention should be performed or not. There are no results of sufficient methodological value to support either approach.

## Conservative Treatment?

Whereas many cases of asymptomatic mild and moderate hip dysplasia will not develop osteoarthritis in early decades [31], it remains unclear whether all symptomatic cases with persistent hip pain will. In the case of periacetabular osteotomy, this potentially could lead to the performance of unnecessary surgery in marginal

**Table 20.1** Summary of studies reporting duration of surgery, blood loss, transfusion requirements, or length of hospital stay

| Author (year) | No. hips | Age, mean (range) | Simultaneous femoral osteotomy (no.hips) | Surgical approach | Duration of surgery, mean (range) | Blood loss, mean (range) | Transfusion (% of procedures) / No. port (range) | Length of hospital stay, mean (range) |
|---|---|---|---|---|---|---|---|---|
| Siebenrock (1999) [14] | 75 | 29.3 years (13–56) | 16 | Modified Smith-Petersen | 3.5 h (2–5) | 2,000 mL (750–4,500) | 100% / 4 port. (1–11 port.) | – |
| Trumble (1999) [6] | 123 | 32.9 years (14–54) | 33 | 56 Modified Smith-Petersen / 67 Ilioinguinal | 4.5 h (–) | 800 mL (–) | – | – |
| Matta (1999) [18] | 66 | 33.6 years (19–51) | – | Modified Smith-Petersen | ÷ fem. osteo. 3.1 h (2–5) / + fem. osteo. 4.1 h (3.2–6) | 939 mL (400–2,000) / 980 mL (500–1,800) | – | 7.9 days (4–29) |
| Davey (1999) [21] | 70 | 36.5 years (16–53) | – | Modified Smith-Petersen | 3.4 h (–) | – | – | – |
| Pogliacomi (2005) [12] | 36 | 35 years[a] (15–55) | 0 | 4 Modified Smith-Petersen / 32 Ilioinguinal | 3.3 h (1.8–7) | 2,300 mL (800–6,900) | – | 8.2 days (7–10) |
| Kralj (2005) [11] | 26 | 34 year (18–50) | – | – | – | 1,400 mL (–) | – | – |
| Peters (2006) [8] | 83 | 28 years (25–47) | 14 | Modified Smith-Petersen | – | 715 mL (–) | – | – |
| Atwal (2008) [28] | 122 | 23.6 years (18–28) | – | – | – | 2,191 mL (1,200–4,021) | – | 5.3 days (4–8) |

– Parameter is not reported
[a]Median years

cases. Conservative treatment might then be a treatment option, but selection criteria are unknown. However, when patients with persistent symptoms are referred, they often suffer moderate or severe pain which affect daily living, and given the ability of periacetabular osteotomy to relieve pain, improve function, and preserve the joint [5, 6, 8, 10, 12, 13], surgery is justified.

## The Minimally Invasive Approach

Classically, surgical treatment of hip dysplasia by means of periacetabular osteotomy has been associated with extensive surgical approaches potentially inducing severe soft tissue damage. This leaves room for advances in the realm of surgical treatment. A safe surgical procedure with achievement of optimal acetabular reorientation is the surgical mainstay of successful periacetabular osteotomy. To improve outcome associated with the surgical approach, a new minimally invasive transsartorial approach for periacetabular osteotomy was developed by the senior author.

## Surgical Technique of the Minimally Invasive Approach

The patient is placed on a radiolucent operating room table in the supine position. The placement of the drapes allows for full mobilization of the lower extremity on the operated side. Fluoroscopic evaluation is necessary throughout the operation, and therefore, the pelvis is kept in a neutral position in order to avoid excessive tilting or rotation. The fluoroscopy equipment is positioned to facilitate obtaining the anterior-posterior and 60° (false profile) views.

The skin incision begins at the anterior-superior iliac spine and continues distally along the sartorius muscle. The length of incision is approximately 7 cm. The fascia is carefully incised, and the lateral femoral cutaneous nerve isolated and carefully retracted. To facilitate transverse retraction of the soft tissues, a semi-flexed position of the hip joint is maintained during performance of the osteotomies. For this purpose, a splint is used. A periosteal elevator is placed subperiosteally along the medial aspect of the ilium starting at the anterior-superior iliac spine, and it is advanced until it lies just below the

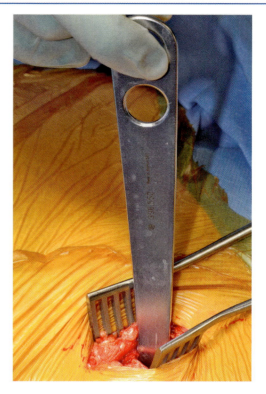

**Fig. 20.2** A blunt retractor positioned along the medial aspect of the ilium to retract the iliopsoas and the medial part of the split sartorius muscles medially

linea terminalis. The inguinal ligament is cut at the attachment to the anterior-superior iliac spine allowing further mobilization of the soft tissues. The periosteal elevator is then pushed medially, splitting the sartorius muscle in the direction of its fibers, and the deep fascia of the muscle is cut. The periosteal elevator is then replaced with a blunt retractor positioned along the medial aspect of the ilium to retract the iliopsoas and the medial part of the split sartorius muscles medially. At this point, the osteotomies are performed (Fig. 20.2). Time spent on the approach is approximately 10 min.

## Performance of Osteotomies

### General Surgical Principles
The acetabular index and center edge angles following reorientation should correspond as closely as possible to the normal anatomy (acetabular index angle 0–10°, center edge angle 30–40°). It is of equal

importance that the surgeon obtains appropriate ante-version of the acetabulum. Assessment of range of motion and joint stability at the end of the procedure will help the surgeon evaluate the change in hip joint mechanics. This description of the minimally invasive approach will give the reader an understanding of soft tissue mobilization, instrument handling, and the performance of the osteotomies. Understanding of the anatomy and utilization of fluoroscopy during surgery are the keys to a safe, minimally invasive periacetabular osteotomy.

## Pubic Osteotomy

Subperiosteal access to the superior ramus of the pubic bone is gained using a periosteal elevator. It is important that the pubic osteotomy is performed medially on the superior ramus since the bone otherwise is too thick, making the osteotomy and mobilization difficult or impossible. A curved blunt retractor is placed in the obturator fossa behind the superior ramus of the pubic bone. It is important that this retractor be placed subperiosteally to protect the obturator artery and nerve. A splined retractor is then placed anteriorly and medially to the site of the osteotomy in order to retract the iliopsoas muscle medially and protect the iliac artery and vein and the femoral nerve (Fig. 20.3). The superior ramus is then osteotomized under direct visualization using a slightly curved osteotome. It is important to advance the osteotome until the osteotomy is complete; otherwise, the repositioning of the splined retractor becomes difficult as it will tend to slide into the osteotomy. The surgeon will often be able to hear and feel (loss of resistance) when the bone is fully osteotomized. This sensory input should be utilized during surgery to avoid both creating an insufficient osteotomy and advancing the osteotome into the soft tissue.

## Ischial Osteotomy

When advancing to the ischial osteotomy, the splined retractor is kept in its position to retract the iliopsoas muscle medially. A large pair of scissors is used to penetrate the interval immediately lateral and distal to the pubic osteotomy, and the scissors are advanced to the ischium below the acetabulum. Keeping the scissors in place, a 30°-angled osteotome can be placed on the ischium. The correct placement of the osteotome is verified using fluoroscopy (anterior-posterior view). The osteotomy begins approximately 5 mm distal to the radiographic teardrop. A 1.5-cm osteotomy is performed

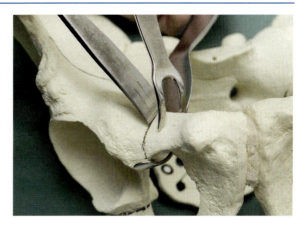

**Fig. 20.3** Site of the osteotomy on the pubic bone and placement of the instruments: a curved blunt retractor is placed behind the pubic bone to protect the obturator nerve and artery. A splined retractor is used for medial retraction of the soft tissues, and a slightly curved osteotome is used to create the osteotomy

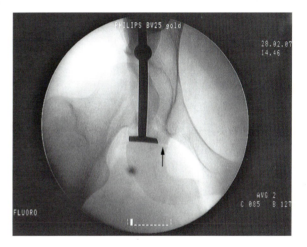

**Fig. 20.4** Fluoroscopic anterior-posterior view showing the lateral placement of the osteotome at the ischial bone below the teardrop. Note the osteotomy performed at the medial edge of the ischium (*black arrow*)

in two steps beginning at the medial edge and then moving the osteotome laterally before the next step (Fig. 20.4). A 30°-angled osteotome is advanced along the inner aspect of the pelvis until it can be placed at the medial aspect of the ischium with one leg of the osteotome in the existing 1.5-cm osteotomy. The placement of the osteotome and the osteotomy itself are performed under strict fluoroscopy control utilizing the so-called false profile view that is angled 60° to the anterior-posterior view (Fig. 20.5). The ischium bone is then osteotomized from the medial to the lateral aspect in a length equal to 2–3 widths of the osteotome (Fig. 20.6).

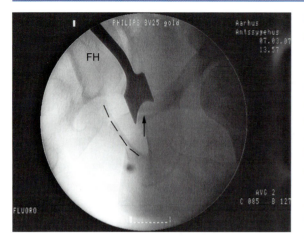

**Fig. 20.5** Fluoroscopic false profile view angled 60° toward the anterior-posterior view. Correct placement of the osteotome with one leg in the existing osteotomy (*black arrow*). The black dashed line marks the border of the pubic bone toward the obturator foramen. *FH* femoral head

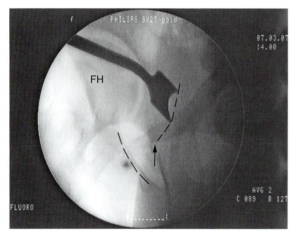

**Fig. 20.6** Correct placement of the osteotome for the last step of the ischial osteotomy. As illustrated by the *black dashed line*, the osteotomy is *slightly curved*. The *black arrow* marks the level of the already performed first step of the osteotomy. The *black dashed* line to the right marks the border of the pubic bone toward the obturator foramen. *FH* femoral head

This osteotomy tends to be slightly curved with the concavity toward the acetabulum. In order to advance in the same plane as the initial 1.5 cm of the osteotomy and to obtain an almost horizontal osteotomy, the handle of the 30°-angled osteotome must be pushed medially. When the posterior aspect of the ischium is osteotomized, the sciatic nerve can be damaged if the osteotome is advanced too far past the bone in the lateral direction.

## Iliac Osteotomy

Initially, a Kirschner wire is inserted along the inner aspect of the pelvis approximately 3 cm cranial to the acetabulum. This is done to secure an appropriate distance away from the joint. From experience, we have found it easier to mobilize and control the acetabular fragment if this distance away from the joint is achieved. The first step of the iliac osteotomy begins between the anterior-superior iliac spine and the anterior-inferior iliac spine at the level of the Kirschner wire. It is performed using an oscillating saw stopping approximately 1 cm before reaching the linea terminalis. In some patients, the distance from the anterior-superior iliac spine to the cranial limit of the joint is relatively short. In these cases, a small oblique osteotomy under the anterior-superior iliac spine is recommended. To protect the structures lateral to the ilium, a blunt retractor is tunneled close to the bone along the outer aspect of the ilium in the area between the anterior-superior and anterior-inferior iliac spines. The blunt retractor must be advanced close to the bone as otherwise the blood supply from the superior gluteal artery can be damaged. A retractor protects the structures medial to the ilium. The first step of the osteotomy is then continued using a wide, straight osteotome. With an anterior open angle of approximately 120°, it is advanced behind the hip joint until it reaches the ischial osteotomy while the posterior column is maintained intact. Fluoroscopy must be used during this last step of the iliac osteotomy (60° angle, false profile view) (Fig. 20.7).

## Reorientation

A bone spreader is placed in the iliac osteotomy. With the osteotomies open, the iliac and ischial osteotomies can in succession be retraced using a 30°-angled osteotome to secure that there are no bony bridges or spikes left, interfering with mobilization of the acetabular fragment. A bone clamp is then applied at the ilium with one leg of the clamp on the inner and outer aspects respectively. On the inner aspect, the ilium is oblique, and a small hole is predrilled to allow secure fixation of the clamp. This gives the surgeon control of the fragment during the reorientation. The first step of the acetabular reorientation is to achieve sufficient lateral coverage. This is done by adducting the fragment. In our experience, this maneuver is sufficient to medialize the hip joint center which in dysplastic hips often is lateralized. As a rule of thumb, the acetabular index

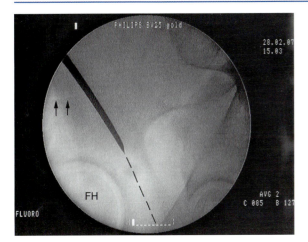

**Fig. 20.7** Fluoroscopic false profile view angled 60° toward the anterior-posterior view, showing the advancement of a straight osteotome in continuation with the first step of the iliac osteotomy (*black arrows*). It is advanced (*black dashed line*) at an anterior open angle of around 120° between the joint and the posterior column until it reaches the ischial osteotomy. *FH* femoral head

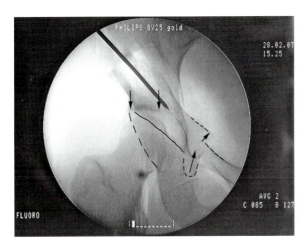

**Fig. 20.8** A large threaded Kirschner wire is temporarily securing the position. Notice the horizontal positioning of the medial and lateral extensions (*arrows*) of the sclerotic acetabular roof, the anteverted configuration of the acetabulum (posterior rim = *dashed line*; anterior rim = *solid line*), the cranial displacement of the superior ramus, and the cranial and medial displacement of the teardrop figure

angle following reorientation should approximate 0° (horizontal positioning of the sclerotic acetabular roof) and never should be less as this will result in over coverage and impingement. The second step of the acetabular reorientation is to achieve sufficient anterior coverage. This is done by extension of the fragment. In our experience, very little movement is needed to create sufficient anterior coverage. The risk of too much anterior coverage and retroversion is great at this point in the reorientation procedure. Version of the acetabulum is evaluated using fluoroscopy in the anterior-posterior view by assessing the relationship between the anterior and posterior acetabular rim. Sufficient anteversion is achieved when the posterior rim is lateral to the anterior rim and the center of the femoral head and the anterior rim is medial to the center of the femoral head and there is no crossover sign. If the acetabular fragment has been properly mobilized and reoriented, cranial displacement of the superior ramus and cranial and medial displacement of the teardrop can be observed in the anterior-posterior fluoroscopic view. If these are not observed, the fragment is hinging probably due to an unfinished osteotomy of the ischium (Fig. 20.8). A large threaded Kirschner wire is then placed from the ilium into the acetabular fragment in order to temporarily secure the new position. A measuring device makes it possible to perform perioperative measurements of the acetabular index and center edge angles using fluoroscopy in the anterior-posterior view. Using small spikes, the measuring device is mounted bilaterally at the anterior-superior iliac spines in order to secure alignment of the pelvis when measuring. Excessive tilt and rotation of the pelvis is avoided through the initial positioning of the patient. On the alignment rod connecting the spikes, two different adjustable angle-measuring discs can be mounted. The angle-measuring disc for the acetabular index angle measurement has to be positioned by recognizing the medial and lateral limits of the sclerotic acetabular roof as landmarks. The angle-measuring disc for the center edge angle measurement has to be positioned by recognizing the center of the femoral head and the lateral limit of the sclerotic acetabular roof as landmarks (Fig. 20.9). The measuring device is easy to use, and it helps the surgeon to assess the achieved acetabular reorientation and thereby avoid undercorrection or overcorrection. The acetabular version cannot be measured and still has to be addressed as described previously. Fine adjustments of the reorientation might be necessary. When no further adjustment is needed, two stainless steel screws are placed from the ilium at the anterior-superior iliac spine into the acetabular fragment to secure its position. The positions of the screws are visualized using fluoroscopy, and the stability of the fixation is tested by applying force on the fragment. The hip range of motion is

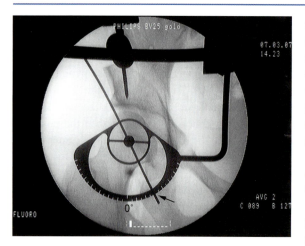

**Fig. 20.9** The angle-measuring disc for the center edge angle measurement. It is positioned by recognizing the center of the femoral head and the lateral limit of the sclerotic acetabular roof as landmarks. The measured angle in this case is 30° (*black arrow*). The "0°" mark is labeled

assessed, and by internally rotating the flexed hip, no impingement should be encountered. By flexing the hip and pushing the knee toward the operating room table, posterior stability of the joint is tested. After irrigation with saline, the inguinal ligament is reattached, and the soft tissues are closed in layers. A suction drain is not used.

### Aftercare
On the day following surgery, the patient is mobilized, walking on crutches with 30 kg of weight-bearing on the operated side. Patients are allowed full range of motion. X-rays are obtained postoperatively and after 8 weeks, and at that time, the patient is allowed full weight-bearing. Using this regimen, there is no risk of secondary displacement or non-union [32].

### Outcome of Surgery

We have assessed the outcome of the minimally invasive approach in two studies [33, 34]. The aims of these two studies were: (1) to assess if the new minimally invasive transsartorial approach for periacetabular osteotomy is safe, allows optimal acetabular reorientation, and minimizes tissue trauma (The length of hospital stay, duration of surgery, intraoperative blood loss, hemoglobin reduction, transfusion requirements, hip joint survival, complications, and achieved acetabular

reorientation were assessed.), and (2) to assess if the new minimally invasive approach produces an outcome similar to that of the "classic" ilioinguinal approach for periacetabular osteotomy. The approaches were compared with respect to the outcome parameters mentioned above to explore if the results supported continued use of the minimally invasive approach. The results of the two studies are shown in Table 20.2.

### Conclusions

Periacetabular osteotomy is applied worldwide and is the joint-preserving treatment of choice in young adults with symptomatic hip dysplasia. The procedure has the potential to relieve pain, improve functions of daily living, and to preserve hip joints by delaying or even preventing development of early osteoarthritis. Periacetabular osteotomy can be considered a major advance in the field of adult joint-preserving hip surgery. However, more reports on the medium and long-term results are needed.

Further surgical advances have been achieved by the development of the minimally invasive approach for periacetabular osteotomy. Using this approach, periacetabular osteotomy can be performed safely, with optimal reorientation of the acetabulum and minimized tissue trauma. Duration of surgery, blood loss, and transfusion requirements are all at a very low level and the short-term hip joint survival is encouraging.

### Appendix

Short outline of the surgical techniques for the modified Smith-Petersen and ilioinguinal approaches as they were performed at our institution:

Specific modifications of the Smith-Petersen approach have been reported [20]. The skin incision was made from the anterior third of the iliac crest to the anterior-superior iliac spine where it curved distally and continued vertically along the tensor fascia latae for approximately 10 cm. The internervous planes between the tensor fasciae latae and sartorius, and the gluteus medius and rectus femoris were developed. In contrast to the previously described modification of the Smith-Petersen approach, the rectus femoris was not detached. In some of the first cases, the origin of

**Table 20.2**  Summary of studies investigating the outcome of the minimally invasive approach for periacetabular osteotomy

| Author (year) | Approach | No. hips | Age | Duration of surgery | Blood loss | Hemoglobin reduction | Transfusion (% of procedures) No. port | Length of hospital stay | Achieved CE and AI angles | Hip joint survival (Kaplan-Meier estimates) |
|---|---|---|---|---|---|---|---|---|---|---|
| Troelsen (2008) [33] | Minimally invasive | 94 | Mean 37 years | Mean 73 min | Median 250 mL | Mean 33 g/L | 3% Median 2 port | Median 8 days | Median CE: 34° AI: 3° | 98% at 4.3 years |
| Troelsen (2008) [34] | Minimally invasive | 165 | Median 35 years | Median 70 min | Median 250 mL | Mean 32 g/L | 4% Median 2 port | Median 7 days | Median CE: 33° AI: 2° | 97% at 4.9 years |
|  | Ilioinguinal | 98 | Median 31 years | Median 100 min | Median 500 mL | Mean 40 g/L | 18% Median 2 port | Median 9 days | Median CE: 31° AI: 9° | 93% at 4.9 years |

the sartorius muscle was detached by means of an osteotomy.

The ilioinguinal approach was performed as previously described [35], but without lateral extension along the iliac crest. The skin incision extended from the anterior-superior iliac spine, along the inguinal ligament, and terminated at the level of the pubic symphysis near the midline. The inguinal ligament was incised, leaving the origins of the abdominal musculature and fascia attached to the proximal part of the split ligament. Further access was created by incising the iliopectineal fascia that separates the lacuna musculorum and lacuna vasorum. This allowed mobilization of the iliopsoas muscle which combined with medial retraction of the external iliac vessels created access to performance of the osteotomies through two windows, one medially and one laterally to the iliopsoas muscle.

# References

1. Tönnis D (1987) Congenital dysplasia and dislocation of the hip in children and adults. Springer, Berlin, Heidelberg, New York
2. Steel HH (1973) Triple osteotomy of the innominate bone. J Bone Joint Surg Am 55:343–350
3. Schramm M, Hohmann D, Radespiel-Troger M, Pitto RP (2003) Treatment of the dysplastic acetabulum with Wagner spherical osteotomy. A study of patients followed for a minimum of twenty years. J Bone Joint Surg Am 85:808–814
4. Ganz R, Klaue K, Vinh TS, Mast JW (1988) A new periacetabular osteotomy for the treatment of hip dysplasias. Technique and preliminary results. Clin Orthop Relat Res 232:26–36
5. Trousdale RT, Ekkernkamp A, Ganz R, Wallrichs SL (1995) Periacetabular and intertrochanteric osteotomy for the treatment of osteoarthrosis in dysplastic hips. J Bone Joint Surg Am 77:73–85
6. Trumble SJ, Mayo KA, Mast JW (1999) The periacetabular osteotomy. Minimum 2 year followup in more than 100 hips. Clin Orthop Relat Res 363:54–63
7. Clohisy J, Barrett S, Gordon J, Delgado E, Schoenecker P (2005) Periacetabular osteotomy in the treatment of severe acetabular dysplasia. J Bone Joint Surg Am 87:254–259
8. Peters CL, Erickson JA, Hines JL (2006) Early results of the Bernese periacetabular osteotomy: the learning curve at an academic medical center. J Bone Joint Surg Am 88:1920–1926
9. Søballe K (2003) Pelvic osteotomy for acetabular dysplasia. Acta Orthop Scand 74:117–118
10. Garras DN, Crowder TT, Olson SA (2007) Medium-term results of the Bernese periacetabular osteotomy in the treatment of symptomatic developmental dysplasia of the hip. J Bone Joint Surg Br 89:721–724
11. Kralj M, Mavcic B, Antolic V, Iglic A, Kralj-Iglic V (2005) The Bernese periacetabular osteotomy: clinical, radiographic and mechanical 7–15-year follow-up of 26 hips. Acta Orthop 76:833–840
12. Pogliacomi F, Stark A, Wallensten R (2005) Periacetabular osteotomy. Good pain relief in symptomatic hip dysplasia, 32 patients followed for 4 years. Acta Orthop Scand 76:67–74
13. Steppacher SD, Tannast M, Ganz R, Siebenrock KA (2008) Mean 20-year follow-up of Bernese periacetabular osteotomy. Clin Orthop Relat Res 466:1633–1644
14. Siebenrock KA, Scholl E, Lottenbach M, Ganz R (1999) Bernese periacetabular osteotomy. Clin Orthop Relat Res 363:9–20
15. Murphy SB, Millis MB (1999) Periacetabular osteotomy without abductor dissection using direct anterior exposure. Clin Orthop Relat Res 364:92–98
16. Hipp JA, Sugano N, Millis NB, Murphy SB (1999) Planning acetabular redirection osteotomies based on joint contact pressures. Clin Orthop Relat Res 364:134–143
17. Trousdale RT, Cabanela ME (2003) Lessons learned after more than 250 periacetabular osteotomies. Acta Orthop Scand 74:119–126
18. Matta JM, Stover MD, Siebenrock K (1999) Periacetabular osteotomy through the Smith-Petersen approach. Clin Orthop Relat Res 363:21–32
19. Clohisy J, Barrett S, Gordon J, Delgado E, Schoenecker P (2006) Periacetabular osteotomy in the treatment of severe acetabular dysplasia. J Bone Joint Surg Am 88(suppl 1): 65–83
20. Hussell JG, Mast JW, Mayo KA, Howie DW, Ganz R (1999) A comparison of different surgical approaches for the periacetabular osteotomy. Clin Orthop Relat Res 363:64–72
21. Davey JP, Santore RF (1999) Complications of periacetabular osteotomy. Clin Orthop Relat Res 363:21–32
22. Hussell JG, Rodriguez JA, Ganz R (1999) Technical complications of the Bernese periacetabular osteotomy. Clin Orthop Relat Res 363:81–92
23. Myers SR, Eijer H, Ganz R (1999) Anterior femoroacetabular impingement after periacetabular osteotomy. Clin Orthop Relat Res 363:93–99
24. Crockarell J Jr, Trousdale RT, Cabanela ME, Berry DJ (1999) Early experience and results with the periacetabular osteotomy. The Mayo Clinic experience. Clin Orthop Relat Res 363:45–53
25. Murphy S, Deshmukh R (2002) Periacetabular osteotomy: preoperative radiographic predictors of outcome. Clin Orthop Relat Res 405:168–174
26. Cunningham T, Jessel R, Zurakowski D, Millis MB, Kim YJ (2006) Delayed gadolinium-enhanced magnetic resonance imaging of cartilage to predict early failure of Bernese periacetabular osteotomy for hip dysplasia. J Bone Joint Surg Am 88:1540–1548
27. Clohisy JC, Nunley RM, Curry MC, Schoenecker PL (2007) Periacetabular osteotomy for the treatment of acetabular dysplasia associated with major aspherical femoral head deformities. J Bone Joint Surg Am 89:1417–1423

28. Atwal NS, Bedi G, Lankester BJ, Campbell D, Gargan MF (2008) Management of blood loss in periacetabular osteotomy. Hip Int 18:95–100

29. van Bergayk AB, Garbuz DS (2002) Quality of life and sports-specific outcomes after Bernese periacetabular osteotomy. J Bone Joint Surg Br 84:339–343

30. Valenzuela RG, Cabanela ME, Trousdale RT (2004) Sexual activity, pregnancy, and childbirth after periacetabular osteotomy. Clin Orthop Relat Res 418:146–152

31. Jacobsen S, Sonne-Holm S, Søballe K, Gebuhr P, Lund B (2005) Joint space width in dysplasia of the hip: a case-control study of 81 adults followed for ten years. J Bone Joint Surg Br 87:471–477

32. Mechlenburg I, Kold S, Rømer L, Søballe K (2007) Safe fixation with two acetabular screws after Ganz periacetabular osteotomy. Acta Orthop 78:344–349

33. Troelsen A, Elmengaard B, Søballe K (2008) A new minimally invasive transsartorial approach for periacetabular osteotomy. J Bone Joint Surg Am 90:493–498

34. Troelsen A, Elmengaard B, Søballe K (2008) Comparison of the minimally invasive and the ilioinguinal approaches for periacetabular osteotomy: 263 single-surgeon procedures in well-defined study groups. Acta Orthop 79:777–784

35. Letournel E (1993) The treatment of acetabular fractures through the ilioinguinal approach. Clin Orthop Relat Res 292:62–76

# Retroverted PAO or Rim Trimming in the Dysplastic Hip with FAI

Philipp Henle and Klaus A. Siebenrock

## Introduction

In contrast to femoral head over coverage in FAI, developmental dysplasia of the hip (DDH) is characterized by an acetabular insufficiency. Although FAI and DDH are distinct pathomorphological entities, they might coincide in specific patients. Li and Ganz were able to show that one in six patients with acetabular dysplasia, in addition, displays retroversion in which the superior one-third of the acetabulum faces posterolaterally [1]. In these patients, anterosuperior impingement (pincer type) might be clinically relevant [2]. In these cases, establishing whether symptoms come from dysplasia or from impingement can be challenging. Leunig et al. [3] were able to show that the pathomorphological labral features seen on MRI can be helpful to differentiate between these two disorders. An enlarged labrum – especially within the anterosuperior quadrant – and the presence of soft tissue ganglia are predictors for the presence of developmental dysplasia. If only degenerative changes are visible on MRI, a FAI constellation can be assumed. Rather frequently, this situation is worsened by the presence of an additional cam impingement component in a clearly nonspherical head [4].

## Therapeutic Options

Theoretically, there are two different surgical therapeutic options available to correct localized femoral head over coverage: to trim the prominent posterior wall or to reorientate the entire acetabulum.

## Anterosuperior Rim Trimming

Trimming of the posterior rim can be achieved by surgical dislocation of the hip. After detachment of the labrum at the affected portion of the acetabulum, the rim can be trimmed to correct the over coverage. Afterward, the labrum will be reattached with bone anchors. In addition, the femoral head-neck offset can be improved by trimming the femoral head-neck transition zone. However, in clearly dysplastic hips, anterior rim trimming is rarely indicated because the already deficient femoral head coverage will be aggravated by this procedure. Trimming might be suitable for patients with borderline dysplasia presenting with clinically relevant acetabular retroversion.

## Periacetabular Osteotomy

If the entire acetabulum has to be reorientated, a periacetabular osteotomy is performed. This technique uses a modified Smith–Petersen approach to allow all acetabular osteotomies to be performed through a single approach. This osteotomy allows an ample acetabular reorientation including medial and lateral displacement.

P. Henle • K.A. Siebenrock (✉)
Department of Orthopaedic Surgery,
Inselspital, Bern University Hospital,
Bern, Switzerland
e-mail: Philipp.Henle@insel.ch;
monika.gempeler@insel.ch

Ó. Marín-Peña (ed.), *Femoroacetabular Impingement*,
DOI 10.1007/978-3-642-22769-1_21, © Springer-Verlag Berlin Heidelberg 2012

The classical PAO procedure for the treatment of dysplasia aims at increasing anterior acetabular coverage. In contrast to that, in PAO, for treatment of combined dysplasia and retroversion, the acetabular reorientation is performed in an anteverting manner. Both techniques have inherent advantages and disadvantages; the dilemma is to decide when to perform which procedure.

## Relevant Issues for Decision Making

### Radiographic Analysis

Proper imaging technique is essential to detect and evaluate localized over coverage or acetabular deficiencies in symptomatic hip joints (see Chap. 19). Notably, pelvic tilt has to be evaluated on radiographs in order to obtain a more accurate judgment of morphological abnormalities. Augmented pelvic tilt will increase the apparent anterior coverage of the femoral head and thus suggest more pronounced retroversion; decreased pelvic tilt will suggest the opposite. Therefore, if the imaging tests are suboptimal, repetition of the radiographs is highly recommended.

A positive crossover sign (see Chap. 19) is only a crude description of an overlap of the anterosuperior rim over the posterior rim, but it may range from a slight overlap to a severe retroversion. Apart from the assessment of the relative length of the crossover area described by Siebenrock et al., a quantitative evaluation of the total area, evaluation of the length or width of anterior overlap has not so far been reported in the literature [5].

Evaluation for a potential deficient posterior wall can be carried out with the help of the posterior wall sign (see Chap. 19). This assessment is crucial since acetabular reorientation in these cases will increase posterior coverage. A positive posterior wall sign indicates small and potentially deficient posterior coverage, which would benefit from acetabular reorientation as the latter decreases anterior coverage and simultaneously increases posterior coverage. In these patients only trimming of the anterior acetabular rim would create a dysplasia-like morphology. In contrast to this, a normal or prominent posterior wall could benefit from trimming of the acetabular rim, which reduces

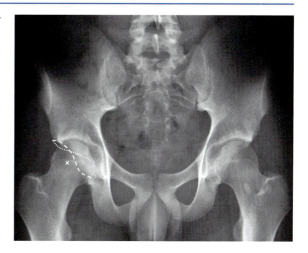

**Fig. 21.1** Preoperative radiograph with a positive crossover sign and a positive posterior wall sign (*dotted line* anterior rim, *dashed line* posterior rim, *X* center of femoral head)

anterior over coverage and the posterior rim prominence at the same time.

In marked retroversion, extensive trimming of the anterior rim would be necessary and might result in insufficient anterolateral coverage. This restricts indications for this specific surgical procedure and favors reorientation – especially in patients with a clear or even marginal dysplastic component.

A helpful decision-making tool during preoperative planning is calculation of the LCE angle (see Chap. 19). After trimming a prominent anterosuperior rim, the LCE angle should not be less than 20°.

### Cartilage Damage

Intra-articular cartilage damage is considered to be a major prognostic factor for clinical outcome after PAO for the treatment of acetabular retroversion especially since acetabular reorientation will rotate the typically damaged peripheral cartilage zone medially toward the more weight-bearing zone. Therefore, clear evidence of extensive cartilage damage favors trimming of the acetabular rim including the damaged cartilage area. Cartilage damage can be visualized by arthro-MRI imaging [6]. In addition, long standing clinical symptoms might also indicate more extensive cartilage damage.

**Fig. 21.2** (**a**) Anterior center edge (ACE) angle on a preoperative false profile view. (**b**) Normal ACE angle postoperatively

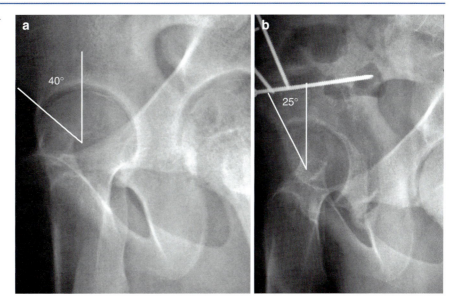

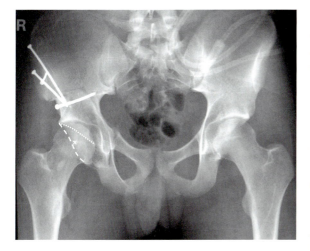

**Fig. 21.3** Postoperative pelvic AP view with negative posterior wall and crossover signs (*dotted line* anterior rim, *dashed line* posterior rim, *X* center of femoral head)

## Summary

Acetabular reorientation may be an adequate treatment in selected cases of acetabular retroversion. At present, the literature does not provide hard-and-fast criteria as to when rim trimming, rather than reorientation of the acetabulum, must be selected. Early and midterm results of PAO for retroversion are encouraging [7], but series are small and long-term outcomes lacking. It seems that the characteristics of an ideal candidate for a PAO would be as follows:

1. An adolescent or young adult
2. Relative short duration of symptoms
3. Minor acetabular cartilage damage or no damage at all
4. Substantial anterior over coverage
5. Small posterior wall (positive posterior wall sign)

   In contrast, if none or only few of these characteristics are present, rim trimming might be the more appropriate surgical treatment for the patient.

## Illustrative Cases

### Case 1

A 25-year-old active male presents with groin pain and a positive anterior impingement sign. The pelvic AP radiograph shows a clear crossover sign, a posterior wall sign, and a prominent ischial spine (Fig. 21.1). The false profile view shows increased anterior coverage (40°) preoperatively (Fig. 21.2a), which was reduced to 25° postoperatively (Fig. 21.2b). The crossover sign has disappeared postoperatively and the acetabulum shows correct anteversion (Fig. 21.3).

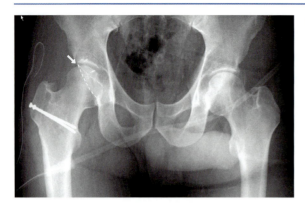

**Fig. 21.4** Compromised lateral coverage (*white arrow*) after trimming of the anterosuperior rim for retroversion (*dotted line* anterior rim, *dashed line* posterior rim, *X* center of femoral head)

## Case 2

Trimming of the acetabular rim in a retroverted acetabulum might result in compromised lateral coverage and create secondary acetabular dysplasia (Fig. 21.4). When anticipated, these hips may be better treated with PAO

## References

1. Li PL, Ganz R (2003) Morphologic features of congenital acetabular dysplasia: one in six is retroverted. Clin Orthop Relat Res 416:245–253
2. Reynolds D, Lucas J, Klaue K (1999) Retroversion of the acetabulum. A cause of hip pain. J Bone Joint Surg Br 81:281–288
3. Leunig M, Podeszwa D, Beck M et al (2004) Magnetic resonance arthrography of labral disorders in hips with dysplasia and impingement. Clin Orthop Relat Res 418:74–80
4. Steppacher SD, Tannast M, Werlen S et al (2008) Femoral morphology differs between deficient and excessive acetabular coverage. Clin Orthop Relat Res 466(4):782–790
5. Siebenrock KA, Kalbermatten DF, Ganz R (2003) Effect of pelvic inclination on determination of acetabular retroversion. A study on cadaver pelvis. Clin Orthop Relat Res 407:241–248
6. Mamisch TC, Bittersohl B, Hughes T et al (2008) Magnetic resonance imaging of the hip at 3 Tesla: clinical value in femoroacetabular impingement of the hip and current concepts. Semin Musculoskelet Radiol 12(3):212–222
7. Siebenrock KA, Schöniger R, Ganz R (2003) Anterior femoroacetabular impingement due to acetabular retroversion. Treatment with periacetabular osteotomy. J Bone Joint Surg Am 85:278–286

# Part V

# Hip Arthroplasty in Young Adult

# Current Arthroplasty Options in the Young Adult Hip

**22**

Eduardo García Cimbrelo, Eduardo Garcia-Rey, and Ana Cruz-Pardos

In considering how THA can be improved, two facts stand out: 1. Failures are essentially long-term. At the first the patient may notice no difference between the artificial head and the living one. Our problem is to make this temporary success permanent. 2. Objectives must be reasonable. Surgeons will never make an artificial hip-joint that will last 30 years and enable the patient to play football at some time in this period.
Sir John Charnley 1961 [1]

Total hip arthroplasty (THA) remains a concern in young patients as a result of the high revision rates associated with the procedure [2, 3]. Although other options have been considered, such as osteotomies, short-stemmed uncemented hip prostheses, and hip resurfacing arthroplasty, THA remains the most frequent indication for a large number of cases and surgeons [4]. Cemented, hybrid, and uncemented implants have been used for the young patient population with substantial variations as regards long-term results and aseptic loosening rates of the acetabular cup [3, 5–10], which most commonly occurs due to polyethylene wear and constitutes the most frequent reason for revision [6–8, 11, 12]. The belief that the osteolysis observed in cemented prostheses more than 10 years postsurgery was caused by cement failure ("cement disease") [13], which led to the recommendation of cementless implants for young patients. Nonetheless, thigh pain, stress shielding, and osteolysis have been reported in association with cementless implants [6, 7].

Polyethylene wear produces osteolysis and loosening in cemented as well as cementless prostheses, especially in young, active patients [14–16]. Different bearing surfaces, including highly cross-linked polyethylene, alumina on alumina, and metal on metal, have been used to prevent these complications. Findings of thigh pain, osteolysis, and stress shielding and the removal problems associated with cementless implants have led to the use of modern conservative implants such as short-stemmed uncemented prostheses and hip resurfacing prostheses [16]. The early designs of resurfacing prostheses were used in the 1980s with little success.

## Current Treatment of Hip Osteoarthritis in the Young Patient

Cemented total hip arthroplasties (THA) are commonly reported to produce poor results in young patients [2]. The poor results with cemented prostheses have been attributed to the greater activity levels that characterize young patients. Most of the series with poor results followed young patients with different implant designs and for only a short time. Using a cemented Charnley arthroplasty, Callaghan reported 20% revision at 20 years [17], 5% for the stem and 19% for the cup; Sochart and Porter reported survival of 89% for the stem and 58% for the cup in patients with CDH [18]; Wroblewski reported survival of 55% for one or both components [10]; and in a worldwide study of 5,089 patients, John Older reported a survival of 83% for the general series, 67% for patients under 40 years old, and 92% for patients over 70 years old [19].

E.G. Cimbrelo (✉) • E. Garcia-Rey • A. Cruz-Pardos
Department of Orthopedic Surgery and Traumatology,
Hospital La Paz, Madrid, Spain
e-mail: gcimbrelo@yahoo.es

Ó. Marín-Peña (ed.), *Femoroacetabular Impingement*,
DOI 10.1007/978-3-642-22769-1_22, © Springer-Verlag Berlin Heidelberg 2012

We assessed 67 Charnley low-friction arthroplasties (LFA) implanted between 1972 and 1977 in patients under 40 years of age [6]. Mean age was 32.4 years, and the mean follow-up until revision or the most recent evaluation was 21.7 years. There were 19 revisions, 18 cup revisions, and 12 stem revisions. The cumulative probability of not undergoing revision of one or both components was 69.9% at 20 years. The cumulative probability of not experiencing cup loosening was 60%. Although primary osteoarthritis is the most frequent diagnosis leading to THA in general series, this diagnosis did not appear in our study. Preoperative diagnoses reflected some bone deficiency in the acetabular structure, such as congenital dysplasia of the hip, acetabular fracture, acetabular protrusio, and rheumatoid arthritis. Technically, a primary THA is usually more difficult in these patients. On the acetabular side, THA requires a complex acetabular reconstruction that increases surgical difficulty and the risk of revision, and thus, the acetabulum must be reconstructed with grafts or metallic devices to ensure sufficient fixation when necessary before a cup can be implanted [6, 8, 11, 20–23].

Polyethylene wear is another major factor in the failure of low-friction arthroplasties. Different alternatives are available for these patients: standard THRs with different bearing surfaces (metal-metal, alumina-alumina, cross-linked polyethylene). Conservative prostheses such as a short-stem prosthesis and hip resurfacing, which also seek to limit wear, could theoretically be used in young patients. The concept of conservative surgery is becoming increasingly well established in the management of active patients with hip arthritis. So, we must analyze the pros and cons of every technique, evaluate its current status, and compare its results with different contemporary techniques.

## Total Hip Arthroplasty in the Young Patient

Poor results in the early cemented prostheses in young patients led to the use of cementless prostheses. Early cementless prostheses like the PCA (Howmedica) or Harris-Galante (Zimmer, Warsaw, IN) produced poor long-term results [14–16]. Early cementless implants obtained reproducible cementless fixation [14, 15]. However, this fixation was associated with thigh pain and proximal stress shielding with proximal stress

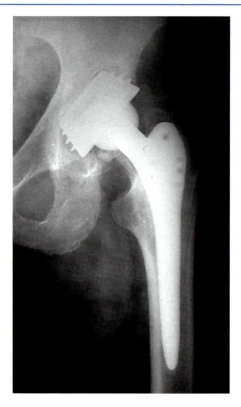

**Fig. 22.1** Anteroposterior radiograph of a hip 18 years after a Zweymüller-Alloclassic prosthesis implantation in a 42-year-old man. Clinical results are excellent and there are no radiographic signs of loosening of any component

protective osteopenia and difficulties in implant removal [24]. New tapered stems like the Zweymüller or Spotorno stems show excellent results with a 100% survival after 10 years (Fig. 22.1) despite varus or valgus malposition [25]. So tapered stems seem to have resolved the issue of bone fixation of the femoral stem.

Although radiographic bone ingrowth is also frequently observed in most hemispheric porous-coated titanium cups [26–28], polyethylene wear is still the most frequent cause of total hip prosthesis failure [29]. Polyethylene wear is the weak link in the long-term results of current THA prostheses. The combination of tapered stems with alternative bearing surfaces has shown excellent results in different series. These encouraging results for femoral stems (Fig. 22.4) [30, 31] would seem to make these appropriate for young patients.

Gamma sterilization in air favors cross-linking but produces free radicals which, in the presence of air, may oxidize and degrade the material's mechanical properties, increasing wear and debris and eventually resulting in osteolysis and prosthetic loosening [29].

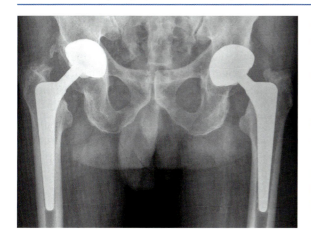

**Fig. 22.2** Anteroposterior radiograph of the pelvis of a 38-year-old man with bilateral uncemented total hip prostheses with alumina on alumina. The right hip was implanted 6 years ago, and the left hip was implanted 8 years ago. Clinical and radiographic results are excellent

Different polyethylenes sterilized in the absence of air (nitrogen, gas plasma, or argon sterilized) have been developed, but these may still oxidize and produce free radicals [32]. Highly cross-linked polyethylenes (HXLPE) are aimed at avoiding these complications [33]. Several HXLPEs are commercially available, but the manufacturing processes are variable, which interferes with material properties and free radical content [34, 35]. In vitro gravimetric analysis has demonstrated that these materials experience substantially less wear than conventional materials: There are even some reports the original machining marks remain after prolonged cycling [33, 36]. Retrieved explants have also confirmed the persistence of machining marks after melt recovery [37]. However, several series [38] reported that the increased radiation dosage necessary for sterilization could have a negative influence on the mechanical properties of UHMWPE, and might compromise the fixation of HXLPE cups [32]. Clinical studies with short and mid follow-ups using RSA measurements [39] or other methods to assess femoral head penetration in different HXLPEs have reported better wear performance than standard polyethylenes [30, 40, 41].

Alumina-on-alumina bearings were introduced by Boutin [42] in France in 1970, and different authors [43–46] have reported good results after 30 years (Fig. 22.2). At the end of the 1970s, cementless prostheses with a threaded ceramic cup were widely used. Published series [47, 48] report no ceramic wear but reveal poor results because of acetabular fixation failure and ceramic fracture. Current ceramics are very different from the old ceramics in terms of porosity, purity, and grain size, their quality having improved considerably, with a decreased risk of fracture [49]. The theoretical advantages of alumina-on-alumina bearings are related to tribologic properties such as scratch resistance and wettability of the material. In addition to superior wear properties, ceramics are biologically inert. These favorable qualities are particularly desirable for implants in young and active patients [31]. Modern third-generation alumina is produced with a finer grain size and fewer impurities than before, thereby improving the material and increasing durability [49]. New generations of alumina-on-alumina couplings have been associated with press-fit metal-backed shells and tapered cementless stems coated with HAP with excellent results [31]. However, alumina fractures and the squeaking associated with the material [50, 51] are still major concerns.

Alumina ceramics are brittle and have no way to deform without breakage. It is difficult to know the exact number of alumina fractures because they are not well recognized and could be underestimated. Fracture risk now stands at approximately one in 2000 for a 10-year period [49]. Liner chipping/fracture could be related to different causes such as cup malposition, neck-cup impingement, and dislocation [50–52]. Alumina fractures can be produced by the propagation of subcritical cracks when subjected to unexpected high-load pressures. Park et al. [53] suggest repetitive impingement can occur in some hips, especially those in which the components are suboptimally positioned and in those with a high range of motion. Stripe wear damage of the head occurs as a result of edge loading and rim wear as a result of subluxation and microseparation. The high frictional torque transmitted across the articulation interface probably occurs during deep flexion or other high-load range-of-motion activities [54]. Subsequent to dislodging, the ceramic liner is completely displaced and will eventually fracture in most cases [52, 54]. A potential solution to ceramic liner displacement is the addition of a geometric irregularity such as a central peg [53]. Hannouche et al. [45] reported three liner fractures in a series using Cerafit and Multicone implants. All these fractures occurred very early (8–16 months postoperatively). These authors point to the need for adequate component positioning and avoidance of small implants

(50 mm/32 mm). Revision surgery for a fracture of an alumina implant is controversial. Failure is infrequent and is easy to solve with a limited revision procedure if performed promptly because osteolysis is rarely encountered. However, early diagnosis of liner fracture is rare, except when ceramic fragments are visible on radiographs. The breakage of a ceramic ball may alter the surface of the Morse taper, which could lead to fracture of the newly implanted head [45]. Toni et al. [51] reported that squeaking in a ceramic-bearing THA can be an early clinical sign of liner chipping, fracture, or stripe wear of the head. They proposed computed tomography to identify cup malposition, ceramic fragments, and low range of mobility and impingement. They also proposed needle aspiration in an attempt to find ceramic fragments. Because the risk of ceramic component fracture still exists, it is mandatory to use a precise surgical technique. Garino [55] suggested placing the cup at 45° or less, increasing anteverted cup placement (greater than 20°), and removing osteophytes and/or part of the anterior wall of the acetabulum to avoid impingement. Patients should also be informed about the potential for this complication before receiving an alumina-on-alumina coupling. Walter et al. [50] report a 0.66% incidence of squeaking in a series of 2,397 ceramic-on-ceramic arthroplasties. Patients with squeaking hips were younger, heavier, and taller when compared with patients without squeaking hips [50]. Toni et al. [52] reported a clinically audible hip noise that may be correlated with ceramic fracture. Hip squeaking is a peculiar phenomenon unique to hard-on-hard total hips. The causes and implications of squeaking are yet to be determined.

Although excellent results have also been reported using a standard metal-on-metal THA [56], there are also potential but unproven problems regarding metal-on-metal wear debris and the effects of ion release, especially in pregnant women and in patients with impaired renal function [57].

## Resurfacing Prostheses

### Causes of Failures in the Early Resurfacing Prostheses

Since polyethylene wear produces loosening and osteolysis and makes revision surgery difficult in young patients, hip resurfacing has been proposed as

an alternative for this group of patients. The theoretical benefits of hip resurfacing include bone stock preservation, physiological loading of the proximal femur, and better options for biomechanical hip reconstruction. These benefits are not new and have been reported previously. In actual fact, hip resurfacing began with of the use of the viscaloid-based mold arthroplasty designed by Smith-Petersen in 1923 to induce the appearance of fibrous material that would replace the altered joint cartilage. Later, in 1938, Smith-Petersen used cups made of vitallium [58]. These cups failed due to axial resorption in 50% of the cases and vertical resorption in a third of the hips, frequently leading to cup subluxation and femoral head fracture. Vitallium cups led to loosening, femoral neck resorption, necrosis, and collapse of the femoral head.

Resurfacing total hip arthroplasties were introduced at the end of the 1970s. It was considered the ideal "conservative" procedure. On the acetabular side, there were no apparent advantages. However, the femoral side advantages were bone stock preservation, physiological loading of the proximal femur, relative ease of revision, and less complications like dislocation and infection than in THR. Different designs were developed in those years: Townley (TARA), Gerard, Paltrineri-Trentani, Furuya, Wagner, Amstutz (THARIES), etc. Steinberg [59] stated that a resurfacing total hip arthroplasty required a meticulous surgical technique, with long periods of rehabilitation and unforeseeable results. The main indication for these prostheses was in patients under 55 years of age, and contraindications were active infection, avascular necrosis with involvement of the total femoral head, and juvenile rheumatoid arthritis.

The first complaint was related to the surgical approaches used. The anterior approach allows a good access, but the loss of blood and strength of abductor force is greater than with the posterior approach. The surgical approach used must supply good visualization of the edges of the acetabular component, a complete view of the edges of the femoral component, and minimized vascular damage of the femoral head.

Really, any approach can be used if the risk of vascular damage is minimized. Steffen et al. [60] inserted an electrode through the femoral neck into the femoral head of patients undergoing a resurfacing arthroplasty through a posterior approach; they found that all patients experienced some compromise to their femoral head blood supply and some suffered a complete

**Fig. 22.3** Wagner resurfacing prosthesis removed at 18 months postsurgery. We can see the thin polyethylene liner, cause of the failure

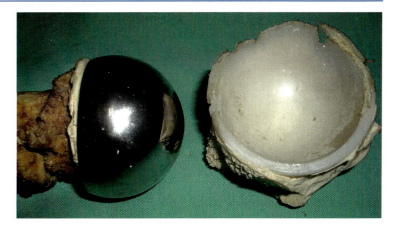

disruption. Kahn et al. [61] using cefuroxime as an indirect measure of blood flow found the posterolateral approach to be associated with a significant reduction in blood supply to the femoral head during resurfacing arthroplasty compared with the transgluteal approach. Beaulé et al. [62] reported that surgeons who perform resurfacing arthroplasty of the hip should pay careful attention to these vessels and avoid excessive dissection around and/or notching of the femoral neck.

Bearing couples with a conventional polyethylene acetabular component combined with large diameter resurfacing components resulted in higher volumetric wear than that of a 28-mm bearing couple. Indeed, very high osteolysis and loosening rates were recorded in the hip resurfacing in the early 1980s. Specific complications of those early prostheses were femoral and cup loosening, avascular necrosis of the femoral head, and femoral neck fractures [63]. Loosening of the prosthetic component was found more frequently in the acetabular cup resulting from polyethylene wear, the PE layer being very thin (Fig. 22.3) in these models, osteolysis, femoral neck fracture, and osteonecrosis of the femoral head [64, 65]. Larger femoral heads required larger and thinner acetabular cups that increased wear. Avascular necrosis of the femoral was also observed. Blood supply to the femoral head may be compromised by capsulotomy, decortication, and reaming of the head. Different series insist on the viability of the femoral head [64, 65], but their results are not conclusive. Femoral neck fractures were frequent (Fig. 22.4) in the late 1970s because of a poor surgical technique (notching of the femoral neck while reaming, or varus placement of the component). Fracture rates vary from 12% in the early designs to 0.7% in the current prostheses [66]. Femoral neck fractures have

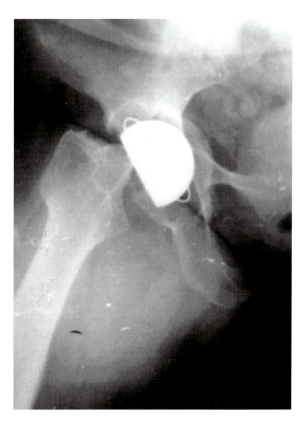

**Fig. 22.4** Radiograph of an old resurfacing prosthesis implanted in a 47-year-old man. The patient presented a femoral neck fracture at 13 months postsurgery

been found more frequently in women (1.91%) than in men (0.98%) ($p<0.001$) [67].

Different long-term studies reported cup loosening as the main cause of failure in the early resurfacing total hip arthroplasties designs [64, 65]. We can conclude that the old surface replacement arthroplasties failed due to polyethylene wear since cups were too thin to be coupled with big femoral heads. However, the metal-on-metal concept foregoes the use of polyethylene and thereby avoids the complications of the early designs. Different series have reported excellent results using contemporary metal-on-metal surface arthroplasties.

## Current Resurfacing Prostheses

The problem of wear has led to the withdrawal of several resurfacing models over the last 30 years. By avoiding the use of polyethylene, the metal-on-metal concept is free of the complications of the early designs. Modern hip resurfacing was reintroduced in Birmingham, UK, in 1991 as a low-wear, bone-preserving option that offered the prospect of a better revision outcome than with a stemmed device [68–70].

Current indications for resurfacing prostheses have increased [71], and excellent results have been published even in patients with severe deformities of the femoral head [72]. Absolute contraindications could be elderly patients with osteoporotic proximal femoral bone, patients with metal hypersensivity, and patients with impaired renal function. Relative contraindications are inflammatory arthropathies, severe acetabular dysplasia, grossly abnormal proximal femoral geometry (slipped capitis femoris epiphysis, Legg-Perthes disease), and large areas of avascular necrosis [67]. Regarding avascular necrosis of the femoral head, Eastaugh-Waring et al. report that if cysts take up less than 25%, grafting plus a resurfacing prosthesis can be indicated [73]. If cysts occupy more than 50%, are larger than 1 cm, or affect the femoral neck outside the confines of the implant (fracture risk), resurfacing is inappropriate. McBryde et al. [74] and McMinn et al. [75] use a resurfacing prosthesis even in hips with a severe congenital dysplasia. Although the surgical technique is more difficult, they report 95% survivorship at 9 years. Different sources, especially in the United Kingdom, consider the resurfacing prosthesis to be the panacea for the surgical treatment of arthritis, particularly in the younger patient who is keen to resume a fully active lifestyle [73].

Factors such as patient selection, surgical technique, and durable component fixation are critical in surface arthroplasty of the hip. Results in specialized centers, the learning curve, serum ion release, etc., must be discussed carefully and honestly. Surgical techniques are extremely important factors in the success of surface

replacement (i.e., preparation of cancellous bone surfaces, cementing technique, positioning of the implant) and are not always reported properly. The clinical significance of elevated serum ion concentrations (i.e., chromium, cobalt, and molybdenum) and the sometimes visible histologic changes seen even around well-functioning implants has not yet been explained [57]. Histologic analyses from retrieved tissue specimens may show chronic synovitis with lymphoplasmacellular infiltrations of different extents in addition to the well-known foreign body reactions, which are a familiar finding in artificial joints in general.

Different studies question some of the theoretical advantages of the resurfacing prosthesis. With regard to offset restoration, Loughead et al. reported that hip resurfacing does not restore hip mechanics as accurately as THA in patients who received a Birmingham Hip Resurfacing prosthesis [76]. Lilikakis et al. [77] reported no benefits in regard to rehabilitation. Crawford and Villar found greater acetabular bone resection than with THR in an in vitro study [78]. The clinical relevance of this study could be the premise that complex acetabular revision surgery requires larger cup sizes than THA [79]. With regard to return to sport after joint replacement, Wilde et al. found no significant differences in the rate of return to sport according to the type of implanted prosthesis [80]. Cutts et al. [81] found 14 revisions (22%) in a series of 65 hips (Corin-HAP) with a mean follow-up of 51 months and a mean age of 55 years. There were femoral neck fractures in six hips (four women over 60 years) with a mean occurrence at 23 weeks, cup loosening in four hips, increased avascular necrosis in one hip, pain in two hips, and infection in one hip. McMinn [68, 69] and Amstutz et al. [72] admit that a learning curve is essential and experience is required. Some authors have reported they had frequent complications during their first cases [72].

## Conservative Hip Prosthesis: Short, Stemless Metaphysis Loading Implants

Our understanding of the role of muscle forces on strain distribution in the proximal femur has increased in recent years [82, 83]. The most outstanding alteration on the pattern of load transfer concerns the metaphyseal region, particularly the proximal lateral femoral cortex. The action of the iliotibial band and the vastus lateralis gluteus medius complex counteracts the varus bending torque of the loads acting on the hip, transforming the tensile stresses in the lateral femur into compressive stresses. According to this new understanding of hip biomechanics, new conservative implants have been designed. The characteristics of these designs are the almost complete absence of a stem, the presence of a well-defined lateral flare intended to conform to the lateral femoral endosteal surface, and the complete preservation of the femoral neck [82].

A conservative implant should preserve bone both at the time of surgery and in the long term by providing more physiological loading [84]. Any implant that makes contact with the diaphyseal cortex or is distally ingrown will offload distally with consequent proximal stress protection [84]. Biomechanical studies have shown that stemless metaphyseal loading implants are not "fit and fill" prostheses [85]. Excellent axial and rotational stability can be achieved within cancellous bone, so the implant is suspended in and moves in consort with the surrounding cancellous bone. This reduces shear stresses at the fixation interface and optimizes load transfer in the metaphysis.

Bone densitometry has demonstrated that the current shorter stems avoided subtrochanteric buttressing and enhanced the load transfer to the proximal femur with consequent bone remodeling. Using DEXA to compare the periprosthetic bone density of the Santori custom-made stem (DePuy, Warsaw, IN) as well as a variety of other commercially available cementless femoral stems, Albanese et al. [86] confirmed that the Proxima stem with complete proximal load transfer produces a homogeneous and more physiological redistribution of bone density, allowing maintenance of proximal periprosthetic bone stock [86]. Santori et al. report that a conservative prosthesis without a stem that effectively loads both medial and lateral proximal flares not only requires less bone removal at the index operation but preserves proximal bone stock over the long term [87].

Westphal et al. report in an in vitro study that initial cyclic motion of the Proxima (DePuy, Warsaw, IN) short-stemmed prosthesis is similar to that for a clinically successful Summit (DePuy, Warsaw, IN) stemmed implant, and therefore, bony ingrowth with long-term consolidation can be expected [88]. The Proxima implant tended to migrate more than the longer shaft prosthesis in the initial phase. Although implant size had no significant effect on migration, implant position and bone geometry might influence migrational characteristics. The lower

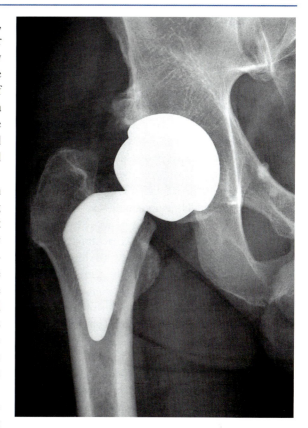

**Fig. 22.5** Anteroposterior radiograph of a hip 2 years after a Proxima cementless stemless metaphyseal loading prosthesis implantation in a 42-year-old man. Clinical results are excellent and there are no radiographic signs of loosening of any component (By courtesy of Dr. J Fernandez-Valencia)

bending stiffness of the Proxima induces more physiological transfer, which may reduce the risk of stress shielding. Large migration and cyclic motion are related to poor bone quality in the Proxima prosthesis. Westphal et al. conclude that only patients with good bone quality should be considered for short-stemmed devices [88].

Santori et al. report their results with an ultrashort custom-made implant implanted in 131 hips with a mean follow-up of 5 years [82]. There was no thigh pain and none of the patients required a femoral stem revision. At 5 years, all implants appeared radiographically stable with well-maintained proximal bone stock. These excellent results attributed to the geometry of this implant have provided significant initial stability, a stability which seemed to be preserved over a long follow-up period. Undersizing the implant, in the presence of good bone quality, appears to be feasible and attractive (Fig. 22.5). Furthermore, the absence of a stem makes this model ideal for less invasive surgery.

## Final Considerations

The reintroduction of hip resurfacing and stemless metaphysis loading implants into total joint replacement warrants reexamination of current treatment recommendations. Although an increasing number of studies provide the results of different conservative hip implants, the data must be viewed with caution. Prostheses have often been evaluated in very experienced single centers with relatively short follow-ups and incomplete radiographic analyses. Surgical techniques are extremely important factors for success, especially since surface replacement (i.e., preparation of cancellous bone surfaces, cementing technique, implant positioning) has not always been reported properly. The clinical significance of elevated serum ion concentrations (i.e., chromium, cobalt, and molybdenum) and sometimes visible histologic changes around even well-functioning implants has not yet been determined.

Carefully performed tribologic studies as well as retrieval analyses do show that the modern generation of conservative hip implants can function very well. It is critical, however, to be aware of the potential hazards and risks associated with the different prostheses. The aim of this presentation is to summarize current literature on clinical success rates and to link the data to recent experimental investigations. This should improve our ability to compare short-stemmed cementless prostheses and surface replacement arthroplasty with "golden standard" joint replacement techniques.

Resurfacing prostheses and short-stemmed cementless prostheses seem to present the following advantages over THA:

1. Failure of total hip arthroplasty in the younger population has been blamed on polyethylene wear. An easy femoral revision is one of the main advantages of a resurfacing prosthesis. However, current tapered stem designs show survival rates of 100% at 10 years, despite a poor surgical technique whereby the stem was implanted in varus or valgus. Thus, bone fixation is not the problem, especially in the femur, with the main cause of failure in THA in young patients being polyethylene wear. If the bearing surface material is switched to ceramics or cross-linked polyethylene, the problem is no longer encountered. Regular results published on total hips with all alumina bearings are currently excellent with 95% survivorship at 10 years. Every sport and all activities are permitted without limitations [80]. The complications and dislocation rate is about 2% with very low recurrence. Aseptic loosening of the socket is the most frequent problem [31], but these sockets are easy to revise. Similarly, excellent results have been reported using standard THA with cross-linked polyethylene [30, 39] or metal-on-metal bearing surfaces [56]. Conservative techniques such as resurfacing and short-stem prostheses have been introduced to solve identical problems and to retain the elastic properties of the femoral head. Some published series with a short-term follow-up have reported a failure rate of up to 7% after 4 years [89]. Some published papers have insisted on problems with leg length discrepancy, difficulties with avascular necrosis, and with the impossibility of performing the procedure through a small incision. The Mac Minn series presented exceptionally good results at 7 years [69]. But there are still some cases of femoral neck fracture. There are also potential but unproven problems regarding metal-on-metal wear debris and serum ion concentrations [90]. Furthermore, no improvement in sport activity level has yet been proven [88].

2. Another theoretical advantage of a short-stemmed or resurfacing prosthesis is a reduction in bone resection. However, this is only true for the femur but not for the acetabulum. The use of large femoral heads requires the use of bigger acetabular cups, measuring at least 54 mm in diameter [79]. The mean acetabular cup diameter used in our institutions is 52 mm. So in cases of acetabular loosening, which is the weak link in most hip arthroplasty designs, acetabular revision surgery will require a large acetabular cup as a result of greater bone deficiency.

3. Good patient selection and adequate surgical technique, after a long learning curve, should provide a survival comparable to THA after 5 years. Although a resurfacing prosthesis has been indicated for young active patients with osteoarthritis and a BMI less than 35, this profile is difficult to find in our clinical practice. In our institutions, osteoarthritis is very infrequent in patients under 40 years of age. On the contrary, avascular necrosis, arthritis secondary to congenital dysplasia, acetabular fractures, juvenile rheumatoid arthritis, arthritis secondary to developmental diseases, etc., are the most frequent diagnoses in this group. Given these young patients'

severe functional impairment, severe deformities, and bone deficiencies, especially in the acetabulum, the use of a resurfacing prosthesis is rarely indicated. Some authors think that a resurfacing prosthesis is actually only indicated in 6% of the patients treated in our institutions, and this paucity makes it difficult to go through the steep learning curve needed in a general hospital where surgeons must treat many different processes.

A resurfacing prosthesis is usually offered to relatively young patients who want to maintain a high activity level. Although the initial experience is satisfactory in different series, controversies regarding the importance of femoral head vascularization, implant design, metallurgical aspects, and cementing technique remain. According to Beaulé and Antoniades [91], the resurfacing prosthesis should not be considered a standard THA that requires experienced surgeons. Surface arthroplasty could be considered a viable alternative to THR, but certain goals must be met: survivorship must be above 90% at 5–10 years; the technique must be proven as reproducible; and ease of conversion to total hip replacement must be confirmed.

# References

1. Charnley J (1961) Arthroplasty of the hip. A new operation. Lancet 1:1129–1132
2. Collis DK (1991) Long-term (twelve to eighteen years) follow-up of cemented total hip replacements in patients who were less than fifty years old: a follow-up note. J Bone Joint Surg Am 73-A:593–597
3. Malchau H, Herberts P, Eisler T et al (2002) The Swedish total hip replacement register. J Bone Joint Surg Am 84(Suppl 2):S2–S20
4. Parvizi J, Campfield A, Clohisy JC et al (2006) Management of arthritis of the hip in the young adult. J Bone Joint Surg Br 88:1279–1285
5. Eskelinen A, Remes V, Helenius I et al (2006) Uncemented total hip arthroplasty for primary osteoarthritis in young patients: a mid- to long-term follow-up study from the Finnish Arthroplasty Register. Acta Orthop 77:57–70
6. García-Cimbrelo E, Cruz-Pardos A, Cordero J et al (2000) Low friction arthroplasty in patients younger than 40 years old: 20- to 25-year results. J Arthroplasty 15:825–832
7. Hallan G, Lie SA, Havelin LI (2006) High wear rates and extensive osteolysis in 3 types of uncemented total hip arthroplasty: a review of the PCA, the Harris-Galante and the Profile/Tri-Lock Plus arthroplasties with a minimum of 12 years median follow-up in 96 hips. Acta Orthop 77: 575–584
8. Kim YH, Kook HK, Kim JS (2002) Total hip replacement with a cementless acetabular component and a cemented femoral component in patients younger than fifty years of age. J Bone Joint Surg Am 84:770–774
9. Singh S, Trikha SP (2004) Hydroxyapatite ceramic coated femoral stems in young patients: a prospective ten-year study. J Bone Joint Surg Br 86:1118–1123
10. Wroblewski BM, Siney PD, Fleming PA (2002) Charnley low-frictional torque arthroplasty in patients under the age of 51 years. Follow-up to 33 years. J Bone Joint Surg Br 84:540–543
11. Ellison B, Berend KR, Lombardi AV Jr et al (2006) Tapered titanium porous plasma-sprayed femoral component in patients aged 40 years and younger. J Arthroplasty 21: 32–37
12. Kearns SR, Jamal B, Rorabeck CH et al (2006) Factors affecting survival of uncemented total hip arthroplasty in patients 50 years or younger. Clin Orthop Relat Res 453:103–109
13. Jones LC, Hungerford DS (1987) Cement disease. Clin Orthop Relat Res 225:192–206
14. Kim YH, Kim VE (1992) Results of the Harris-Galante cementless hip prosthesis. J Bone Jont Surg Br 74:83–87
15. Cruz-Pardos A, García-Cimbrelo E (2001) The Harris-Galante total hip arthroplasty. A minimum 8-year follow-up. J Arthroplasty 16:586–597
16. Thanner J, Kärrholm J, Malchau H et al (1999) Poor outcome of the PCA and Harris-Galante hip prostheses. Randomized study of 171 arthroplasties with 9-year follow-up. Acta Orthop Scand 70:155–162
17. Callaghan JJ, Forest EE, Sporer SM et al (1997) Total hip arthroplasty in the young adult. Clin Orthop Relat Res 344:257–262
18. Sochart DH, Porter ML (1997) The long-term results of Charnley low-friction arthroplasty in young patients who have congenital dislocation, degenerative osteoarthrosis, or rheumatoid arthritis. J Bone Joint Surg Am 11:1599–1617
19. Older J (2002) Charnley low-friction arthroplasty. A worldwide retrospective review at 15 to 20 years. J Arthroplasty 17:675–680
20. Nizard R, Pourreyron D, Raould A et al (2008) Alumina-on-alumina hip arthroplasty in patients younger than 30 years old. Clin Orthop Relat Res 466:317–323
21. Schreurs BW, Busch VJ, Welten ML et al (2004) Acetabular reconstruction with impaction bone-grafting and a cemented cup in patients younger than fifty years old. J Bone Joint Surg Am 86:2385–2392
22. García-Cimbrelo E, Díaz-Martin A, Madero R et al (2000) Loosening of the cup after low-friction arthroplasty in patients with acetabular protrusion. The importance of the position of the cup. J Bone Joint Surg Br 82:108–115
23. Spangehl MJ, Berry DJ, Trousdale RT et al (2001) Uncemented acetabular components with bulk femoral head autograft for acetabular reconstruction in developmental dysplasia of the hip: results at five to twelve years. J Bone Joint Surg Am 83:1484–1489
24. Engh CA Jr, Claus AM, Hopper RH Jr et al (2001) Long-term results using the anatomic medullary locking hip prosthesis. Clin Orthop Relat Res 393:137–146
25. Garcia-Cimbrelo E, Cruz-Pardos A, Madero R et al (2003) Total hip arthroplasty with use of the cementless Zweymuller Alloclassic system. A ten to thirteen-year follow-up study. J Bone Joint Surg Am 85-A:296–303

26. Kim Y-H, Oh S-H, Kim J-S (2003) Primary total hip arthroplasty with a second-generation cementless total hip prosthesis in patients younger than fifty years of age. J Bone Joint Surg Am 85:109–114

27. Grobler GP, Learmonth ID, Bernstein BP et al (2005) Ten-year results of a press-fit porous-coated acetabular component. J Bone Joint Surg Br 87:786–789

28. Sychterz C, Claus A, Engh C (2002) What we have learned about long-term cementless fixation from autopsy retrievals. Clin Orthop Relat Res 405:79–91

29. Harris WH (2001) Wear and periprosthetic osteolysis. The problem. Clin Orthop Relat Res 393:66–70

30. García-Rey E, García-Cimbrelo E, Cruz-Pardos A et al (2008) New polyethylenes in total hip replacement. A prospective comparative clinical study of two types of liner. J Bone Joint Surg Br 90-B:149–153

31. García-Cimbrelo E, García-Rey E, Murcia-Mazón A et al (2008) Alumina-on-alumina in THA: a multicenter prospective study. Clin Orthop Relat Res 466:309–316

32. McKellop HA, Shen FW, Lu B et al (2000) Effect of sterilization method and other modifications on the wear resistance of acetabular cups made of ultra-high molecular weight polyethylene. A hip-simulator study. J Bone Joint Surg Am 82:1708–1725

33. Muratoglu OK, Bragdon CR, O'Connor DO et al (2001) A novel method of cross-linking UHMWPE to improve wear, reduce oxidation, and retain mechanical properties. J Arthroplasty 16:149–160

34. Rieker CB, Konrad R, Schön R et al (2003) In vivo and in vitro surface changes in a highly cross-linked polyethylene. J Arthroplasty 18(Suppl 1):48–54

35. Greenwald AS, Bauer TW, Ries MD (2001) Committee on biomedical engineering, committee on hip and knee arthritis: new polys for old: contribution or caveat? J Bone Joint Surg Am 83(Suppl 2):27–31

36. Collier JP, Currier BH, Kennedy FE et al (2003) Comparison of cross-linked polyethylene materials for orthopaedic applications. Clin Orthop Relat Res 414:289–304

37. Crowninshield RD, Laurent MP, Yao JQ et al (2002) Cross-linking to improve THR wear performance. Hip Int 12:103–107

38. Muratoglu OK, Greenbaum ES, Bragdon CR et al (2004) Surface analysis of early retrieved acetabular polyethylene: a comparison of conventional and liners highly crosslinked polyethylenes. J Arthroplasty 19:68–77

39. Digas G, Kärrholm J, Thanner J et al (2003) Highly cross-linked polyethylene in cemented THA. Randomized study of 61 hips. Clin Orthop Relat Res 417:126–138

40. Manning DW, Chiang PP, Martell JM et al (2005) In vivo comparative wear study of traditional and highly cross-linked polyethylene in total hip arthroplasty. J Arthroplasty 20:880–886

41. Dorr LD, Wan Z, Shahrdar C et al (2005) Clinical performance of a Durasul highly cross-linked polyethylene acetabular liner for total hip arthroplasty at five years. J Bone Joint Surg Am 87:1816–1821

42. Boutin P (2000) Total hip arthroplasty using a ceramic prosthesis. The classic. Clin Orthop Relat Res 379:3–11

43. Bizot P, Nizard R, Hamadouche M et al (2001) Prevention of wear and osteolysis. Alumina-on-alumina bearing. Clin Orthop Relat Res 393:85–93

44. Hamadouche M, Boutin P, Daussange J et al (2002) Alumina-on-alumina total hip arthroplasty. A minimum 18.5-year follow-up study. J Bone Joint Surg Am 84:69–77

45. Hannouche D, Nich C, Bizot P et al (2003) Fractures of ceramic bearings. History and present status. Clin Orthop Relat Res 417:19–26

46. Sedel L, Kerboull L, Christel P (1990) Alumina on alumina hip replacement results and survivorship in young patients. J Bone Joint Surg Br 72:658–663

47. García-Cimbrelo E, Martínez-Sayanes JM, Minuesa A et al (1996) Mittelmeier ceramic-ceramic prosthesis after ten years. J Arthroplasty 11:773–781

48. Huo MH, Martin RP, Zatorsky LE et al (1996) Cementless total hip arthroplasties using ceramic-on-ceramic articulation in young patients: a minimum 5-year follow-up study. J Arthroplasty 11:673–678

49. Bizot P, Hannouche D, Nizard R et al (2004) Hybrid alumina total hip arthroplasty using press-fit metal-backed socket in patients younger than 55 years. A six- to 11-year evaluation. J Bone Joint Surg Br 86:190–194

50. Walter WL, O'Toole GC, Walter WK et al (2007) Squeaking in ceramic-on-ceramic hips. The importance of acetabular component orientation. J Arthroplasty 22:496–503

51. Toni A, Traina F, Stea S et al (2006) Early diagnosis of ceramic liner fracture. Guidelines based on a twelve-year clinical experience. J Bone Joint Surg Am 88(Suppl 4): 55–63

52. D'Antonio J, Capello W, Manley M et al (2002) New experience with alumina-on-alumina ceramic bearings for total hip arthroplasty. J Arthroplasty 17:390–397

53. Park Y-S, Hwang S-K, Choy W-S et al (2006) Ceramic failure after total hip arthroplasty with an alumina-on-alumina bearing. J Bone Joint Surg Am 88:780–787

54. Poggie RA, Turgeon TR, Coutts RD (2007) Failure analysis of a ceramic bearing acetabular component. J Bone Joint Surg Am 89:367–380

55. Garino J (2000) Modern ceramic-on-ceramic total hip systems in the United States. Clin Orthop Relat Res 379:41–47

56. Delaunay CP, Bonnomet F, Clavert P et al (2008) THA using metal-on-metal articulation in active patients younger than 50 years. Clin Orthop Relat Res 466:340–346

57. Brodner W, Bitzan P, Meisinger V et al (2003) Serum cobalt levels after metal-on-metal total hip arthroplasty. J Bone Joint Surg Am 85-Am:2168–2173

58. Smith-Petersen MN (1948) Evolution of the mould arthroplasty of the hip joint. J Bone Joint Surg Br 30-B:59–75

59. Steinberg ME (1982) Evolution and development of surface replacement arthroplasty. Orthop Clin North Am 13: 661–666

60. Steffen RT, Smith SR, Urban JPG et al (2005) The effect of hip resurfacing on oxygen concentration in the femoral head. J Bone Joint Surg Br 87:1468–1474

61. Khan A, Yates P, Lovering A et al (2007) The effect of surgical approach on blood flow to the femoral head during resurfacing. J Bone Joint Surg Br 89:21–25

62. Beaulé PE, Campbell PA, Hoke R, Dorey F (2006) Notching of the femoral neck during resurfacing arthroplasty of the hip. J Bone Joint Surg Br 88-B:35–39

63. Bierbaum WN, Sweet R (1982) Complications of resurfacing arthroplasty. Orthop Clin North Am 13:761–775

64. Howie DW, Cornish BL, Vernon-Roberts B (1993) The viability of the femoral had after resurfacing hip arthroplasty in humans. Clin Orthop Relat Res 291:171–184

65. Amstutz HC, Gregoris P (1996) Metal-on-metal bearings in hip arthroplasty. Clin Orthop 329:S11–S34

66. Treacy RB, McBryde CW, Pynsent PB (2005) Birmingham hip resurfacing arthroplasty. A minimum follow-up of five years. J Bone Joint Surg Br 87:167–170

67. Shimmin AJ, Bare J, Back DL (2005) Complications associated with hip resurfacing arthroplasty. Orthop Clin North Am 36:187–193

68. McMinn D, Treacy R, Lin K et al (1996) Metal on metal surface replacement of the hip. Experience of the McMinn prosthesis. Clin Orthop Relat Res 329(Suppl):S89–S98

69. McMinn DJW (2003) Development of metal/metal hip resurfacing. Hip Int 13:41–53

70. Daniel J, Pynsent PB, McMinn DJW (2004) Metal-on-metal resurfacing of the hip in patients under the age of 55 years with osteoarthritis. J Bone Joint Surg Br 86:177–184

71. De Smet KA (2005) Belgium experience with metal-on-metal surface arthroplasty. Orthop Clin North Am 36:203–213

72. Amstutz HC, Su EP, Le Duff MJ (2005) Surface arthroplasty in young patients with hip arthritis secondary to childhood disorders. Orthop Clin North Am 36:223–230

73. Eastaugh-Waring SJ, Seenath S, Learmonth DS et al (2006) The practical limitations of resurfacing hip arthroplasty. J Arthroplasty 21:18–22

74. McBryde CW, Shears E, O'Hara JN et al (2008) Metal-on-metal hip resurfacing in developmental dysplasia. A case-control study. J Bone Joint Surg Br 90:708–714

75. McMinn DJW, Daniel J, Ziaee H et al (2008) Results of the Birmingham Hip resurfacing dysplasia component in severe acetabular insufficiency. A six- to 9.6-year follow-up. J Bone Joint Surg Br 90:715–723

76. Loughead JM, Chesney D, Holland JP et al (2005) Comparison of offset in Birmingham hip resurfacing and hybrid total hip arthroplasty. J Bone Joint Surg Br 87:163–166

77. Lilikakis AK, Arora A, Villar RN (2005) Early rehabilitation comparing hip resurfacing and total hip replacement. Hip Int 15:189–194

78. Crawford JR, Palmer SJ, Wimhurst JA et al (2005) Bone loss at hip resurfacing: a comparison with total hip arthroplasty. Hip Int 15:195–198

79. De Haan R, Campbell PA, Su EP et al (2008) Revision of metal-on-metal resurfacing arthroplasty of the hip. The influence of malpositioning of the components. J Bone Joint Surg Br 90:1158–1163

80. Wylde W, Blom A, Dieppe P et al (2008) Return to sport after joint replacement. J Bone Joint Surg Br 90:920–923

81. Cutts S, Datta A, Ayoub K et al (2005) Early failure modalities in hip resurfacing. Hip Int 15:155–158

82. Santori FS, Manili M, Fredella N et al (2008) Ultra-short stems with proximal load transfer: clinical and radiographic results at five-year follow-up. Hip Int 16(Suppl 3): S31–S39

83. Bitsakos C, Kerner J, Fisher I et al (2005) The effect of muscle loading on the simulation of bone remodelling in the proximal femur. J Biomech 38:133–139

84. Kulkarni M, Wylde V, Aspros D et al (2006) Early clinical experience with a metaphyseal loading implant: why have a stem? Hip Int 16(Suppl 3):S3–S8

85. Learmonth ID (2008) Conservative hip implant. Foreword. Hip Int 16(Suppl 3):S1

86. Albanese CV, Rendine M, De Palma F et al (2006) Bone remodelling in THA: a comparative DXA scan study between conventional implants and a new stemless femoral component. A preliminary report. Hip Int 16(Suppl 3): S9–S215

87. Santori N, Albanese CV, Learmonth ID et al (2008) Bone preservation with a conservative metaphyseal loading implant. Hip Int 16(Suppl 3):S16–S21

88. Westphal FM, Bishop N, Püschel K et al (2008) Biomechanics of new short-stemmed uncemented hip prosthesis: an in-vitro study in human bone. Hip Int 16(Suppl 3): S22–S30

89. Kim PR, Beaulé PE, Laflamme GY et al (2008) Causes of early failure in a multicenter clinical trial of hip resurfacing. J Arthroplasty 23(Suppl 1):44–49

90. Pandit H, Glyn-Jones S, McLardy-Smith P et al (2008) Pseudotumors associated with metal-on-metal hip resurfacings. J Bone Joint Surg Br 90:847–851

91. Beaulé P, Antoniades J (2005) Patient selection and surgical technique for surface arthroplasty of the hip. Orthop Clin North Am 36:177–185

# Resurfacing Arthroplasty for Femoroacetabular Impingement

**23**

Matías J. Salineros and Paul E. Beaulé

## Introduction

Femoroacetabular impingement (FAI) is a recently described pathology in which an abnormal shape of the femoral head–neck junction and/or a retroverted acetabulum causes a pathological femoroacetabular contact, chiefly during hip flexion and internal rotation. Repetition of this abnormal contact provoked by impingement could constitute an important cause of osteoarthritis of the hip [1].

Having completed its initial evaluation phase, hip resurfacing arthroplasty has become an alternative to total hip replacement that is particularly suitable for young and active patients [2, 3]. Improvements related to design and metallurgy technologies have addressed many of the problems previously associated to these kinds of implants [4, 5]. As is also the case with other joint-preserving procedures [6–8], appropriate patient selection is fundamental since this avoids complications and eventual failure of the technique [9, 10].

The potential advantages of resurfacing arthroplasty over traditional total hip replacement are as follows:
Preservation of femoral bone stock [11]
More physiological bone transfer in the proximal femur [11]
Near-normal hip joint kinematics [12]
Low dislocation rate

More straightforward revision tan with conventional implants [13]
Better tolerance of high-demand activity, which improves patients' perception as to regaining former quality of life
Disadvantages include:
Extensive surgical approach
Technically demanding
Indication contingent on the levels of bone stock remaining in the femur
Lack of modularity
Limited recovery of limb length in certain cases
Risk of femoral neck fracture [14]
Release of metal ions [15, 16]

As regards the results of this technique, medium-term survivorship rates between 97% and 99% have been reported [9, 10, 17, 18]. In all but one of these series [9], some sort of selection was prospectively applied that included the presence of osteoarthritis, absence of osteopenia, and the absence of large cysts in the femoral head. The main two failure modes for this technique are femoral component loosening and femoral neck fractures [19, 20]. The reported prevalence of femoral neck fractures ranges between 0.8% and 1.45% [10, 14]; these fractures tend to occur within the first 6 months postoperatively. Femoral head osteonecrosis together with notching the upper portion of the femoral neck while reaming the head have been reported as events associated to femoral neck fracture [19–21]. On the basis of the findings obtained in last generation metal-on-metal components, Campbell et al. [19] report wide variations in terms of cement penetration in the femoral head. In certain cases, cement takes up 89% of the head, leading to necrotic

M.J. Salineros • P.E. Beaulé (✉)
Division of Orthopaedic Surgery, Ottawa Hospital,
University of Ottawa, Ottawa, ON, Canada
e-mail: pbeaule@ottawahospital.on.ca

Ó. Marín-Peña (ed.), *Femoroacetabular Impingement*,
DOI 10.1007/978-3-642-22769-1_23, © Springer-Verlag Berlin Heidelberg 2012

**Table 23.1** Surface arthroplasty risk index (SARI) [25]

| Cyst in the femoral head >1 cm | 2 points |
|---|---|
| Body weight <82 kg | 2 points |
| Previous hip surgery | 1 point |
| UCLA activity score >6 | 1 point |

lesions in the femoral head. In these cases, the interface becomes exceedingly stiff, which may result in failure of the technique.

Much in the same way as any other new technique, appropriate intraoperative implant placement greatly affects their survivorship and proper functioning. Correct implant placement is of particular significance in metal-on-metal hip resurfacing surgery since much like unicompartmental knee replacement [22], it is characterized by unique technical features. These prostheses were abandoned for a long period of time and were subsequently reintroduced as a result of improvements made in the surgical technique. This means that the new surgeon generations interested in this technique need specific training that is different from that required for conventional arthroplasty.

## Patient Selection

As is the case with the uncemented designs in hip replacement [23], the metal-on-metal bearing surface is not the only reason for the success of resurfacing arthroplasty [24]. When reviewing the short-term results of patients under 40 years of age subjected to metal-on-metal resurfacing arthroplasty, Beaulé et al. [25] identified certain factors that played a significant role in the premature failure of this technique. This is how the SARI (surface arthroplasty risk index) score was established, whereby the subjects assessed can obtain a maximum of 6 points (Table 23.1). A SARI score above 3 indicates a four times higher-than-normal possibility of premature failure or adverse radiological changes, associated with 89% survivorship at 4 years [9]. The SARI score also contributed significant information as regards the final results of cemented McMinn (Corin, Circentester, England)-type implants at a mean follow-up of 8.7 years. In this series, failed implants or those presenting with evident radiological loosening in the femoral component obtained a markedly higher SARI score (3.9 vs. 1.9), with average survivorship ranging between 80% and 93%, respectively [26].

## Selecting and Placing the Implant

Even if patient selection is appropriate, resurfacing arthroplasty poses several technical challenges in terms of the position and the size of the implant [3]. The structural abnormalities associated to certain conditions increase the difficulties inherent in correct component placement, orientation, and fixation. A clear example of this is a patient with a dysplastic hip where an acetabular deficiency combined with the impossibility of placing screws through the acetabular component make initial implant stability unforeseeable. Given that this deformity is compounded by significant leg length discrepancy and that a valgus femoral neck could compromise the functional result of the resurfacing procedure, a total hip replacement is recommended in these cases [27].

Because of the conservative nature of this procedure and our goal to reproduce the proximal femoral anatomy as closely as possible, implant position will have fundamental importance for the survivorship and function of the implant. On the coronal plane, varus positioning should be avoided at all costs, with 5–10° valgus being the ideal, minimizing the tensile stress on the superior bone-prosthesis interface [28, 29]. For example, a comparison of implant placement at 130° with placement at 140° reveals that the former inclination leads to an increase in tensile stress of 31%. As regards the sagittal/axial plane, it is essential to restore anterior head–neck offset.

## Femoroacetabular Impingement in Conservative Arthroplasty

Several reports have recognized the existence of impingement in total hip replacement and its relationship with decreased range of motion [30]; some reports even state that such impingement could also result in instability [31]. The risk of impingement could even be higher following resurfacing arthroplasty since the head–neck junction is preserved. Beaulé et al. [32] reported that 56% of hips treated with hip resurfacing presented with decreased anterior head–neck offset preoperatively. Within the group of patients with decreased anterior head–neck offset, the most frequent preoperative diagnosis was osteoarthritis and osteonecrosis, with associated femoroacetabular impingement in many cases [1, 33]. FAI has been described as a frequent cause of osteoarthritis. Authors believe that the anatomical alteration that leads to anterolateral contact between the femoral head–neck junction and the anterolateral acetabular rim causes progressive articular damage [34, 35].

If this pathology is not appropriately diagnosed at the time of indicating and carrying out a hip resurfacing procedure, impingement-derived symptoms will persist. In this case, abnormal contact will occur between the rim of the acetabular component and the femoral component or the junction between the component and the femoral neck, restricting range of motion [36].

Verticalization of the acetabular component must be avoided as it will lead to a considerable increase in wear [37]. Ideally, the component should be positioned at an angle of 40–45°. Excessive component horizontalization must also be avoided as it could lead to anterior impingement during flexion [38].

Femoral components used in hip resurfacing are not modular, which means that specific techniques are required to achieve an optimal relationship between the femoral head and neck. An alternative approach could be to modify the position of the femoral component by changing its version or shifting the component anteriorly or posteriorly. The problem with such a technique is that it does not provide an overall improvement of the head–neck relationship; it only changes it partially. For example, if we orient the angle of the component anteriorly, or if we translate it, we shall obtain a better head–neck relationship anteriorly but at the expense of the posterior head–neck relationship, with impingement on the acetabular rim in that area. These techniques should only be used after careful preoperative planning that guarantees preservation of head–neck offset on both planes. When applying this technique, it must be remembered that guide wire positioning is of the essence in this procedure. If an increase in anteversion is pursued, the guide wire must be placed from anterior to posterior in relation to the femoral neck; for increased retroversion, the opposite is required. In order to achieve anterior translation, the entry site for the needle must be placed more anteriorly and placement must occur parallel to the femoral neck. It should be remember that excessive translation or a change in version could result in reaming the anterior or posterior cortex of the neck at its base, so extreme care and meticulousness are paramount (Fig. 23.1).

Another useful technique to prevent postoperative impingement is removal of anterior and lateral osteophytes from the femoral neck in order to restore the sphericity of the femoral head. This is useful both to prevent postoperative impingement and to improve the surgeon's appreciation of the position of the guide wire. Failure to perform this maneuver makes it difficult to correctly identify the axis of the neck, which normally results in overly posterior implant placement since the posterior head–neck offset is more prominent than anterior head–neck offset. All of this result in a reduction in anterior head–neck offset, leading to postoperative anterolateral impingement [39, 40]. Failure to resect the osteophytes and to restore sphericity to the femoral head may also result in oversizing of the implant, which will in turn require a larger acetabular implant, undermining the bone-preserving feature of this technique [41]. Osteophyte removal should be performed meticulously and taking care not to weaken the femoral neck, thereby avoiding the feared periprosthetic fractures [42] (Fig. 23.2).

Even if postoperative impingement is a multifactorial pathology [43, 44], D'Lima et al. have shown that there is a complex interaction between anteroposterior orientation of the acetabular component, the anteversion of the acetabular component, and the anteversion of the femoral component. Such a relationship will determine the maximum range of motion of the joint as well as the point during the range of movement at which impingement is more likely. Eccentric wear in the joint has been reported following impingement in up to 84% of prostheses extracted as a result of aseptic loosening [36]. Thus, it is important maximize the amount of anterior head–neck offset by appropriate selection and placement of components, particularly femoral ones [32].

The senior author (PB) prefers anterior dislocation of the femoral head in the event of deformities associated with FAI since this permits appropriate visualization of the anteromedial, anterolateral, and posterolateral head–neck junction. For this reason, this author normally uses an anterior surgical approach through the Hueter interval or carrying out a controlled hip dislocation if joint preservation is at all possible [39, 45].

There is one situation that is worth analyzing. It is that of patient under 45 years of age whose clinical history and physical and immunological exam are compatible with FAI and moderate hip osteoarthritis (Tonnis II–III) [46]. Alternatives in this case are open or arthroscopic treatment of FAI, resurfacing arthroplasty if certain conditions are met, and total hip replacement. Our recommendation in these cases is to conduct a controlled hip dislocation [39, 47], which preserves blood supply to the femoral head and allows direct observation of the status of articular cartilage. If the articular cartilage is seen to be in good condition, an acetabuloplasty can be performed with detachment and reattachment of the labrum if it is a pincer-type FAI. If the impingement is of the cam-type, we carry out an osteoplasty of the head–neck junction. In the event of combined FAI, both procedures are performed (Fig. 23.3). In addition, if on dislocating the joint we realize that the joint surface is worn and presents with moderate to severe osteoarthritis, we can use the same approach to carry out a resurfacing procedure with adequate exposure of the joint in one single surgical event [48].

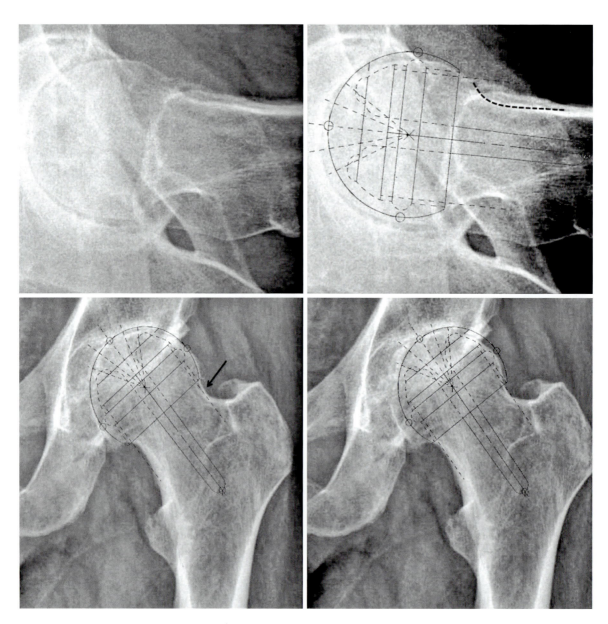

**Fig. 23.1** Preoperative radiographs: *Above left*: cross-table view showing an anterior bump. *Above right*: cross-table view where the anterior template was shifted anteriorly to avoid postoperative impingement. The *dotted line* represents the bone resection of the head–neck junction. *Middle left*: AP radiograph with a template in the center of the neck. *Arrow* indicates an area of potential notching. *Middle right*: AP radiograph where the template has been shifted superiorly to avoid notching. *Below right and left*: postoperative result in line with preoperative plan

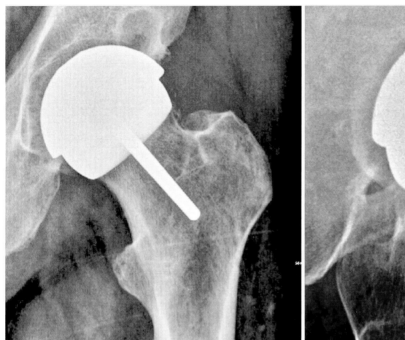
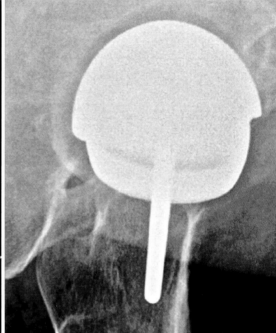

**Fig. 23.1**   (continued)

## Summary

Given that resurfacing hip arthroplasty preserves the femoral head–neck junction, care must be taken during implant placement, avoiding the repetition of pre-existing malformations. As regards resurfacing arthroplasty, removal of anterior osteophytes will help reconstruct an appropriate anterior head–neck offset, reducing the risk of impingement, in addition to contributing to adequate femoral implant selection, which will in turn preserve the acetabular bone stock. Another favorable consequence of osteophyte removal and reconstruction of the head–neck anatomy is correct guide wire placement. This maneuver will determine the appropriate position of the femoral implant, avoiding damage to the femoral neck and the resulting fracture risk.

Surgeons taking their first steps in hip resurfacing should visit experienced centers in an effort to try and prevent the complications inherent in an inappropriate learning curve.

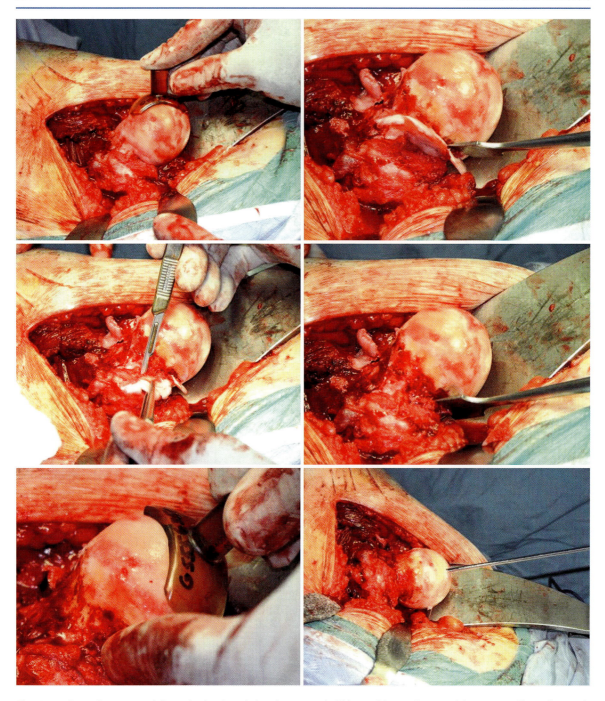

**Fig. 23.2** Osteophyte removal from the head–neck junction. *Above left*: estimated size of femoral head and anterolateral bump. *Above right*: partial removal of anterolateral bump, preserving soft tissue and avoiding encroachment on femoral neck. *Middle left*: bump removal is carefully completed; detachment of soft tissues. *Middle right*: removal of lateral bump avoiding damage to the femoral neck, which increases fracture risk. This maneuver is performed after releasing the anterolateral femoral neck. This provides a reference of the amount of bone that needs to be resected. *Below left*: final result, testing of head sphericity, and determination of femoral implant size. *Below left*: insertion of guide wire at the center of the femoral neck. This maneuver becomes easier once the osteophytes have been removed from the head–neck junction as these distort perception of real location of the neck

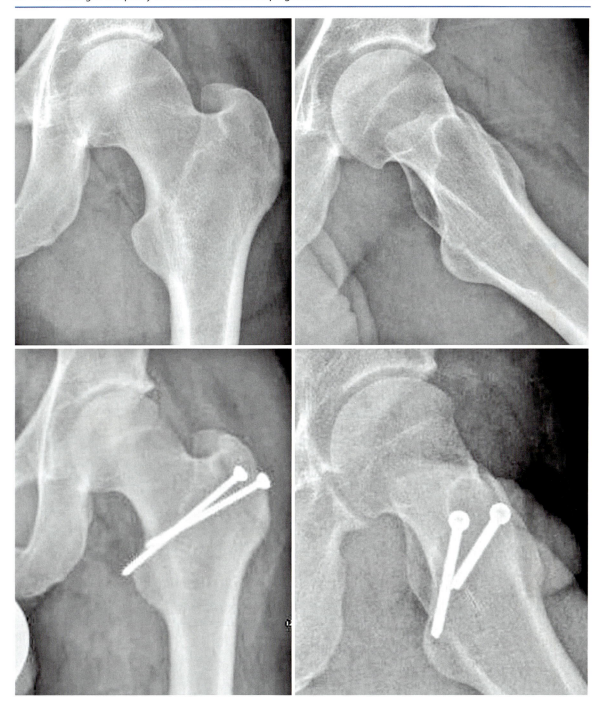

**Fig. 23.3** *Above*: AP and Dunn views showing anterolateral bump, subchondral sclerosis, and reduction of joint space. *Below*: Postoperative radiographs following controlled dislocation of the hip, performed together with resection of anterolateral bump. Quality of articular cartilage was good enough to preserve the joint. If needed, this approach allows implantation of a resurfacing prosthesis

# References

1. Ganz R et al (2003) Femoroacetabular impingement: a cause for osteoarthritis of the hip. Clin Orthop 417(417): 112–120
2. Grigoris P et al (2005) The evolution of hip resurfacing arthroplasty. Orthop Clin North Am 36(2):125–134
3. Beaule PE, Antoniades J (2005) Patient selection and surgical technique for surface arthroplasty of the hip. Orthop Clin North Am 36(2):177–185
4. Treuting RJ et al (1997) Prohibitive failure rate of the total articular replacement arthroplasty at five to ten years. Am J Orthop 26(2):114–118
5. Amstutz HC, Grigoris P, Dorey FJ (1998) Evolution and future of surface replacement of the hip. J Orthop Sci 3:169–186
6. Trousdale RT et al (1995) Periacetabular and intertrochanteric osteotomy for the treatment of osteoarthrosis in dysplastic hips. J Bone Joint Surg Am 77(1):73–85
7. Siebenrock KA et al (1999) Bernese periacetabular osteotomy. Clin Orthop 363:9–20
8. Beck M et al (2004) Anterior femoroacetabular impingement. Part II. Midterm results of surgical treatment. Clin Orthop 418:67–73
9. Amstutz HC et al (2004) Metal-on-metal hybrid surface arthroplasty: two to six year follow-up. J Bone Joint Surg 86A(1):28–39
10. Daniel J, Pynsent PB, McMinn DJW (2004) Metal-on-metal resurfacing of the hip in patients under the age of 55 years with osteoarthritis. J Bone Joint Surg 86B(2):177–184
11. Kishida Y et al (2004) Preservation of the bone mineral density of the femur after surface replacement of the hip. J Bone Joint Surg 86B(2):185–189
12. Mont MA et al (2006) Hip resurfacing arthroplasty. J Am Acad Orthop Surg 14(8):454–463
13. Ball ST, Le Duff MJ, Amstutz HC (2007) Early results of conversion of a failed femoral component in hip resurfacing arthroplasty. J Bone Joint Surg Am 89(4):735–741
14. Amstutz HC, Le Duff MJ, Campbell PA (2004) Fracture of the neck of the femur after surface arthroplasty of the hip. J Bone Joint Surg 86A(9):1874–1877
15. Brodner W et al (2003) Serum cobalt levels after metal-on-metal total hip arthroplasty. J Bone Joint Surg 85A(11): 2168–2173
16. Jacobs JJ et al (1996) Cobalt and chromium concentrations in patients with metal on metal total hip replacements. Clin Orthop Relat Res 329S:S256–S263
17. Back DL et al (2005) Early results of primary Birmingham hip resurfacings. An independent prospective study of the first 230 hips. J Bone Joint Surg Br 87(3):324–329
18. Treacy R, Pynsent P (2005) Birmingham hip resurfacing arthroplasty. A minimum follow-up of five years. J Bone Joint Surg 87B(2):167–170
19. Campbell P et al (2006) The John Charnley Award: a study of implant failure in metal-on-metal surface arthroplasties. Clin Orthop Relat Res 453:35–46
20. Little CP et al (2005) Osteonecrosis in retrieved femoral heads after failed resurfacing arthroplasty of the hip. J Bone Joint Surg 87B(3):320–323
21. Beaule PE et al (2006) Vascularity of the arthritic femoral head and hip resurfacing. J Bone Joint Surg Am 88(Suppl 4):85–96
22. Lindstrand A et al (2000) The introduction period of unicompartmental knee arthroplasty is critical: a clinical, clinical multicentered, and radiostereometric study of 251 Duracon unicompartmental knee arthroplasties. J Arthroplasty 15(5): 608–616
23. Jones LC, Hungerford DS (1987) Cement disease. Clin Orthop 225:192–206
24. Beaule PE, Amstutz HC, Sinha RJ (2002) Surface arthroplasty of the hip revisited: current indications and surgical technique. In: Hip replacement: current trends and controversies. Marcel Dekker, New York, pp 261–297
25. Beaule PE et al (2004) Risk factors affecting outcome of metal on metal surface arthroplasty of the hip. Clin Orthop 418(418):87–93
26. Beaule PE et al (2004) Metal-on-metal surface arthroplasty with a cemented femoral component: a 7–10 year follow-up study. J Arthroplasty 19(8 Suppl 3):17–22
27. Silva M et al (2004) The biomechanical results of total hip resurfacing arthroplasty. J Bone Joint Surg 86A(1):40–41
28. Beaule PE et al (2004) Orientation of femoral component in surface arthroplasty of the hip: a biomechanical and clinical analysis. J Bone Joint Surg 86A(9):2015–2021
29. Freeman MAR (1978) Some anatomical and mechanical considerations relevant to the surface replacement of the femoral head. Clin Orthop Relat Res 134:19–24
30. Amstutz HC, Markolf KL, Harris WH (1974) Design features in total hip replacement. In: Harris WH (ed) The hip society. CV Mosby, St. Louis, pp 111–124
31. Bartz RL et al (2000) The effect of femoral component head size on posterior dislocation of the artificial hip joint. J Bone Joint Surg 82(9):1300–1307
32. Beaule PE et al (2007) The femoral head/neck offset and hip resurfacing. J Bone Joint Surg Br 89(1):9–15
33. Kloen P, Leunig M, Ganz R (2002) Early lesions of the labrum and acetabular cartilage in osteonecrosis of the femoral head. J Bone Joint Surg 84B(1):66–69
34. Ito K et al (2001) Femoroacetabular impingement and the cam-effect. J Bone Joint Surg 83B(2):171–176
35. Beaule PE et al (2005) Three-dimensional computed tomography of the hip in the assessment of femoroacetabular impingement. J Orthop Res 23(6):1286–1292
36. Wiadrowski TP et al (1991) Peripheral wear of Wagner resurfacing hip arthroplasty acetabular components. J Arthroplasty 6(2):103–107
37. De Haan R et al (2008) Correlation between inclination of the acetabular component and metal ion levels in metal-on-metal hip resurfacing replacement. J Bone Joint Surg Br 90(10):1291–1297
38. Beaule PE, Poitras P (2007) Femoral component sizing and positioning in hip resurfacing arthroplasty. Instr Course Lect 56:163–169
39. Beaule PE (2004) A soft tissue sparing approach to surface arthroplasty of the hip. Oper Tech Orthop 14(4):16–18
40. Harty M (1982) Surface replacement arthroplasty of the hip. Anatomic considerations. Orthop Clin North Am 13(4): 667–679
41. Loughead JM et al (2006) Removal of acetabular bone in resurfacing arthroplasty of the hip: a comparison with hybrid total hip arthroplasty. J Bone Joint Surg Br 88(1):31–34
42. Mardones RM et al (2005) Surgical treatment of femoroacetabular impingement: evaluation of the effect of the size of the resection. J Bone Joint Surg Am 87(2):273–279

43. D'Lima DD et al (2000) The effect of the orientation of the acetabular and femoral components on the range of motion of the hip at different head-neck ratios. J Bone Joint Surg 82A(3):315–321
44. Scifert CF et al (1998) A finite element analysis of factors influencing total hip dislocation. Clin Orthop 355:152–162
45. Siguier T, Siguier M, Brumpt B (2004) Mini-incision anterior approach does not increase dislocation rate: a study of 1037 total hip replacements. Clin Orthop Relat Res 426:164–173
46. Tonnis D (1976) Normal values of the hip of the hip joint for the evaluation of x-rays in children and adults. Clin Orthop 119:39–47
47. Ganz R et al (2001) Surgical dislocation of the adult hip. A new technique with full access to the femoral head and acetabulum without the risk of avascular necrosis. J Bone Joint Surg 83B(8):1119–1124
48. Beaule PE et al (2009) The young adult with hip impingement: deciding on the optimal intervention. J Bone Joint Surg Am 91(1):210–221

# How to Do Resurfacing in Hip Dysplasia

Koen De Smet

Recently, a new generation of metal-on-metal total hip resurfacing arthroplasty devices has been introduced with the aim of preserving proximal femoral bone stock, minimizing the risk of postoperative dislocation of large femoral heads and reducing wear of the articulation for longer prosthetic survivorship. Resurfacing arthroplasty also has the advantage of ensuring a more biomechanical loading pattern of the proximal femur.

Osteoarthritis secondary to developmental dysplasia of the hip (DDH) is one of the main reasons for hip arthroplasty. Total hip replacement in patients with DDH presents the surgeon with a challenge. Taking into account that resurfacing is more technically demanding, resurfacing in dysplasia needs to be addressed carefully. Most patients in this demographic group are young and active, they require improved hip range of motion as well as pain relief, and they may even expect to recover the ability to run and jump after the arthroplasty. The outcomes of metal-on-metal hip resurfacing in dysplasia are encouraging, although some studies and surgeons report significantly poorer medium-term results in patients with dysplasia than in those with primary osteoarthritis [1–5]. This difference in outcome can be explained by the greater technical difficulty, the more pervasive anatomical abnormalities and the higher percentage of females encountered in dysplastic surgery. Smaller, narrower, markedly anteverted and often valgus femurs and deformed or eccentric acetabula are some of the anatomical challenges in dyspla-

sia. The degree of dysplasia will affect the difficulty of the surgery or may even rule out resurfacing as an option. Special dysplasia resurfacing cups can assist the surgeon in getting sufficient fixation in the pelvis.

In this chapter, we shall give some advice on 'how to do resurfacing in dysplasia'. The various potential problems in this indication group will be discussed in detail. Reasons for failure in dysplasia are femoral neck fractures, cup loosening, aseptic loosening of the femoral component and a higher wear rate of the metal-on-metal bearing couple because of the use of smaller components and the higher risk of cup inclination. The coverage angle of the resurfacing cup, which is design related [6], has an increased importance in dysplasia cases because of the potentially increased risk of high wear, as discussed below. Fortunately, it is still not clear whether serum or blood metal ion levels can be used as a surrogate measurement of prosthetic wear [7].

## Approach

Only the posterolateral approach is advised for treatment of severe dysplasia where leg lengthening is also needed. The exposure of the acetabulum and the possibility of lengthening the leg without interfering with the greater trochanter or destroying the abductor mechanism are far superior with this approach. The flexion contracture or inability to extend the hip that is often seen after reduction of the hip is related to the tightness of tendons and muscles resulting from leg lengthening. This condition tends to disappear in a couple of weeks without major exercise and without excessive physical therapy. In the posterior approach, the anteversion of the cup is used to prevent dislocation and impingement.

K. De Smet
Department of Orthopaedic Surgery,
AMC (ANCA Medical Center for Hip Surgery),
Ghent, Belgium
e-mail: dr.desmet@heup.be

Ó. Marín-Peña (ed.), *Femoroacetabular Impingement*,
DOI 10.1007/978-3-642-22769-1_24, © Springer-Verlag Berlin Heidelberg 2012

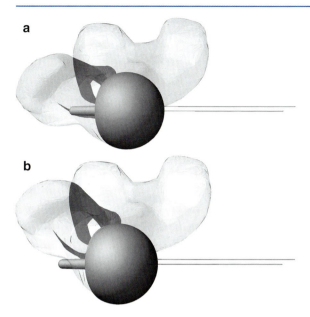

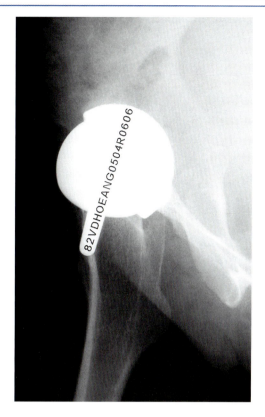

Drawing 24.1 (a) Resurfacing femoral head in neutral position to normal femoral anteversion (15°). (b) Resurfacing femoral head in neutral position to high femoral anteversion (35°). Protrusio of the stem

In dysplasia, it is sometimes better to place the cup in less anteversion so as to correlate it with the high anteversion of the femur. With the anterolateral approach, this can be done with less risk of posterior dislocation. However, this small advantage does not beat the specific advantages offered by the posterolateral approach.

## Anteversion

The femoral component of a hip resurfacing implant is normally placed in a neutral position relative to the femoral neck. In normal osteoarthritis, there is no problem to correct the normal anteversion in the femoral neck to a neutral angle on the head. With this position, the natural anteversion angle of the femoral neck is not changed; the implant is placed in a neutral position on an anteverted neck (Drawing 24.1a). Maximum correction of anteversion possible is 20–25°. The greater the correction of anteversion, the higher the risk of protrusion of the stem from the anterior aspect of the femoral neck and the higher the risk that the femoral neck may get notched by reaming and subsequent impingement (Drawing 24.1b). In some resurfacing designs, the stem is smaller and thinner, resulting in a lower risk of protrusion. Stem protrusion from the

Fig. 24.1 Protrusio with BHR through the femoral neck

bone does not necessarily indicate a higher risk of failure. In designs with a large stem, stress shielding, a higher risk of neck narrowing and fracture may be of concern. In my practice, I have not yet observed any problems with protrusion of the stem (Fig. 24.1).

If the femoral neck anteversion is higher than 35–40°, i.e. beyond correction, either a higher anteversion position of the head implant should be accepted in relation to cup anteversion or a different technique should be chosen. If the anteversion cannot be accepted in relation to the cup, and resurfacing is still preferred, a derotation osteotomy should be performed. In these cases, the femoral prosthesis is implanted first in line or parallel with the existing anteversion of the neck, and then, the osteotomy is performed. Because the hip will not be reduced before 8 min and there should be no insertion of a cannula in the lesser trochanter to avoid weakening of the bone, setting of the cement and subsequent heat production in the bone will occur; therefore, the prosthesis should be washed continuously with cool water to prevent thermal damage [8]. In a second stage, the femoral osteotomy is performed distally from the lesser trochanter at a level where an 8-hole AO plate can be

**Fig. 24.2** (**a**) Preop x-ray left hip female 30 years of age. High hip dislocation Crowe 4. (**b**) AP x-ray at 2 years. BHR dysplasia resurfacing with subtrochanteric shortening osteotomy with 8-hole plate and screws. Restored centre of rotation. (**c**) Lateral x-ray at 2 years, rotation of the leg shows subluxation of the prosthesis. No derotation was done in this case

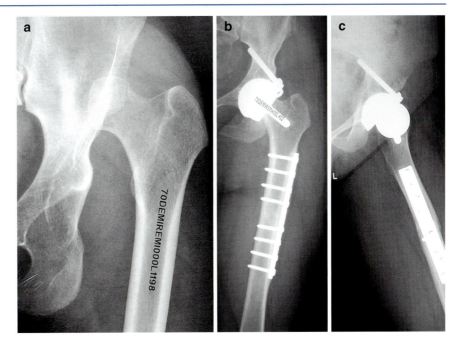

**Fig. 24.3** (**a**) AP view of a right hip looks like a lateral femur. (**b**) Lateral view of a right hip looks like AP femur

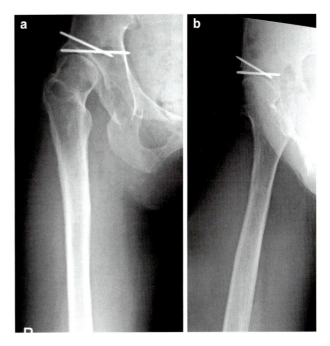

applied. Four screws above the osteotomy and four screws below the osteotomy are essential for solid fixation. With this technique, 6 weeks plantar touch and 6 weeks partial weight-bearing are prescribed for the patients' rehabilitation. In Crowe IV dysplasia with severe dislocation and excessive leg lengthening, derotation can be combined with a shortening osteotomy (Fig. 24.2).

The anteversion angle of the femur can best be measured on a CT-scan [9]. If on a radiographic profile view femoral anteversion appears to be very large (>45°), a derotation osteotomy is obligatory (Fig. 24.3).

If the anteversion is not sufficiently corrected and there is also a corresponding high anteversion angle of the femur, the risk of subluxation with high wear or dislocation will increase (see Fig. 24.2c).

Fig. 24.4 (a) Preop x-ray right hip, female 18 years of age. Deformed femur because of several surgeries for dysplasia with also a femoral osteotomy. (b, c) AP and lateral x-ray of BHR at 2 years

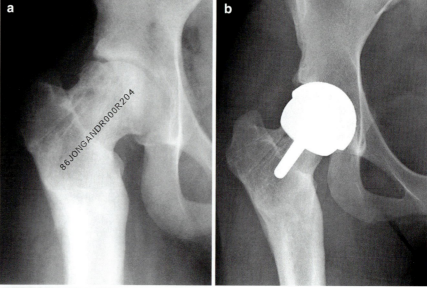

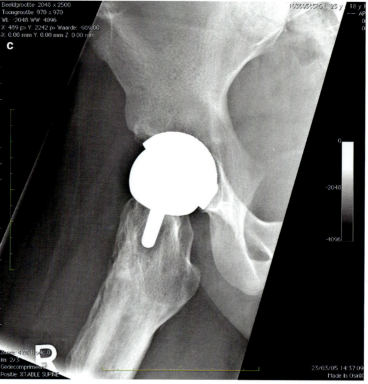

## Valgus

The high valgus seen on x-rays is often overestimated because of the combined anteversion or rotation of the femur. If the anteversion is corrected with the rotation of the leg on the x-ray, a lower value will be obtained for the angle. If the anteversion of the femur is not changed with an osteotomy, the objective is again to place the prosthesis in as normal an anatomic position as possible without increasing

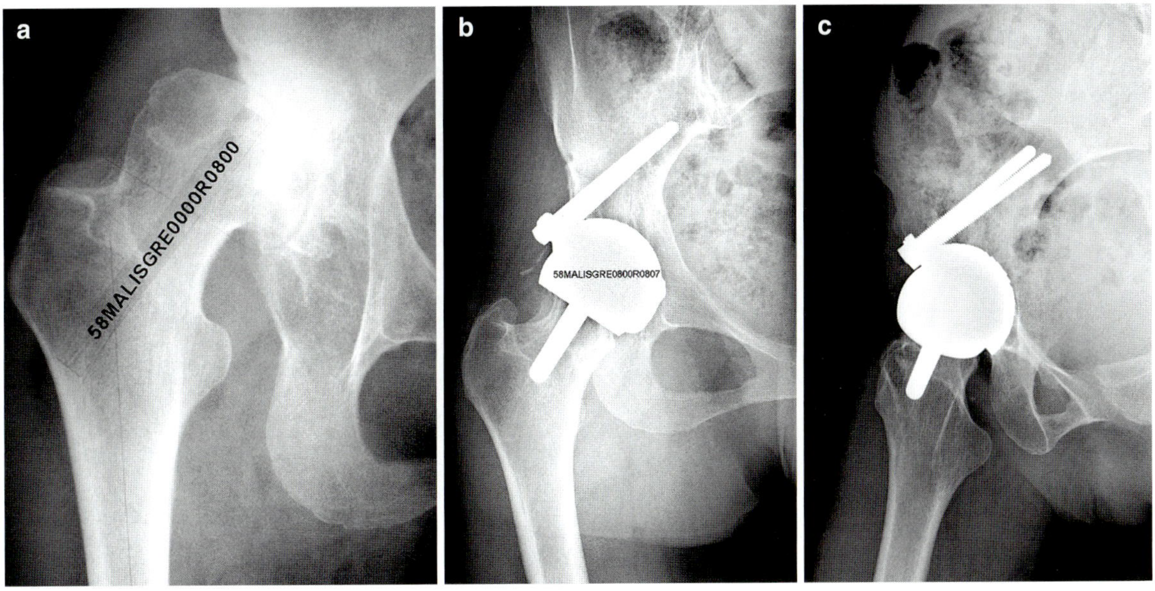

**Fig. 24.5** (**a**) Female 42 years, right hip dysplasia. (**b, c**) AP and lateral view of BHR dysplasia at 7 years

the risk of notching or shifting the prosthesis into excessive varus. The normal anatomic position entails a varus/valgus angle of around 140° and neutral femoral anteversion. A slightly higher valgus angle up to 145° and anteversion up to 15° are acceptable.

## Proximal Femoral Deformity

Some dysplastic patients have had a previous femoral osteotomy with destruction or deformation of the proximal femur and the endosteal canal. This makes placement of a total hip prosthesis difficult. These cases could be considered specific indications for resurfacing, which allow circumvention of the difficulties posed by a narrow and often curved proximal femoral canal (Fig. 24.4).

## Femoral Bone Deficiency or Cysts

Because of the dysplasia, differences in load transfer may result in large cysts or osteopenic areas in the femoral head (Fig. 24.5). Care to avoid thermal necrosis and overpenetration of the bone should decrease the risk of failure.

## Acetabular Deficiency and Angle

The kind of acetabular deficiency depends on the grade of dysplasia. Crowe classified dysplastic hips into four classes using the acetabular angle and the amount of proximal migration as the significant features [10]. In dysplasia, the acetabular angle ranges from 41° to 63°, with an average of 52°. The higher the abduction angle, the higher the risk of steep cup positioning leading to edge loading and early wear of the prosthesis. Implanting the cup at the ideal 40° abduction angle implies that the superolateral edge of the cup will not be covered by bone. Cup implantation with full bony coverage in that area entails malpositioning and hence early failure and an increased risk of dislocation. This lack of coverage at the superolateral area can be accepted because it does not cause any clinical symptoms. If the cup is not covered anteriorly, it can cause groin pain, often mistakenly called iliopsoitis. If the cup is positioned at an excessively low abduction angle or too flat, it can impinge laterally on the femoral neck. Bone coverage deficiency decreases the press fit fixation area of the implant. It is precisely the size of this area that determines if a normal cup can be used, if the extent of dysplasia is compatible with resurfacing, or if a special dysplasia cup with additional screw fixation is needed. Press fit can be increased

**Fig. 24.6** (**a**) Female patient, Down's syndrome, 19 years, left hip dysplasia. Triple osteotomy with overcorrection 35° of retroversion. (**b**) AP x-ray, BHR dysplasia with two screws at 2 years

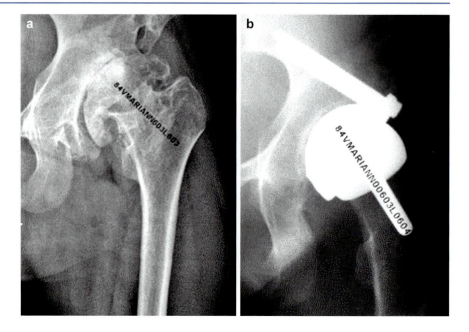

or obtained by reaming the floor of the acetabulum to make it deeper so that the cup can be seated deeper. If the pelvic bone stock is poor, performance of hip resurfacing rather than a total hip procedure, where a smaller cup with screws can be used, should be seen as a relative contra-indication. Resurfacing should always be a bone preserving procedure. If this is not achieved, the most important advantage of resurfacing is lost.

When using a resurfacing device in dysplastic patients, conversion to either a total hip prosthesis or a dysplasia resurfacing implant should be possible. Dysplasia cups are always one size bigger than a normal cup, increasing bone removal from the acetabular rim and increasing the risk of leaving an uncovered area anteriorly. These cups also have a flange or a similar construct at the edge that increases the risk of impingement with the femoral neck. Differences between the cups are discussed in the dysplasia cup design section. Dysplasia cups can prevent overly steep cup placement, or an excessively deep placement for adequate press fit, but they are associated with a higher risk of peripheral bone removal, leaving larger uncovered regions and causing impingement.

## Acetabular Deformity

In this section, we wish to focus on anatomical deformities, not on the shallowness, high abduction or deficiency of the acetabulum discussed in the previous paragraph. Rotation or anteversion of the acetabulum in a previously unoperated pelvis is more open, with a deficient anterior wall. To prevent uncovered regions and groin pain, two techniques can be used. The cup can be placed deeper with more bone removal; the capsule and even the labrum can be maintained to avoid conflict with the anterior muscles or tendons. Placement in excessive anteversion should be avoided because of the increased risk of higher wear of the metal-on-metal bearing and of dislocation, particularly because it is always be combined with high femoral anteversion. A CT scan can be used to assess the bone stock antero-posteriorly, which is the most important parameter in the deformed acetabulum. The inferosuperior range is less important in the decision-making process for the use of resurfacing: it is the antero-posterior width of the acetabulum that determined whether the surgeon can restore the hip centre.

Patients who have undergone previous surgery on the acetabulum can be a challenge. When reorientation of the acetabulum matches the normal anatomy, the acetabular procedure should be easier than the previous one. A particular problem arises when the pelvis (triple pelvic osteotomy) or the acetabulum (Ganz-periacetabular osteotomy) has been tilted too anteriorly, resulting in a neutral or even a retroverted acetabulum. If this is the case, then the cup will stick out posteriorly, which can lead to pain when sitting on hard surfaces. Loss of press fit is another problem. Deepening out the medial floor or enhanced fixation with a dysplasia cup can solve this problem (Fig. 24.6). Removal of all excess anterior bone is necessary to prevent impingement and restore good mobility, especially flexion. Sometimes bone must be removed from the antero-inferior iliac spine, interfering with the attachment of rectus and quadriceps. The same time-consuming bone removal procedure is needed in cases where a shelf osteotomy is performed and the anterior roof prevents normal hip flexion. In these cases, anterior impingement should be checked at the end of the procedure placing a finger on the femoral neck, and testing for posterior subluxation. If there is any concern, the hip should be dislocated again and more bone should be removed.

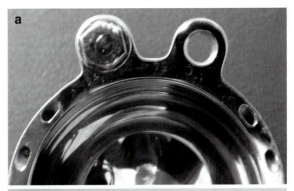
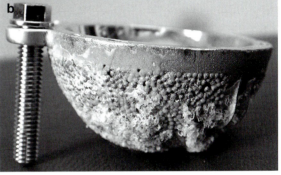

**Fig. 24.7** Mickey Mouse ears/screw holes and screw in BHR dysplasia. (**a**) Front view and (**b**) side view

## Impingement with Greater Trochanter

At the end of the resurfacing procedure and following reduction of the hip, the surgeon must evaluate for the presence of impingement anteriorly at 90° flexion and internal rotation. In addition, it is also important to assess dysplastic patients with the leg in extension and external rotation. The higher anteversion of the femoral neck and the medialisation of the cup to obtain press fit and bone coverage can result in the greater trochanter abutting on the ischial bone posteriorly. Because a higher offset cannot be obtained by lengthening the femoral head as is done with a total hip prosthesis, the only solution to this abutment is to reduce the bulk of the ischial bone or the greater trochanter at the point where the contact occurs. As the bone is removed, impingement should be tested until an acceptable situation is obtained. Impingement will lead to discomfort in certain movements, subluxation and eventual wear of the prosthesis. Dislocation can occur early or late, often because of wear, swelling from excessive fluid production and destruction of surrounding soft tissues.

## Dysplasia Cup Designs

Only four of the designs currently available include a dysplasia cup. The Birmingham Hip Resurfacing System (Smith & Nephew, Warsaw, US), the Adept Resurfacing System (Finsbury, Essex, UK), the Cormet 2000 System (Corin, Cirencester, UK) and the Conserve Plus System (Wright Medical, Memphis, US). The Adept and Conserve Plus designs take into consideration that the screws should be angled to engage the bone. The Adept, BHR and Corin design

can only be used in dysplasia, while the Conserve Plus design, because of the offset of the flange with the screws from the rim of the cup, can also be used in non-dysplasia cases needing enhanced fixation. The BHR dysplasia cup has two so-called Mickey Mouse ears (screw holes) that are threaded and on the same plane as the cup; both "ears" are on the same plane, with no angle to the neutral plane for anteversion (Fig. *24.7*).

The Conserve Plus dysplasia cup design (QUADRAFIX) has a flange with three holes (one cup for both sides) where there is a narrow flange (Fig. *24.8*). The screws are angled 20° towards the acetabular bone in abduction, and 20° of retroversion to neutralize the anteversion of the cup. The second screw is neutral to the anteversion angle of the cup. These improved screw angles direct the screws into the bone with a well-positioned cup. In the BHR dysplasia cup, the screws often fail to engage the bone. With the two screws of BHR design, there is a risk of placing the socket too steep and/or failing to place it in anteversion, which leads to wear and impingement with the edge loading wear mechanism described above.

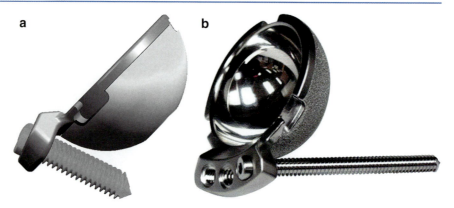

**Fig. 24.8** Quadrafix
Conserve Plus cup.
(**a**) drawing detail of the screws
obliquity. (**b**) real implant

## Grafting

The superolateral edge of the uncovered cup can be grafted with autografts obtained by reaming the pelvis or the femoral head. Radiographic follow-up of these cases shows very good healing of these grafts [4].

## Conclusion

The anatomic abnormalities associated with the dysplasia of the hip make total hip arthroplasty a very complex and challenging procedure. The new generation of metal-on-metal hip resurfacing arthroplasty provides good stability and low risk of dislocation in young active patients. There are, however, very few studies currently available that examine the use of a metal-on-metal hybrid resurfacing system for the treatment of severe osteoarthritis secondary to developmental dysplasia of the hip.

Knecht et al. [1] reported on a small series of 54 patients managed with resurfacing who had good functional results at 1–4 years' follow-up. Nishii et al. [2] in their series show that although 70% of the patients had developmental dysplasia of the hip, the survival rate, with the time to failure for any reason used as endpoint, was 96% at 5 years.

Amstutz et al. described a series of patients with hip dysplasia – Crowe I (88%), Crowe II (12%) – treated with Conserve plus hip resurfacing using a normal resurfacing cup design [11]. Seven of the 59 hips needed reoperation at a mean follow-up of 6 years; the conclusion was that the fixation of the porous-coated acetabular components without additional fixation was excellent despite incomplete lateral acetabular coverage of the socket. Rigorous patient selection and meticulous bone

preparation are essential to minimize femoral neck fractures and loosening after this procedure.

McMinn et al. [4] in 2008 published the results of 110 consecutive dysplasia resurfacing arthroplasties in 103 patients (55 men and 48 women) performed between 1997 and 2000, with a minimum follow-up of 6 years. The dysplasia cup permitted early weight-bearing and allowed incorporation of morcellised autograft without the need for structural bone grafting.

McBryde et al. [5] performed metal-on-metal hip resurfacing for developmental dysplasia in 96 hips, of which 17 (18%) were classified as Crowe grade III or IV. There were 5 (5.2%) revisions in the dysplasia group and none in the osteoarthritic patients.

## Summary

In my personal experience, a posterolateral approach is advised for treatment of severe dysplasia where leg lengthening is also needed. Correction of anteversion in the femur should be matched to the acetabular position. If needed, a derotation osteotomy should be performed.

The cup position is challenging, and a correct position is needed to prevent accelerated wear of the metal bearing. Positioning of the resurfacing prosthesis and correct bone removal to prevent impingement can lead to good clinical results even with this indication. The use of a dysplasia cup can help when press fit is lost or when deeper placement of the cup would not be conservative to the bone stock.

In summary, resurfacing should only be done by a surgeon with experience of hip arthroplasty. Resurfacing in dysplastic patients should only be done by a surgeon experienced in hip resurfacing.

# References

1. Knecht A, Witzleb WC, Beichler T, Günther KP (2004) Functional results after surface replacement of the hip: comparison between dysplasia and idiopathic osteoarthritis. Z Orthop Ihre Grenzgeb 142(3):279–285
2. Nishii T, Sugano N, Miki H, Takao M, Koyama T, Yoshikawa H (2007) Five-year results of metal-on-metal resurfacing arthroplasty in Asian patients. J Arthroplasty 22(2):176–183
3. Amstutz HC, Antoniades JT, Le Duff MJ (2007) Results of metal-on-metal hybrid hip resurfacing for Crowe type-I and II developmental dysplasia. J Bone Joint Surg Am 89(2): 339–346
4. McMinn DJ, Daniel J, Ziaee H, Pradhan C (2008) Results of the Birmingham hip resurfacing dysplasia component in severe acetabular insufficiency: a six- to 9.6-year follow-up. J Bone Joint Surg Br 90(6):715–723
5. McBryde CW, Shears E, O'Hara JN, Pynsent PB (2008) Metal-on-metal hip resurfacing in developmental dysplasia: a case-control study. J Bone Joint Surg Br 90(6):708–714
6. De Haan R, Pattyn C, Gill HS et al (2008) Correlation between inclination of the acetabular component and metal ion levels in metal-on-metal hip resurfacing replacement. J Bone Joint Surg Br 90(10):1291–1297
7. De Smet K, De Haan R, Calistri A et al (2008) Metal ion measurements as a diagnostic tool to identify problems with metal-on-metal hip resurfacing. J Bone Joint Surg Am 90(Suppl 4):202–208
8. Gill HS, Campbell PA, Murray D et al (2007) Reduction of the potential for thermal damage during hip resurfacing. J Bone Joint Surg Br 89(1):16–20
9. Amstutz HC, Le Duff MJ, Su EP (2008) Childhood disorders. In: Amstutz HC (ed) Hip resurfacing: principles, indications, technique and results. Saunders Elsevier, Los Angeles, pp 181–202
10. Crowe J, Mani V, Ranawat C (1979) Total hip replacement in congenital dislocation and dysplasia of the hip. J Bone Joint Surg Am 61-A:15–23
11. Amstutz HC, Le Duff MJ, Harvey N, Hoberg M (2008) Improved survivorship of hybrid metal-on-metal hip resurfacing with second-generation techniques for Crowe-I and II developmental dysplasia of the hip. J Bone Joint Surg Am 90(Suppl 3):12–20

# Part VI

# Postoperative Management (POM)

# Rehabilitation Following Femoroacetabular Impingement Surgery

# 25

Lafayette de Azevedo Lage

## Introduction and General Considerations

The purpose of hip rehabilitation is to restore the level of function the patient had prior to the occurrence of the lesion and/or the onset of the symptoms. Rehabilitation of the hip after the surgery for femoroacetabular impingement (FAI) by arthroscopy, minimally invasive surgery [1], or safe surgical dislocation of the femoral head [2–4] is very important. Treatment of FAI was introduced in 1936 by Smith-Petersen [5] who addressed the condition by means of femoral and acetabular osteoplasty. However, his results were not successful since his subjects were already afflicted with advanced arthritis. The physical therapist must remember this and refrain from insisting on administering physical therapy to patients who do not evolve adequately. Practitioners should forge a close relationship with orthopedic surgeons since only the latter can provide information on the degree of improvement that can be expected and verify the progress achieved. Imaging techniques, even MRI, may provide false negatives [6, 7], with the surgeon's notes being critical for the estimation of how much patients may improve and of whether they will be totally or partially symptom-free. There are few data and few research studies to support any specific kind of rehabilitation. It is a fact that rehabilitation following arthroscopic surgery by an experienced surgeon tends to be faster, but the final result is usually the same as that of minimally invasive surgery. A study by Sadrih et al. [8] is the only one where good results were obtained with both techniques. This work suggests that arthroscopy drastically minimizes the risks of open surgery. Lage reports that arthroscopy has the advantage of repairing small lesions that are hard to fix by open surgery as it provides an enlarged image and undersize instruments specially designed to fix minimal lesions [9, 10]. The physical therapist must know what specific surgical procedures the patient was subjected to as this information will help in the design of an individualized rehabilitation program. This information must be collated prior to designing the rehabilitation program. The surgeon must provide as many details as possible of what he found and what he did during the surgery so as to prevent deterioration of the patient's clinical status or even destruction of the surgery by the rehabilitation protocol. The concomitant surgical procedures in the treatment of femoroacetabular impingement by any of the three methods mentioned (open, minimally invasive, or arthroscopic) may be several, namely:

- Partial or total resection of the labrum
- Reinsertion of the labrum with anchors
- Reconstruction of the labrum with a segment of autologous graft
- Acetabular chondroplasty with radiofrequency probe
- Acetabular chondroplasty with microfractures. In such cases the non-weight-bearing period should extend for 6–8 weeks
- Chondroplasty of the femoral head in a weight-bearing area or not
- Partial resurfacing arthroplasty of the femoral head

L. de Azevedo Lage
Department of Orthopedic Surgery,
Clínica Lage, São Paulo, Brazil
e-mail: lafayette@clinicalage.com.br

Ó. Marín-Peña (ed.), *Femoroacetabular Impingement*,
DOI 10.1007/978-3-642-22769-1_25, © Springer-Verlag Berlin Heidelberg 2012

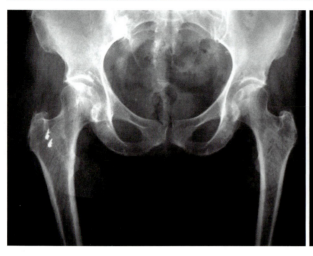
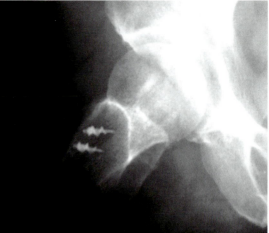

**Fig. 25.1** Muscular reattachment with bone anchors

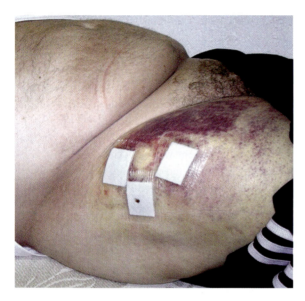

**Fig. 25.2** Postoperative hematoma after hip arthroscopy

- Capsule suturing and extension of capsulotomy that should force to use temporary brace
- Shrinking the capsule shrinkage by radiofrequency at the end of surgery by radiofrequency makes it too tight. This procedure, common in hip arthroscopy, is not performed in the Ganz or Ribas procedure, where the capsule is tightened at the end of the procedure
- Partial or total debridement of the ligamentum teres
- Reconstruction of the ligamentum teres
- Osteoplasty of femoral head for removal of the cam deformity

- Osteoplasty of acetabular edge in pincer-type impingement with removal of the calcified or degenerated labrum or reinsertion of the labrum with anchors
- Removal of the cam- and pincer-type deformities
- Removal of adhesions surgery
- Removal of loose bodies
- Muscular reattachment with anchors (Fig. 25.1)
- Presence of important swelling or hematoma (Fig. 25.2)

The physical therapist should ask if the patient is satisfied, and how he/she feels. Unreasonable expectations regarding the surgery may harm the perception of the result obtained, especially considering that not all patients manage to rid themselves of all their symptoms. It is important to ask patients about their symptoms before the surgery since the effects of hip pathology and femoroacetabular impingement may vary from patient to patient (Fig. 25.3). FAI patients find it hard to pinpoint the origin of their pain. At first, pain may be diffuse (just lumbar discomfort when seated for long periods, for example). Hip surgeons see many patients who have already been subjected to other surgical treatments such as spine surgery, laparoscopy, urinary tract surgery, and even surgery for hemorrhoids.

The visual analog pain scale and patient satisfaction are also important aspects to be considered when assessing progress along the rehab program. Carlioz [11] was probably the first to perform an osteoplasty of the femoral neck deformity by resecting the "bump" that characterizes cam-type impingement in 1968.

**Fig. 25.3** Pain location drew by the patient: localized pain (*red*), location of pain (*orange*), irradiated pain (*yellow*), pain irradiates when exerting pressure(*green*), sporadic pain (*purple*),and constant pain (*stripe purple*)

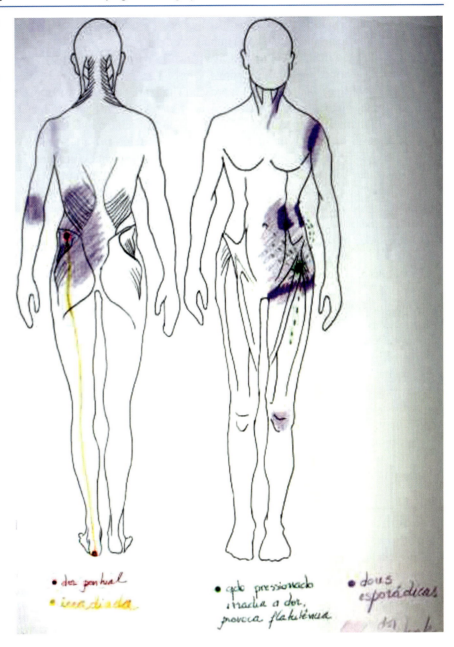

Ganz reported that a 90° flexion maneuver associated to internal rotation was painful in hips with FAI. The physical therapist should avoid performing that maneuver in the immediate post-op period.

The physical therapist should pay attention to the fact that not all the surgeries for femoroacetabular impingement are successful. Hayworth et al. [12] retrospectively reviewed 24 cases of arthroscopic hip revision in 23 patients (14 women and 9 men) of a mean age of 33.6 years (1 case was bilateral). Only in

13 out of the 24 cases (54%) did patients show significant pain improvement some time after the first arthroscopy. Philippon [13] reports that 34 of 37 patients subjected to an arthroscopic hip revision performed in other hospitals showed no improvement in terms of pain. Although his study does not refer only to femoroacetabular impingement, it clearly proves that hip arthroscopy is still a developing technique. In other words, it may or may not be effective, depending on the surgeon's skills. The authors of this study on revision

hip arthroscopy concluded that patients usually need revision hip arthroscopy due to persistent impingement symptoms. May and Beaulé [14] revised five patients that had been submitted to hip arthroscopy for resection of labral lesions using Ganz's approach with osteotomy of the greater trochanter. Pain persisted. In all of the cases, during the procedure, a cam-type lesion was found, which was removed using the spherometer to accurately verify the sphericity of the femoral head. All patients obtained some degree of pain relief, but in three of them, despite an improvement in function, pain persisted and anti-inflammatory drugs were occasionally required.

Rehabilitation protocols should follow some basic principles:

- Limitation of certain movements that could interfere with soft tissue healing
- Control of swelling and pain to prevent muscular atrophy and movement limitation
- Immediate start of ROM exercises
- Progressive increase of weight bearing (this increase is specific to each kind of surgery)
- Start neuromuscular control and muscular activity exercises soon
- Progressive strengthening of the lower limbs and restoration of proprioception to the operated limb
- Cardiovascular rehabilitation and conditioning
- Customized training for a fast return to sport practice

## Preoperative Rehabilitation

Griffin et al. [15] underlined the importance of preoperative rehabilitation in patients due to be subjected to hip arthroscopy. This treatment should start right after the appointment with the surgeon. Its goals are:

- Improvement of range of motion (this should be done gradually so as not to worsen the patient's clinical status and avoiding forceful movements, i.e., flexion associated to internal rotation and adduction).
- Strengthening of musculature.
- Improvement of resistance.

Preoperative physical therapy also allows the physical therapist to explain to the patient the multiple aspects of the postoperative rehabilitation process. The patient is informed about weight-bearing restrictions as well as the duration and the frequency of the therapy.

## Postoperative Rehabilitation

### Hip Arthroscopy

We based our work on the studies performed by Stalzer et al. [16] and Philippon et al. [17, 18] who drew up specific protocols for each arthroscopic procedure. Before providing details on specific rehabilitation exercises, some considerations should be made for a better understanding of the rehabilitation process as such.

*Osteoplasty with or without resection of the acetabular rim*: In these cases, passive movements should start as soon as possible after surgery and be performed 2–3 times a day to prevent adhesions. The removal of the femoral bump and/or the acetabular rim causes bleeding and swelling due to an accumulation of blood; this facilitates adhesion of the capsule to the acetabular rim. Passive movements should be taken to the limits of pain resistance. Passive rotation movements should reach at least 70° to avoid adhesion of the circular fibers of in the zona orbicularis of the femoral neck. Partial weight bearing (20% of body weight) should start with the feet flat on the ground and be maintained for 2 weeks in order to minimize the risk of fracture of the femoral neck and the risk of inflammation. Heel strike should be avoided to prevent excessive use of hip flexors and creation of shear forces.

*Chondroplasty*: After chondroplasty, the patient may gradually bear weight as tolerated. During this period, the patient may just ambulate with the feet flat on the ground (flat foot weight bearing). Continuous passive motion (CPM) exercises should be done 4 h a day for 2 weeks. Following CPM, the patient should lie face down 2 h a day to stretch out the hip flexors to avoid flexor contraction. Passive motion on all planes must be achieved within 6–8 weeks.

*Microfracture*: After microfracture, the patient should ambulate with the feet flat on the ground (flat foot weight bearing) for 8 weeks. CPM exercises should be done from 6 to 8 h a day for 6–8 weeks. Following CPM, the patient should lie face down 2 h a day to stretch out the hip flexors to avoid flexor contraction. Passive motion on all planes must be achieved within 6–8 weeks.

*Labral debridement or reattachment*: There are no specific limitations in terms of range of motion since no muscles attach directly to the labrum. However, active movements should be avoided due to the large volume of soft tissue structures (capsule and muscles) around the hip joint. Passive movements are recommended to prevent

**Fig. 25.4**  Quadruped rocking

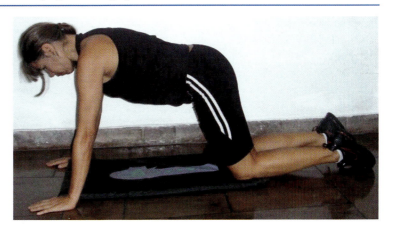

adhesions between the capsule and the labrum; there is limitation to flexion. Abduction above 45° is only permitted after 10–21 days. There are no weight-bearing restrictions. Forcible stretching is forbidden in patients with FAI due to the forces acting in the labrum. Appropriate maintenance of force and muscular balance inside and around the hip is essential to protect the joint from injury. Early treatment of the femoroacetabular impingement may prevent or limit the extent of the labral lesion.

*Capsule shrinkage with radio frequency or capsule suturing (capsulorrhaphy)*: External rotation and stretching should be limited during the first 14–21 days. Contraction of the hip flexors is common, and the neutral stretching is recommended until the end of the first week. There are no weight bearing restrictions. Appropriate maintenance of force and muscular balance around the hip is essential to reduce the excessive capsule tension, especially when the labrum is injured.

The rehabilitation protocol is divided into four phases. The first and second phases are obligatory for all patients, while the third and fourth phases are for athletes or patients wishing to return to sporting activities.

## Phase I: Mobility and Protection

The goals of phase 1 are: tissue healing, recovery of (albeit restricted) range of motion, reduce pain and inflammation, and enhance muscular control. This phase lasts from 6 to 8 weeks, with soft tissue healing occurring during this period. Immobilization, which is largely responsible for forming tissues adhesions, should be avoided. Passive movements should be indicated, preferably CPM, taking into account the weight-bearing and ROM restrictions discussed above. Lying face down 2 h a day stretches the flexors and prevents flexion contractures. Weight bearing is permitted with the foot flat on the ground up to a maximum of 10 k for 2–8 weeks depending on the procedure performed (microfracture needs 8 weeks of just 10 kg weight bearing). Passive movements with total flexion and abduction up to 45° must be performed from the 7th to the 14th or 21st day. External rotation of the lower limbs should be avoided in all cases, regardless of the procedure carried out (capsulorrhaphy, RF capsule shrinkage, or open procedure). Anti-rotating boots should be worn during the first 2 or 3 postoperative weeks. During the passive movement period, the patient must be asked if he/she can feel anything pushing or biting; should that be the case, ROM must not be forced. Philippon et al. use a brace to block motion from 0° to 105° in the first 14–21 days with the option of increasing abduction in cases where greater joint congruity is desired. Walking in the swimming pool with water chest high may be initiated in the first postoperative day (waterproof bandages are placed at the arthroscopic portals). By walking in the swimming pool during the first few days after surgery, the patient can practice symmetrical ambulation in a virtually weightless environment.

Initial muscle strengthening exercises should focus on the gluteus medius muscle, the flexors, extensors, rotators and gluteus minimus, and maximus, taking care not to stress to the labrum. Isometric exercises for the gluteus, quadriceps, hamstrings, and transverse abdominals should start immediately after the procedure. Other exercises such as quadruped rocking, active internal rotation, and isometric hip exercises should be started on the second week. Side-lying clam exercises, double-leg bridging, lateral three-way leg raises, and short-lever hip flexion start on third week (Figs. 25.4–25.7).

**Fig. 25.5** Side-lying clams

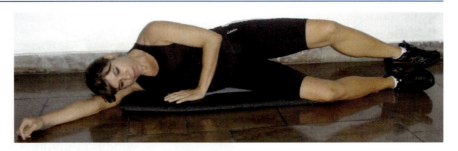

**Fig. 25.6** Double-leg bridging

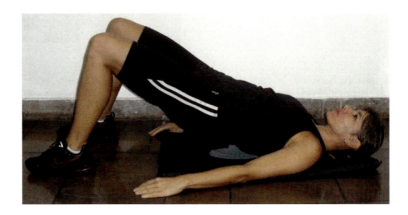

**Fig. 25.7** Short-lever hip flexion

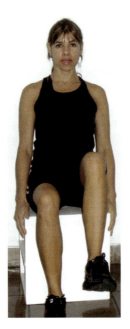

caveat that in microfracture cases, the use of crutches is obligatory for 8 weeks). In week 5, it is possible to start rotation exercises on a rotary disk, advanced bridging, lateral bridging, rotation on a lower limb, sidewalking against resistance, and crouching on one knee. Single-leg windmills and rapid sidewalking movements are added in week 6 (Figs. 25.8–25.10).

Cardiovascular conditioning is developed through stationary bicycle cycling against resistance starting from the week 3 (in cases of microfracture, these exercises should only begin in week 7 to avoid stress to the newly formed cartilage). The elliptic bicycle and the stepper are added in week 5 (in cases of microfracture, these exercises should begin only in week 13 to avoid stress to the newly formed cartilage).

## Phase II: Stabilization and Ambulation

Phase 2 stabilization exercises may start during the second week simultaneously with the phase 1 exercises and be maintained thereafter with due caution. Phase 2 exercises are introduced in three stages. The first stage comprises the neuromuscular control exercises, which are introduced while patients are still on their phase 1 exercises, so the weight bearing and ROM restrictions are the same as those for phase 1. The second

Straight-leg raises, double one-third knee bends, and double-leg cord rotation start on the fourth week. More vigorous strengthening and proprioception exercises should increase progressively until crutches are abandoned and full weight bearing is started (with the

**Fig. 25.8** Advanced bridging

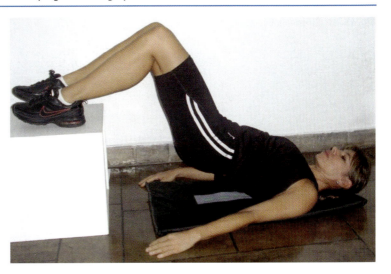

**Fig. 25.9** Sidewalking against resistance

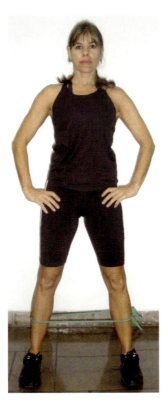

collective sports, skating, and dancing movements may be started. Conventional underwater treadmills should not be used by the patient at this point as these devices give rise to shear forces in the anterior hip (the automatic movement of the treadmill stresses the anterior hip joint area which interferes with rehabilitation). The surgical precautions discussed previously are unnecessary in this phase, but emphasis must be laid on achieving a normal gait pattern, good stability, and muscular control. Development of the functional aspects related to the patient's sport is important at this stage. Golf players may start with swing practice (proper stance, long distance drives). In order to move forward to phase 3, patients must have attained the goals of phase 1 – correction of muscular imbalances and gait abnormalities, and ability to perform certain simple functional activities. Patients must be pain-free, have full range of motion, and ambulate normally.

**Phase III: Strengthening**

This phase should only be started when the patient has achieved excellent stability and control of functional movements. Tests for the functional movements include ambulation, single-leg bridging, planks in all positions, and single-knee bends. These movements should be made without compensation of any kind (Figs. 25.11 and 25.12).

The goals of phase 3 are developing patients functional activity until the muscular force on the operative side is the same as that on the non-operated side. Before advancing to phase 4, the patient must pass the sport test. Patients that do not intend to return to a

stage of phase 2 is ambulation. Patients without microfracture may abandon their crutches after 2 weeks, while those with microfracture should use them for 8 weeks. Stabilization exercises in this phase should be performed by patients without signs of irritation of adductors, piriformis, or hip flexors. The third stage of phase 2 includes individualized exercises related to the specific sport the patient wishes to go back to. Running,

**Fig. 25.10** Single-leg windmills

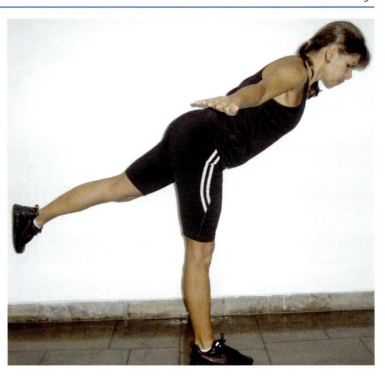

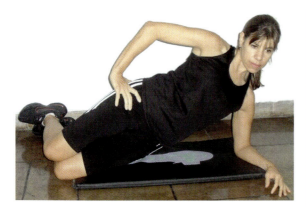

**Fig. 25.11** Side supports

high-level sport do not need to take the sport test and should return to their usual activities as tolerated.

The Sport Test includes four exercises with a total of 20 points that evaluate the resistance and functional strength of the lower limb. The exercises are based on a good burst (the ability to dynamically start a race in a controlled and fast manner with 70° knee flexion) and stop and absorption (the ability to land in a soft and controlled way on the operative lower limb in a lateral and rotational direction, and the ability to flex and

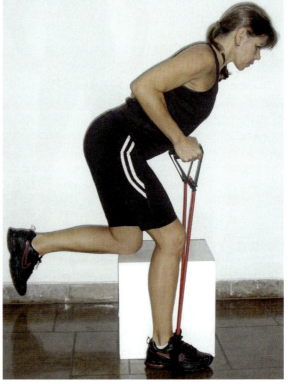

**Fig. 25.12** Single-knee bends

extend the limb from a lunge position without pain, fatigue, or compensation). The four exercises are:

(a) *Single-knee bends* should be done for 3 min,1 s downward, and 1 s upward without pelvic tilt or rotational movements (medial rotation/adduction) of the lower limb (1 point for every 30 s up to a total of *6 points*).

(b) *Side-to-side lateral movement* where the patient bursts the operated limb outward against the resistance of an elastic tension band tied to the waist at the level of the navel and later brings the operated leg back gently, with good absorption and 70° knee flexion. The patient makes this movement for 100 s without any compensation (medial rotation/adduction). For this second test, 1 point is given for every 20 s of correct and painless accomplishment up to a total of *5 points*.

(c) *Diagonal side-to-side movement*. This is very similar to the previous exercise, but it is accomplished at a 45° angle on the front plane and 45° angle on the back plane. Scoring is identical to the previous test up to a total of *5 points*.

(d) *Forward box lunges* on a chair to evaluate the hip's capacity to bend and to extend without pain. It is done for 2 min against the resistance of an elastic band. One point is awarded for each 30 s without pain or compensation up to a total of *4 points*.

To succeed in the sport test, it is necessary to achieve a total score equal to or higher than 17 points. This test is used as a presurgical functional exam and also to decide whether a given patient should go back to training or sports practice. Once the patient passes the sport test, he can start training and eventually returning to sports. The sporting test is an important complement to the patient's clinical exam and subjective impressions because it helps quantify the patient's functional level. A maintenance program including stabilization exercises, strengthening the external rotators is recommended to maintain the muscular groups balanced. Crouching in excess of 70° must be avoided once the patient has been allowed to return to his/her previous sport activity.

## Phase IV: Gradual Introduction of Sport Activities

Introduction of linear run, elliptic bicycle, and intensification of aerobic training, and gradual introduction of regular sport activities, except for impact sports involving continuous flexion such as kickboxing, soccer,

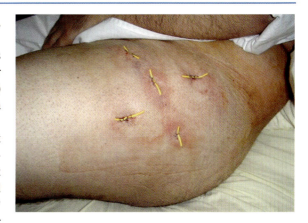

**Fig. 25.13** Stitching 1 day after the use of the external distractor for hip arthroscopy

tae kwon do, karate, and some contemporary ballet exercises. For these activities, we suggest waiting 4 months or more, depending on the evolution of each patient.

## Rehabilitation Protocol of Hip Arthroscopy Done with a Specialized Hip External Distractor

Sadri developed a special external fixator for hip arthroscopy that is fixed to the hip through special metal pins similar to Schanz's pins that are screwed to the bone to distract the hip without any compression of the perineal region. In this way, the unpleasant complications caused by the perineal post such as scrotum or labia majora ulcer and edema or neuropraxia are avoided (Fig. 25.13).

The protocol is the following: partial weight bearing (5–10 kg for 6 weeks) is necessary to avoid neck fractures. No mobility restrictions are imposed. Hip flexion and extension exercises performed in bed with the heel resting on the bed (heel sliding exercises) are useful to prevent adhesions (10/h from day 1). Abductor strengthening exercises should be started at the end of the third week post-op. Competition sports can be resumed after 6 months.

## Rehabilitation After Open Surgery

Rehabilitation following the Ganz's procedure [2] (osteochondroplasty with trochanteric osteotomy) or the Siebenrock-Ganz's procedure [19] (periacetabular osteotomy due to acetabular retroversion) is similar to that following surgical osteotomy of the proximal femur or of the acetabulum. Patients remain in bed for about 1 week starting nonweight-bearing ambulation and partial weight-bearing ambulation after 8 weeks and, gradually, full weight bearing, and abandonment of crutches is authorized. Postoperative rehabilitation is similar to that for conventional proximal femoral osteotomy.

## Rehabilitation After a Mini-anterior Approach

If osteochondroplasty without labral detachment is performed, risks through a minimal invasive access are minimized with this approach. The rehabilitation period is shortened to 2 weeks [1, 20]. The patient is hospitalized for 48–72 h until the drainage can be removed. Eventually, the patient may need one more day in hospital. Prophylaxis with antibiotics and anti-thromboembolic and anti-inflammatory drugs (indomethacine) is recommended to prevent heterotopic calcification. The patient walks with crutches for at least 2 weeks; functional recovery exercises must be performed for 4 or 5 weeks. After this, the patient can progressively resume his/her physical-sport activities. Closed-chain exercises can be introduced from the third week. Care must be taken to prevent the formation of a retractile scar during the 5 weeks that the patient does physical therapy. During the first 2 weeks, a weekly ultrasound scan is taken to rule out the presence of effusion in the hip joint.

If osteochondroplasty with labral detachment and reattachment is performed, patients ambulate with crutches (partial weight bearing) during the first 10 days. If the retrolabral ulcerative lesion microfractures, partial weight bearing should extend to 3 weeks.

- *1st week*: Rest, cryotherapy every 2 h during the first 48 h after surgery. Use of an elastic compression garment is indicated. Soft kinetic therapy must be initiated in order to achieve 90° of flexion, 60° of abduction, 60° of external rotation, 10° of adduction, and 10° of internal rotation (pendulum movements and isometric quadriceps, gluteus maximus and medius exercises).
- *2nd week*: Suspension therapy must be introduced to achieve the ROM levels mentioned above. Ultrasound therapy and electrostimulation are applied to the quadriceps and gluteal muscles to promote stretching. Free ambulation is allowed once stitches are removed. ROM should be maintained.
- *3rd week*: Active resistance exercises and ultrasound therapy for the adductors and anterior hip muscles are introduced. Electrostimulation and stretching of quadriceps and gluteal muscles are carried out. Concentric exercises are resumed at the end of the 3rd week (cycling with a high-seat bicycle to reach maximum flexion of 90°, which can be supplemented by crawl/freestyle swimming).
- *4th to 6th week*: Assisted active and passive kinetic therapy. Progressive use of gluteus medius, gluteus maximus, and quadriceps muscles. At the 4th week, the anterior hip joint should be treated. This treatment should be identical to the standard treatment of rectus femoris avulsions (once the muscle is reattached at the end of surgery). The patient can start using just one crutch and start ambulating without crutches on the following week. Aerobic closed-chain exercises must be continued (e.g., cycling with a high-seat bike and swimming).
- *7th to 12th week*: For 2 weeks, kinetic therapy must be increased to achieve more than 90° flexion, internal rotation, adduction of 20°, abduction, and 70° external rotation. Closed-chain exercises are maintained. Cycling to achieve flexion >90° is encouraged depending on patient's clinical-functional evolution. Balanced proprioception exercises and exercises involving single-limb support at 20° of flexion and 30°–40° adduction and internal rotation are introduced.
- *12th week and further*: Introduction of the linear run, elliptic bicycle, intensification of aerobic training, and gradual introduction of usual sporting activities except for impact sports involving flexion such as kickboxing, soccer, tae kwon do, karate, and some exercises of contemporary ballet. These exercises should be deferred by at least 4 months, depending on evolution.

## Use of Pulsed Signal Therapy (PST) in Postoperative Rehabilitation

PST is a noninvasive way of treating musculoskeletal dysfunctions, such as osteoarthritis, osteoporosis, tendon lesions, herniated discs, stress fractures, and all kinds of muscle- and joint-related problems.

**Fig. 25.14** Pulsed signal therapy (PST) is applied just after surgery

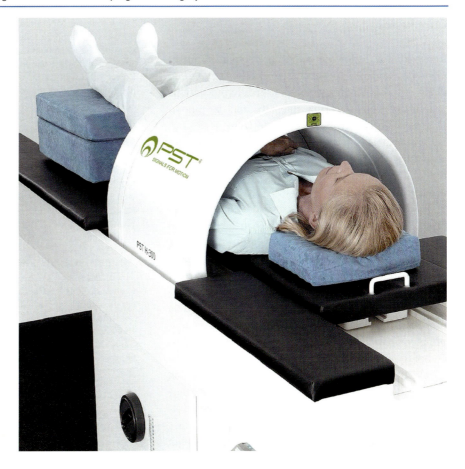

Studies show pain reduction of 70–80% after nine 1-h sessions a day, applied directly around the cervical spine or knee articulation [21, 22]. Fioravanti et al. studied the effects of the PST waves on osteoarthritic chondrocytes cultured in alginate gel with and without interleukin 1 β (ILI β) and analyzed the proteoglycan concentration (PGs) in the culture medium and the chondrocytes' morphology after exposure to PST. They observed a significant increase in proteoglycan concentration (PGs) in the cultured cells exposed to PST. They explain that PST could possibly simulate a normal articulation in living beings. The cartilage is fixed, and as far as negative loads are concerned, when the cartilage is squeezed, it releases these negative loads toward the adjacent areas that have positive loads. When the compression is eased, e.g., during ambulation, these positive loads are attracted to the negative loads, giving rise to what is known as "streaming potential." The "potential of the electrical field

flow" is a well-known term in Physics. It determines the incentive for regeneration and stimulation reactions, in other words, for maintaining and repairing tissue [23–25].

We have used PST mainly in patients having chondral lesions (submitted or not to microfractures) and noticed a beneficial effect of PST waves in these patients. Nevertheless, double-blind randomized studies are needed to confirm our preliminary findings. Besides, PST's healing and regenerating effect on connective tissue (the waves act directly on the pain-transmitting C-fibers reducing their intensity) seems to persist for months in these patients who, apparently, have a better prognosis as compared with treatments that do not use this drug-free and painless therapy that is exempt from side effects. Sessions must be held every day, soon after the physical therapy. The patient remains inside a PST OSTEO coil for 1 h a day up to a total of 12 sessions is completed (Fig. 25.14).

## Conclusion

Rehabilitation following femoroacetabular impingement is associated to specific restrictions regarding range of movement, as well as to specific precautions in terms of weight-bearing, intensity, and the time to resume activities involving strength. General postoperative rehabilitation protocols following total hip arthroplasty are not suited to every patient undergoing hip joint arthroscopy or open surgery to treat femoroacetabular impingement.

Postoperative rehabilitation should be based on the principles of tissue healing, as well as on the individual characteristics of the patient. Both arthroscopic and open procedures may vary widely due to the complexities involved in treating labral lesions [26] and their associated pathologies. Physical therapists are essential to develop specific rehabilitation protocols for each procedure performed to address femoroacetabular impingement. Indeed, FAI may be considered the most complex pathology of the hip joint, which demands absolute precision and timely intervention, and which can give the surgeon an unpleasant surprise since current imaging techniques still provide inadequate information about the degree of cartilage damage present.

Finally, it must be said that unreasonably high patient expectations may, in some cases, interfere with the postoperative outcome since it is not always possible to fully eradicate patients' symptoms and allow them to fully resume their usual sporting activities. Our knowledge of the hip musculature and biomechanics will continue to develop as so will our rehabilitation programs.

## References

1. Ribas M, Ginebreda I, Candioti L, Vilarrubias JM (2005) Surgical treatment of the anterior femoroacetabular impingement syndrome of the hip. J Bone Joint Surg Br 87(Suppl 1):84
2. Ganz R, Gill TJ, Gautier E, Ganz K, Krügel N, Berlemann U (2001) Surgical dislocation of the adult hip a technique with full access to the femoral head and acetabulum without the risk of avascular necrosis. J Bone Joint Surg Br 83(8):1119–1124
3. Ganz R, Leunig M, Leunig-Ganz K, Harris WH (2008) The etiology of osteoarthritis of the hip: an integrated mechanical concept. Clin Orthop Relat Res 466(2):264–272
4. Ganz R, Parvizi J, Beck M, Leunig M, Nötzli H, Siebenrock KA (2003) Femoroacetabular impingement: a cause for osteoarthritis of the hip. Clin Orthop Relat Res 417:112–120
5. Smith-Petersen MN (1936) Treatment of malum coxae senilis, old slipped upper femoral epiphysis, intrapelvic protrusion of the acetabulum, and coxa plana by means of acetabuloplasty. J Bone Joint Surg Am 18:869–880
6. Edwards DJ, Lomas D, Villar RN (1995) Diagnosis of the painful hip by magnetic resonance imaging and arthroscopy. J Bone Joint Surg Br 77(3):374–376
7. Leunig M, Podeszwa D, Beck M, Werlen S, Ganz R (2004) Magnetic resonance arthrography of labral disorders in hips with dysplasia and impingement. Clin Orthop Relat Res 418:74–80
8. Sadri H, Hoffmeyer P. Treatment of femoroacetabular impingement by hip arthroscopy compared to open surgery with a minimum 2 year follow-up Orthop Traumatol Surg Res 2005;3(suppl I):55
9. Lage LA, Costa RC (1995) Artroscopia do quadril: indicações e técnica. Rev Bras Ortop 30(8):555–558
10. Lage LA, Costa RC, Villar RN (1996) A importância do "labrum" acetabular: revisão da literatura. Rev Bras Ortop 31(10):792–796
11. Carlioz H, Pous JG, Rey JC (1968) Les epiphysiolyses femorales superieures. Rev Chir Orthop Reparatrice Appar Mot 54(5):387–491
12. Heyworth BE, Shindle MK, Voos JE, Rudzki JR, Kelly BT (2007) Radiologic and intraoperative findings in revision hip arthroscopy. Presented at the annual meeting of the American Academy of Orthopaedic Surgeons, San Diego, California, Feb 2007
13. Philippon MJ, Schenker ML, Briggs KK, Kuppersmith DA, Maxwell RB, Stubbs AJ (2007) Revision hip arthroscopy. Am J Sports Med 35(11):1918–1921. Epub Aug 16, 2007
14. May O, Matar WY, Beaul PE (2007) Treatment of failed arthroscopic acetabular labral debridement by femoral chondro-osteoplasty: a case series of five patients. J Bone Joint Surg Br 83(B):595–598
15. Griffin DR, Villar RN (1999) Complications of arthroscopy of the hip. J Bone Joint Surg Br 81:604–606
16. Stalzer S, Wahoff M, Scalan M, Draovitch P (2005) Rehabilitation after hip arthroscopy. Oper Tech Orthop 15(3):280–289
17. Walhoff M, Briggs KK, Philippon MJ (2009) Hip arthroscopy rehabilitation: evidence-based practice. In: Ben W, Kibler MD (eds) Orthopaedic knowledge update: Sports Medicine 4. American Academy of Orthopaedic Surgeons, Rosemont, Chapter 23, pp 273–281
18. Enseki KR, Martin RL, Draovitch P, Kelly BT, Philippon MJ, Schenker ML (2006) The hip joint: arthrosocopic procedures and postoperative rehabilitation. J Orthop Sports Phys Ther 36(7):516–525
19. Siebenrock KA, Schoeniger R, Ganz R (2003) Anterior femoro-acetabular impingement due to acetabular retroversion. Treatment with periacetabular osteotomy. J Bone Joint Surg Am 85-A(2):278–286
20. Ribas MV, Vilarrubias JM, Ginebreda I, Silberberg J, Leal J (2005) Atrapamiento o choque femoroacetabular. Rev Ortop Traumatol 49:390–403
21. Trock DH, Bollet AJ, Dyer RH Jr, Fielding LP, Miner WK, Markoll R (1993) A double-blind trial of the clinical effects of pulsed eletromagnetic fields in osteoarthritis. J Rheumatol 20(3):456–460

22. Trock DH, Bollet AJ, Markoll R (1994) The effect of pulsed electromagnetic fields in the treatment of osteoarthritis of the knee and cervical spine. Randomized, double blind, placebo controlled trials. J Rheumatol 21(10): 1904–1911

23. Fioravanti A, Nerucci F, Collodel G, Markoll R, Marcolongo R (2002) Biochemical and morphological study of human articular chondrocytes cultivated in the presence of pulsed signal therapy. Ann Rheum Dis 61: 1032–1033

24. Krueger I, Faensen M (2006) Effects of pulsed signal therapy (PST) on gene expression in three-dimensional chondrocyte cultures. University Medical Centre Charité of Humboldt University, Department of Rheumatology & DRK-Klinik Westend-Tissue Engineering Group

25. Markoll R (2002) Pulsed signal therapy: a practical guide for clinicians. American Academy Of Pain Management, 6th edn, Chapter 57, pp 715–728

26. Lage LA, Patel JV, Villar RN (1996) The acetabular labral tear: an arthroscopic classification. Arthroscopy 12(3):269–272

# Postoperative Management of Hip Resurfacing

# 26

Alfonso Valles and Carlos Gebhard

Surgical technique is the most crucial aspect affecting clinical outcome following total hip replacement and hip resurfacing. However, postoperative management is also an important factor for successful patient outcome. It can determine things like patient comfort, length of hospitalization, number of complications, and maybe even an earlier or improved return to activity.

## Introduction

In many hospitals, there is no difference between postoperative management after hip resurfacing (HR) and following total hip arthroplasty (THA). Many centers use guidelines or clinical pathways, which facilitate the work of the staff involved in patient care. They also allow more uniform treatment and an easier decision-making process.

Patients subjected to HR are usually younger and more active than those treated with THA. This could positively influence the patient recovery by reducing medical comorbidities and complications and permitting an earlier return to ambulation. However, other factors associated to the surgical technique specific to HR could neutralize these advantages. OR time is usually slightly longer for HR than for THA as reported

by many authors. The incision needed for surgical approach is also longer, and a complete capsulotomy is required for good exposure. All these factors could lead to increased bleeding and more pain in the postoperative period.

## Postoperative Analgesic Treatment

The effectiveness of postoperative pain treatment will affect not only patient comfort but also speed of recovery and length of hospital stay. The early mobilization favored by effective pain control could prevent such complications as deep venous thrombosis (DVT) and pulmonary embolism (PE).

The different options for postoperative pain relief include epidural anesthesia, nerve blocks, intra- and postoperative infiltration of the wound, and administration of analgesic drugs, either intravenously or orally.

Continuous epidural analgesia affords excellent pain relief but is associated with substantial side effects. It may cause urinary retention, nausea, hypotension, and diminished muscle control, delaying patient mobilization. If at all used, this technique should not be continued after the first 24 h.

Preoperative and postoperative wound infiltration has been hailed recently as a very effective method of pain relief, which also shortens hospital stay. A combination of a local anesthetic, an anti-inflammatory drug and adrenalin, is commonly used for this purpose. Andersen [1] compared wound infiltration at the end of surgery and through an intra-articular catheter 24 h postoperatively in two randomized groups. One of the groups was injected with local anesthetic and the other

A. Valles (✉) • C. Gebhard
Department of orthopedic surgery and Traumatology,
Hospital Universitario Príncipe de Asturias,
Alcalá de Henares-Madrid, Spain
e-mail: jvalles.hupa@salud.madrid.org

Ó. Marín-Peña (ed.), *Femoroacetabular Impingement*,
DOI 10.1007/978-3-642-22769-1_26, © Springer-Verlag Berlin Heidelberg 2012

**Table 26.1** AAOS clinical guideline on prevention of symptomatic pulmonary embolism in patients undergoing total hip or knee arthroplasty

| Chemoprophylaxis | | |
|---|---|---|
| Preoperative assessment of risk | Normal PE risk | Elevated PE risk |
| Normal bleeding risk | Aspirin, warfarin, LMWH, SP | Warfarin, LMWH, SP |
| Elevated bleeding risk | Aspirin, warfarin, none | Aspirin, warfarin, none |

*AAOS additional recommendations*

- Preoperative assessment of all patients for elevated risk of PE
- Preoperative assessment of all patients for elevated risk of bleeding
- Patients with known contraindications to anticoagulation should be considered for vena cava filter replacement
- Patients should be considered for intraoperative and/or immediate postoperative mechanical prophylaxis
- In consultation with the anesthesiologist, patients should be considered for regional anesthesia
- Postoperatively, patients should be considered for continued mechanical prophylaxis until discharge to home
- Postoperatively, patients should be mobilized as soon as feasible to the full extent of medical safety and comfort
- Routine screening for DVT or PE postoperatively in asymptomatic patients is not recommended
- Patients should be encouraged to progressively increase mobility alter discharge to home
- Patients should be educated about the common symptoms of DVT and PE

*DVT* deep venous thrombosis, *PE* pulmonary embolism, *LMWH* low-molecular-weight heparin, *SP* synthetic pentasaccharides

with placebo. Patients receiving the analgesic solution had less pain up to 2 weeks postoperatively. They also used less analgesia during the first week and were more satisfied.

Infiltration with a local anesthetic around the hip was compared [2] with continuous epidural infusion during the first 20 h. Pain was similar in both groups on the first day but lower in the next few days in patients treated with wound infiltration. Patients used fewer narcotics, improved their early walking ability, and had a shorter hospital stay.

The "local infiltration analgesia" (LIA) technique was first described by Kerr and Kohan [3] and is based on systematic intraoperative infiltration of all structures subjected to surgical trauma with 150–200 mL of a mixture of ropivacaine (2 mg/mL; maximal dose 300 mg), ketorolac (30 mg), and adrenalin (10 μg/mL). A fine catheter is left in place, and top-ups of this solution (RKA) can be delivered in the first few hours if needed. Finally, extensive reinjection is performed after 20 h (on the morning of the day after surgery), and the catheter is withdrawn.

This technique includes compression and cooling of the wound for the first 4 h to minimize drug absorption and systemic toxicity and increase its analgesic effect. Most patients treated with this method were mobilized on a walking frame 4 h postoperatively and discharged from hospital on the first postoperative day (89%). The present paper compares the results between patients treated with HR and THR. Length of stay is

shorter in HR group than THR (1.3 days vs. 4.3), but the mean age is lower too.

If analgesia with an epidural catheter or a local anesthetic is not used in the first 24–48 h, an intravenous infusion with different systemic analgesics can be employed (dexketoprofen, ketorolac, metamizol…). Opioids can be used regularly or as a rescue drug. The possibility of side effects such as nausea, vomiting, and delay in mobilization patient cannot be forgotten. To minimize these side effects, avoidance of opioids at daytime [3] and the use of antiemetic drugs (ondansetron) have been recommended.

Oral analgesics are continued beyond the first 24 h. Different drugs can be used. Most reports refer to the use of paracetamol, tramadol, codeine, and ibuprofen. The use of ibuprofen should be discontinued after the first 3 days, and residual pain be treated only with paracetamol as soon as possible

## Thromboembolic Prophylaxis

Thromboembolic prophylaxis includes taking different measures and administering different drugs. There is consensus about the importance of early mobilization and walking, but determination of the best drug therapy is still a moot point. The recommendations of the AAOS [4] are summarized in Table 26.1.

The effectiveness of low-molecular-weight heparin, fondaparinux, ximelagatran, and synthetic pentasaccharides in lowering the incidence of pulmonary embolism (PE) has been questioned in a recent publication [5]. The authors found a slightly higher mortality with the use of these drugs, probably associated to a higher frequency of hemorrhagic complications. They conclude that multimodal prophylaxis, including the use of regional anesthesia, postoperative pneumatic compression, chemoprophylaxis with aspirin, and selective use of anticoagulants, would be safer. Other reports [6, 7] support this kind of prevention. Multimodal prophylaxis is commonly used in centers with a high number of patients [3, 8], and their good results (accurate technique, lower surgical time, earlier mobilization) could be influenced by factors related to their vast experience.

## Prevention of Heterotopic Ossification

Prevention of heterotopic ossification (HO) with the administration of nonsteroidal anti-inflammatory drugs (NSAIDs) is not mentioned in most of the articles reviewed. In some of them [9], only high-risk patients (with a prior acetabular fracture) are treated with indomethacin (25 mg every 12 h for 5 days). In other reports [10], NSAIDs are mentioned but without providing details on the drug used and length of administration. Amstutz [11] treats all his patients with indomethacin (50 mg before surgery and 25 mg every 8 h for 3 days). Patients undergoing simultaneous bilateral replacement get a single dose of radiation therapy (700 rads).

In a randomized clinical trial, Rama [12] compared the incidence and severity of HO in cohorts of patients who had undergone either HR or THR. HR was associated with a significantly higher rate of severe HO. Patients with severe HO had lower functional outcome scores. Patients received oral celecoxib (200 mg in the morning of the operation and 200 mg twice a day for 3–5 days) as part of postoperative analgesia. A conclusion of the study is that routine prophylaxis against HO should be considered in HR.

## Physical Therapy

As in THR, early mobilization and ambulation are keenly advised following HR by all authors, but the studies that discuss postoperative function mention none or just a few details of the rehabilitation protocols used.

Patients undergoing HR are usually younger and more physically active than standard THR patients. They often have greater expectations and tend to be more compliant with exercise programs. However, exercise programs and rehabilitation protocols for HR and for THA patients are, in many hospitals, the same. Lack of a specific protocol for these patients has been suggested to be related with suboptimal recovery [13]. We believe that treatment should be adapted to the specific characteristics of HR (lower dislocation rate) and of each patient (previous physical status and activity level, expectations). The aims of any exercise program are gait reeducation and progressive range of motion and muscular strength recovery.

As mentioned by many studies, assisted weight-bearing gait with a walking frame must be started on the first postoperative day [3, 4, 8–11]. With slight differences, most authors advise the use of two crutches for the first 2 or 3 weeks with gradual progression toward full weight-bearing, using one crutch or a cane for another 3 or 4 weeks. Some authors propose keeping weight-bearing restriction for longer [9] when femoral neck notching has occurred.

Controversy exists about range of motion after HR. Some studies have reported increased range of motion when compared with THR [14], but others have reported no difference or even a lower range of motion for HR [13].

Limited range of motion following HR could be explained by the reduced head-neck ratio of HR vs. conventional prostheses. The difference would be higher if a standard stem was associated to a large head. In a recent study [15] with a computer-aided design (CAD), none of the resurfacing prostheses were able to provide flexion of 90° without impingement of the femoral neck against the acetabulum. The average range of motion of HR implants was below the range of motion of a stemmed THR. Another study [16] with an in vitro model showed similar results.

Beaulé [17] has emphasized that most hips undergoing HR have an abnormal femoral head-neck ratio that could go uncorrected during surgery, leading to impingement and pain. To avoid this complication, an optimal technique with restoration of the anterior offset is required.

As the dislocation rate is lower in HR than in conventional THR, the precautions contained in different HR protocols to prevent them could be relaxed, promoting instead the gradual introduction of activities that might

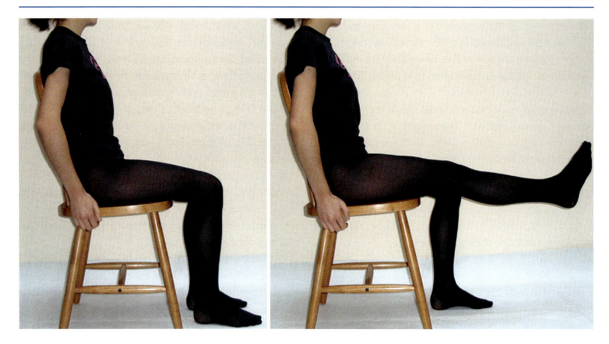

**Fig. 26.1** Knee extension while sitting on a chair

**Fig. 26.2** Active hip flexion

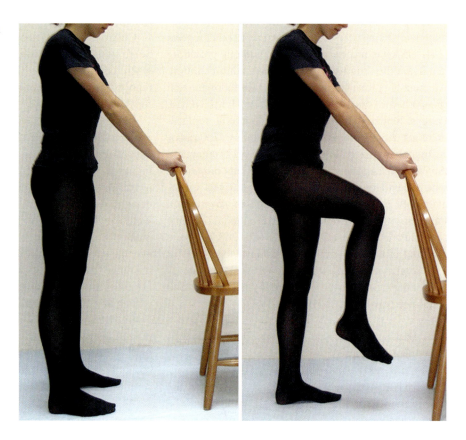

**Fig. 26.3** Hip extension

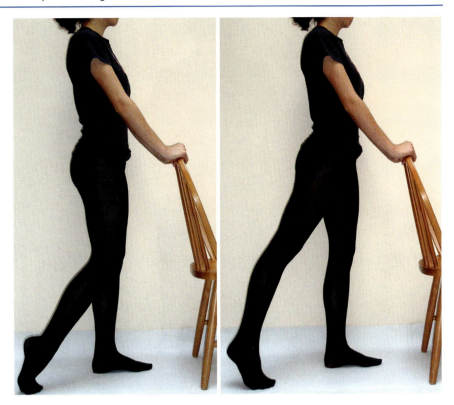

assist patients in speeding up achievement of a greater range of motion [13].

Most programs include active hip flexion, extension, and abduction exercises as well as knee and ankle mobilization for the first few weeks (Figs. 26.1–26.4). After, the sixth week exercises should progressively facilitate a better range of motion and muscle strengthening. McMinn [8] recommends that patients should swim or exercise in a pool and to do either no-impact or low-impact exercises at a fitness center. He also recommends stretching exercises to optimize range of motion [18].

Return to high-impact activity has to be carefully planned in a gradual manner and should be delayed a few months [11]. Starting too soon could provoke a fracture of the femoral neck. With time, periarticular osteopenia is reversed, and the protective effects of muscle tone, strength, and coordination return to normal. Patients are then able to safely undertake more strenuous activities [19].

Theoretical advantages of HR compared with conventional THR include a safer return to sports and an achievement of a higher level of athletic ability; however, some controversy still exists.

There are some studies that report on patients' sport activity after HR. Naal [20] reported high participation in sports in his 112 patients. The number of patients engaged in sports increased after surgery. This study showed a shift away from such contact sports as football and highly weight-bearing sports like tennis or jogging to more joint-sparing sports such as walking, cycling, and swimming, but over 50% of patients participated in downhill skiing.

A debate exists as to whether the higher activity level and sports activity referred to in many studies depended on the advantages related to the implant (a bigger head, enhanced load-transmission pattern, bone preservation) or on the fact that patients undergoing HR are usually younger and more active. In a study comparing HR and conventional THR patients with a similar preoperative activity level, Lavigne [21] observed a greater degree and intensity of postoperative sports activity in the HR group.

Pollard [22] compared the results of HR and THR in two groups. More patients with HR ran, participated in sport, and carried out heavy manual work than those with THA. In another study [23], high-level functional outcome measures for the hip joint were compared in two groups of HR and conventional THR patients. Balance, coordination, speed, and directional change in the affected hip were evaluated and significantly better results were

**Fig. 26.4** Hip abduction

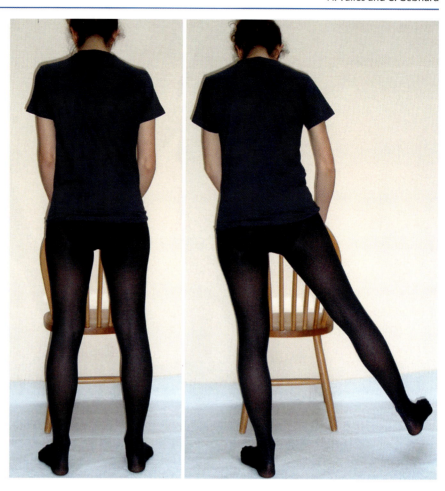

**Table 26.2** Start of different activities and sports McMinn

| Month | 1 | 2 | 3 | 4 | 5 | 6 | 7 | 8 | 9 | 10 | 11 | 12 |
|---|---|---|---|---|---|---|---|---|---|---|---|---|
| Activity | Walking | Driving | | Gardening | | | | | | | | |
| Sport | | Swimming | | | Golf | | Tennis | | | | Running | Jogging |
| | | | | | | | | | | | | Ski |
| | | Gymnastic | | | | | | | | | | Impact sports |

Driving: Start at the 6th week (3rd week if the operated hip is left and it is an automatic car). Tennis: Start with double-match. Running: Start on a treadmill

found in the HR group. The authors concluded that HR allows patients to return to higher levels of function and that existing outcome measures are not discriminating enough to highlight the potential benefits of HR over conventional THR.

We can conclude that there is evidence that after HR, patients can perform heavy labor and sports activities more competently than after THR. Appropriate return time to different activities should be decided individually for each patient, taking into consideration facts such as previous health status, expectations, and desired activity level. Continuing sport activity is a common concern of HR patients that should be considered. Specific recommendations on this subject are scarce in scientific articles. However, written recommendations given in many centers to their patients are more informative [24]. McMinn [18] discusses the appropriate return time to different activities and sports (Table 26.2).

## Conclusions

Effective treatment of postoperative pain can improve patients' ability for early mobilization and help decrease complications and shorten length of hospital stay. New techniques such as those described in this chapter could change traditional postoperative management. Thus, classic thromboembolic prophylaxis in use in many centers should be reconsidered. Advantages of HR over THR increase patient confidence when following their exercise programs and contribute to a speedier return to different activities after the operation. Patients undergoing HR, usually younger and more active, can expect a functional and sport activity level that is probably better than that obtained with THR. To achieve this with a low risk of complications, they should participate in an appropriate exercise program. The aims of such programs and their progression should be discussed with every patient.

## References

1. Andersen LJ, Poulsen T, Krogh B et al (2007) Postoperative analgesia in total hip arthroplasty. A randomized double-blinded, placebo-controlled study on peroperative and postoperative ropivacaine, ketorolac, and adrenaline wound infiltration. Acta Orthopaedic 78(2):187–192
2. Andersen KV, Pfeiffer-Jensen M, Haradsteldt V et al (2007) Reduced hospital stay and narcotic consumption, and improved mobilization with local and intraarticular infiltration after hip arthroplasty. A randomized clinical trial of and intrarticular technique versus epidural infusion in 80 patients. Acta Orthop 78(2):180–186
3. Kerr DR, Kohan L (2008) Local infiltration analgesia: a technique for the control of acute postoperative pain following knee and hip surgery: a case study of 325 patients. Acta Orthop 79(2):174–183
4. American Academy of Orthopaedic Surgeons clinical guideline on prevention of symptomatic pulmonary embolism in patients undergoing total hip or knee arthroplasty. Rosemont (IL): American Academy of Orthopaedic Surgeons (AAOS); 2007. 63 p.
5. Sharrock NE, González Della Valle A, Go G et al (2008) Potent anticoagulants are associated with a higher all-cause mortality rate after hip and knee arthroplasty. Clin Orthop 466:714–721
6. Lotke P, Lonner J (2006) The benefit of aspirin chemoprofilaxis for thromboembolism after TKA. Clin Orthop 452:175–180
7. Shepard M et al (2006) Fatal pulmonary embolism following THA and TKA. A study of 2153 cases using routine mechanical profilaxis and selective chemoprofilaxis. Hip Int 16:53–56
8. McMinn DJ, Daniel J, Pynsent PB et al (2005) Mini-incision resurfacing arthroplasty of hip through the posterior approach. Clin Orthop 441:91–98
9. Back DL, Dalzield R, Young D et al (2005) Early results of primary Birmingham hip resurfacings. An independent prospective study of the first 230 hips. J Bone Joint Surg Br 87:324–329
10. Treacy RB, McBryde CW, Pynsent PB (2005) Birmingham hip resurfacing arthroplasty. A minimum follow-up of five years. J Bone Joint Surg Br 87:167–170
11. Amstutz HC, Beaulé PE, Dorey FJ et al (2004) Metal-on-metal hybrid surface arthroplasty: two to six-year follow-up study. J Bone Joint Surg Am 86:28–39
12. Rama KR, Vendittoli PA, Ganapathi M et al (2009) Heterotopic ossification after surface replacement arthroplasty and total hip arthroplasty. A randomized study. J Arthroplasty 24:256–262
13. Newman MA, Barker KL, Pandit H et al (2008) Outcomes after metal-on-metal hip resurfacing: could we achieve better function? Arch Phys Med Rehabil 89:660–666
14. dela Rosa MA, Silva M, Heisel C et al (2007) Range of motion alter hip resurfacing. Orthopaedics 5:352–357
15. Kluess D, Zietz C, Lindner T et al (2008) Limited range of motion of hip resurfacing arthroplasty due to unfavorable ratio of prosthetic head size and femoral neck diameter. Acta Orthop 79:748–754
16. Bengs B, Sangiorgio S, Ebramzadeh E (2008) Less range of motion with resurfacing arthroplasty than with total hip arthroplasty. In vivo examination of 8 designs. Acta Orthop 79:755–762
17. Beaulé PE, Harvey N, Zaragoza E et al (2007) The femoral head/neck offset and hip resurfacing. J Bone Joint Surg Br 89:9–15
18. The McMinn Centre (2005–2006) http://www.mcminncentre.co.uk/flash/
19. Daniel J, Pynsent PB, McMinn DJ (2004) Metal-on-metal resurfacing of the hip in patients under the age of 55 years with osteoarthritis. J Bone Joint Surb Br 86:177–184
20. Naal FD, Maffiuletti NA, Munzinger U et al (2007) Sports after hip resurfacing arthroplasty. Am J Sports Med 35:705–711
21. Lavigne M, Masse V, Girard J et al (2008) Activités sportives après resurfaçage et prothèse totale de hanche: une étude prospective randomisée. Revue de Chirurgie Orthopédique el Réparatrice de l´Appareil Locomoteur 94:361–367
22. Pollard TC, Raker RP, Eastaugh-Waring SJ (2006) Treatment of the young active patient with osteoarthritis of the hip: a five- to seven year comparison of hybrid total hip arthroplasty and metal-on-metal resurfacing. J Bone Joint Surg Br 88:592–600
23. Bull J, Soler J, Haddad F (2008) Hip resurfacing has sustained functional outcomes when compared to total hip arthroplasty. Hip Int 18:185
24. Schmalzried TP, Ball S. JRI high performance hips. Post-operative guidelines. http://www.jri-docs.com/JRI_Prospective_Post_Hip.html

# Part VII

# Outcome in FAI Treatment

# Clinical Scores in Femoroacetabular Impingement

# 27

Néstor Moreno and Óliver Marín-Peña

## Introduction

Clinical scores are used by orthopedic surgeons as a way of monitoring their patients' evolution. Surgeons can use these scores to follow the evolution of a given condition in time and to determine the effect exerted by different therapeutic procedures on such pathologies and on their patients.

Surgeons must be able to find out whether a certain surgical technique is beneficial or rather detrimental for their patients. In this way, they can quantify the results they obtain with different techniques. Likewise, it is essential for surgeons to understand their results and report them to the orthopedic community.

In the last few decades, use of clinical scores has become widespread in different kinds of clinical studies, particularly in randomized controlled studies, as a result of a growing interest in evidence-based medicine. This has led to the development of a large number of clinical scores, which are employed with ever-increasing frequency.

Beaton [1] compares clinical scores with "windows" that make it possible to determine the impact on a certain condition on a patient, so each window provides just one single perspective on the problem with several "windows" being necessary to command a complete view. But, what are these "windows"?

In the first place, there are the quality-of-life scores. The commonest scores in this category are the SF-36 questionnaire and its abridged version and the SF-12 questionnaire. Even if these scales allow comparisons between populations with different health problems, they are less sensitive to overall changes in the status of an orthopedic patient than specific scores.

Specific clinical scores may focus on a specific condition or a specific anatomical region (a specific joint in the case of orthopedics); these scores are designed to analyze health-related factors that are directly relevant to the population of interest. Thus, different types of scores have been developed for different pathologies; in the case of the hip, osteoarthritis has naturally been the subject of different scores aimed at determining the effects that different types of treatment have upon the condition. As regards anatomical regions, scales have been designed that measure the effect of a condition on the hip or the whole of the lower limb.

## Hip Joint-Specific Clinical Scores

In the hip joint, the most common clinical scores used to quantify surgical results have been the Merle d'Aubigne and Postel scale [2], the Harris Hip Score [3], the Oxford Hip Score [4], the WOMAC (Western Ontario and McMaster Universities) osteoarthritis index [5], the Lower Extremity Functional Scale [6] (LEFS), the Nonarthritic Hip Score [7] (NHS), the Lower Limb Questionnaire of the American Academy of Orthopaedic Surgeons [8] (AAOS), the Hip disability and Osteoarthritis Outcome Score [9] (HOOS), the McMaster-Toronto Arthritis Patient

N. Moreno (✉)
Department Orthopedic Surgery and Traumatology,
Hospital Universitario de Gran Canaria " Dr Negrin",
Las Palmas de Gran Canaria, Spain
e-mail: rotsenonerom@terra.es

Ó. Marín-Peña
Department of Orthopedic and Traumatology,
University Hospital Infanta Leonor (Madrid-Spain),
e-mail: olivermarin@yahoo.es

Ó. Marín-Peña (ed.), *Femoroacetabular Impingement*,
DOI 10.1007/978-3-642-22769-1_27, © Springer-Verlag Berlin Heidelberg 2012

Preference Disability Questionnaire (MACTAR) [10] and the Patient-Specific Index [11].

More recently, a series of scores have been developed which tend to be more specific in terms of patient type and, especially, expectations of patients suffering from femoroacetabular impingement. These are the modified Harris Hip Score [12, 13] (mHHS) and the Hip Outcome Score (HOS) with its activities of daily living (ADL) and sports subscales [14, 15].

## Clinical Scores and Femoroacetabular Impingement

Although a detailed description of all the scales above does not fall within the scope of the present chapter, we shall make a few considerations about them in connection to the pathology under discussion. Femoroacetabular impingement is a mechanism that damages the hip joint causing early articular deterioration. This process combines varying proportions of anatomical deformity and overuse. This means that in the majority of cases, patients seeking our help are people with high levels of physical/sports activity; most patients are symptomatic only during performance of such intense activity. This makes essential to ask the patient to rate his/her level of functional impairment or limitation. In addition, at this stage, solution to the pathology is not usually hip replacement but rather some variant of non-prosthetic surgery. These two characteristics make it difficult to clinically evaluate this condition with the conventional scales used for assessment of hip arthritis and prosthetic surgery.

The Merle d'Aubigné and Postel scale [2], the Harris Hip Score [3], and the Oxford Hip Score [4] were designed to measure the effect of total hip replacement on hip arthritis in elderly patients. Their use is common for this type of pathology in Europe, USA, and UK, respectively. Also, the Harris Hip Score [3] was developed to be administered by qualified health care professionals and not to be self-administered by the patient him/herself. So these are scales designed for the hip joint but which do not appropriately assess femoroacetabular impingement.

Other scores have been developed for the subjective assessment of patients with a hip condition. The WOMAC [5], the HOOS [9], the MACTAR [10], and the Patient-Specific Index [11] are some of such

scores. Specific scales have also been developed for the lower limb such as the LEFS score [6] and the AAOS Lower Limb Questionnaire [8]. However, neither the origin of these scores nor the purpose for which they were developed seems adapted to the specific pathology present in femoroacetabular impingement or to the patients having this condition. In spite of this, some of these scores, in particular the WOMAC [5] and the HOOS [9] scales, can be used to evaluate the evolution of the disease in time as well as its possible evolution to hip arthritis.

In the last few years, the need has arisen to design tools to assess the efficacy of the recent developments in hip surgery, in particular conventional hip joint preserving surgery and hip arthroscopy. In 2003, Christensen presented a clinical score to assess nonarthritic hips (Nonarthritic Hip Score, NHS) [7]. This score was developed and validated for young patients (33 years old on average) with high functional and treatment-related expectations. The scale is of remarkable simplicity since it comprises only 20 sports-related questions that can be answered in 5 min.

As hip pathologies evolved, it became necessary to evaluate a larger number of patients, which resulted in a series of changes being introduced into the Harris Hip Score. This process led to the development of the modified Harris Hip Score (mHHS). In 2000, Byrd [16] introduced this new score, which retained questions relative to pain and function and removed those relative to motion and deformity since the latter were not relevant to patients subjected to hip arthroscopy. The new questionnaire could be filled in by patients themselves without the help of a physician.

Martin [14, 15] states that the mHHS does not contain questions related to the ability to participate in sports activities. After a review of the existing evaluation tools, Martin argued for the need to develop a new clinical score that is better adapted to patients undergoing hip arthroscopy and to the pathologies amenable to that treatment. This is how the Hip Outcome Score (HOS) came into existence. This new score contains two subscales: one relative to activities of daily living and the other relative to sports practice. Its simplicity makes this score easy to apply in the course of the surgeon's everyday consultations.

**Table 27.1** Different scales used for clinical outcomes in hip surgery

| | Valued aspects | Items number | Self-administer by patient | Anatomic area evaluated | Pathology specific designed | Maximum score | Sport-related questions |
|---|---|---|---|---|---|---|---|
| Merle D'Aubigne | • Pain<br>• Mobility<br>• Gait ability | 3 | No | Hip | Hip arthroplasty | 18 | No |
| Harris hip score | • Pain<br>• Function<br>• Deformity<br>• Range of motion | 16 | No | Hip | Hip arthroplasty | 100 | No |
| Oxford hip score | • Pain<br>• Function<br>• Activity | 12 | Yes | Hip | Hip arthroplasty | 48 | No |
| WOMAC | • Pain<br>• Rigidity<br>• Function<br>• ADL | 32 | Yes | Hip/knee | Osteoarthritis | 100 | No |
| HOOS | • Pain<br>• Rigidity<br>• Function<br>• Ability ADL<br>• Live quality | 40 | Yes | Hip | Osteoarthritis | 100.00% | 4(40) |
| LEFS | • Function | 20 | Yes | Lower Limb | Lower limb pathology | 100.00% | 4(20) |
| Lower limb questionnaire AAOS | • Rigidity<br>• Swelling<br>• Pain<br>• Walk aids | 7 | Yes | Hip/knee | Lower limb pathology | | No |
| MACTAR | • Ability ADL | 25 | Yes | Whole body | Rheumatoid arthritis | | No |
| Patient-specific index | • Main complaint | 22 | Yes | Whole body | Hip arthroplasty | 100.00% | No |
| NHS | • Pain<br>• Mechanical symptoms<br>• Function<br>• Activity | 20 | Yes | Hip | Young patient without osteoarthritis | 100 | 4(20) |
| mHHS | • Pain<br>• Function | 8 | Yes | Hip | Hip arthroscopy | 100 | No |
| HOS ADL | • Ability ADL | 17(2) | Yes | Hip | Hip arthroscopy | 100.00% | No |
| HOS sport | • Ability sport activities | 9 | Yes | Hip | Hip arthroscopy | 100.00% | 9(9) |

Table 27.1 contains a schematic representation of the different clinical scores mentioned above. Some of their chief characteristics are described, which could make the surgeon choose one rather than another in his/her daily practice. In my view, an ideal scale would be a simple and succinct one which could be filled out by the patient in only a few minutes. Designing a scale for each pathology and patient type would be both difficult and unpractical as it would multiply the number of available scores and complicate their use. However, it is important to distinguish basic functional needs from the desire to carry out intense physical activity. I do not think that we should evaluate nonarthritic patients on the same scales as those with an established

degenerative pathology. Likewise, it must be remembered that sports practice has, in many cases, become part of our lifestyles or even a profession in its own right.

## Current Use of Clinical Scores in Femoroacetabular Impingement

A review of the papers published in the last 2 years reveals that there is no consensus in terms of the clinical scores used by the different authors to measure the outcomes of their interventions. In 2009, Philippon [17] published a paper where he uses the mHHS in a group of professional hockey players. Kang [18] also published a paper where he also applies the HHS and the sports subscale of the HOS to a group of athletes. These two authors perform arthroscopic treatment for femoroacetabular impingement.

Two further studies were published by Peters [19] and Yun [20] in 2009 in which femoroacetabular impingement was treated by surgical dislocation of the hip; in both of them, the conventional HHS was used. On the other hand, Sekiya [21] evaluated cartilage repair in femoroacetabular impingement with the mHHS and the HOS, the latter with both subscales. In two different studies on arthroscopic treatment, Horisberger [22] and Bruner [23] used the NHS (Nonarthritic Hip Score).

In studies also published this year, Byrd [24] and Villar [25] used the modified Harris Hip Score to assess arthroscopic treatment, and Laude [26] used the NHS for open surgery through an anterior approach. In turn, Mast [27] and Beck [28] used the Merle d'Aubigne score for hip dislocation surgery; the latter scale was the one used by the Ganz group to assess their outcomes in the first few years of this decade [29].

In a presentation at the Santander Hip Meeting earlier 2010, Griffin [30] explained that he uses four clinical scores in his daily practice, which he has his patients fill out prior to consultation; these are the modified Harris Hip Score, the NHS score, the HOS with its two subscales and the HOOS score.

## Conclusions

Surgeons must have a set of clinical scores that enable them to measure the effects of their interventions on the pathologies they treat. The scales traditionally used in the field of hip surgery are not appropriate for patients with femoroacetabular impingement.

Development of a universally accepted scale specifically aimed at assessing these patients is necessary in order to allow uniform interpretation of the different studies published.

## References

1. Beaton DE, Schemitsch E (2003) Measures of health-related quality of life and physical function. Clin Orthop Relat Res 413:90–105
2. D'Aubigne RM, Postel M (1954) Functional results of hip arthroplasty with acrylic prosthesis. J Bone Joint Surg Am 36:451–475
3. Harris WH (1969) Traumatic arthritis of the hip after dislocation and acetabular fractures: treatment by mold arthroplasty. An end-result study using a new method of result evaluation. J Bone Joint Surg Am 1:737–755
4. Dawson J, Fitzpatrick R, Carr A et al (1996) Questionnaire on the perceptions of patients about total hip replacement. J Bone Joint Surg Br 78-B:185–190
5. Bellamy N, Buchanan WW, Goldsmith CH et al (1988) Validation study of WOMAC: a health status instrument for measuring clinically important patient relevant outcomes to antirheumatic drug therapy in patients with osteoarthritis of the hip or knee. J Rheumatol 15:1833–1840
6. Binkley JM, Stratford PW, Lott SA et al (1999) The Lower Extremity Function Scale (LEFS): scale development, measurement properties, and clinical application. North American Orthopaedic Rehabilitation Research Network. Phys Ther 79:371–383
7. Christensen CP, Althausen PL, Mittleman MA et al (2003) The nonarthritic hip score: reliable and validated. Clin Orthop Relat Res 406:75–83
8. Hunsaker FG, Cioffi DA, Amadio PC et al (2002) The American Academy of Orthopaedic Surgeons outcomes instruments: normative values from the general population. J Bone Joint Surg Am 84:208–215
9. Nilsdotter AK, Lohmander LS, Klassbo M et al (2003) Hip disability and osteoarthritis outcome score (HOOS) – validity and responsiveness in total hip replacement. BMC Muskuloskelet Disord 4:10
10. Tugwell P, Bombardier C, Buchanan WW et al (1987) The MACTAR Patient Preference Disability Questionnaire – an individualized functional priority approach for assessing improvement in physical disability in clinical trials in rheumatoid arthritis. J Rheumatol 14:446–451
11. Wright JG, Young NL (1997) The patient-specific index: asking patients what they want. J Bone Joint Surg Am 79:974–983
12. Irrgang JJ, Lubowitz JH (2008) Measuring arthroscopic outcome. Arthroscopy 24(6):718–722
13. Martin RL (2005) Hip arthroscopy and outcome assessment. Oper Tech Orthop 15:290–296
14. Martin RL, Philippon MJ (2007) Evidence of validity for the hip outcome score in hip arthroscopy. Arthroscopy 23(8):822–826

15. Martin RL, Kelly BT, Philippon MJ (2006) Evidence of validity for the hip outcome score. Arthroscopy 22: 1304–1311
16. Byrd JW, Jones KS (2000) Prospective analysis of hip arthroscopy with 2-year follow up. Arthroscopy 16: 578–587
17. Philippon MJ, Weiss DR, Kuppersmith DA, Briggs KK, Hay CJ (2010) Arthroscopic labral repair and treatment of FAI in professional hockey players. Am J Sports Med 38(1): 99–104
18. Kang C, Hwang DS, Cha SM (2009) Acetabular labral tears in patients with sports injury. Clin Orthop Surg 1(4): 230–235
19. Peters CL, Schabel K, Anderson L et al (2010) Open treatment of FAI is associated with clinical improvement and low complication rate at short term follow-up. Clin Orthop Relat Res 468(2):504–510
20. Yun HH, Shon WY, Yun JY (2009) Treatment of FAI with surgical dislocation. Clin Orthop Surg 1(3):146–154
21. Sekiya JK, Martin RL, Lesniak BP (2009) Arthroscopic repair of delaminated acetabular articular cartilage in FAI. Orthopedics 32(9):692p.
22. Horisberger M, Brunner A, Herzog RF (2010) Arthroscopic treatment of FAI of the hip: a new technique to access the joint. Clin Orthop Relat Res 468(1):182–190
23. Brunner A, Horisberger M, Herzog RF (2009) Evaluation of a computed tomography-based navigation system prototype for hip arthroscopy in the treatment of FAI. Arthroscopy 25(4):382–391
24. Byrd JW, Jones KS (2009) Arthroscopic femoroplasty in the management of cam-type FAI. Clin Orthop Relat Res 467(3):739–746
25. Bardakos NV, Vasconcelos JC, Villar RN (2008) Early outcome of hip arthroscopy for FAI: the role of femoral osteoplasty in symptomatic improvement. J Bone Joint Surg Br 90(12):1570–1575
26. Laude F, Sariali E, Nogier A (2009) Femoroacetabular impingement treatment using arthroscopy and anterior approach. Clin Orthop Relat Res 467(3):747–752
27. Graves ML, Mast JW (2009) FAI: do outcomes reliably improve with surgical dislocations. Clin Orthop Relat Res 467(3):717–723
28. Beck M (2009) Groin pain after open FAI surgery: the role of intraarticular adhesions. Clin Orthop Relat Res 467(3):769–774
29. Clohisy JC, St John LC, Schutz AL (2010) Surgical treatment of FAI: a systematic review of the literature. Clin Orthop Relat Res 468(2):555–564
30. Griffin D (2009) Proceedings from hip arthroscopy and sports Meeting, Santander(Spain) 2009

# Index

Ó. Marín-Peña (ed.), *Femoroacetabular Impingement*,
DOI 10.1007/978-3-642-22769-1, © Springer-Verlag Berlin Heidelberg 2012